SARCOIDOSIS DIAGNOSIS AND MANAGEMENT

Edited by **Mohammad Hosein Kalantar Motamedi**

Sarcoidosis Diagnosis and Management
Edited by Mohammad Hosein Kalantar Motamedi

Published by InTech

Janeza Trdine 9, 51000 Rijeka, Croatia

Publishing Process Manager Martina Blecic

Technical Editor Teodora Smiljanic

Cover Designer InTech Design Team

Additional hard copies can be obtained from orders@intechopen.com

Sarcoidosis Diagnosis and Management, Edited by Mohammad Hosein Kalantar Motamedi
p. cm.
ISBN 978-953-307-414-6

For EU product safety concerns:
IN TECH d.o.o., Prolaz Marije Krucifikse Kozulić 3, 51000 Rijeka, Croatia,
info@intechopen.com or visit our website at intechopen.com.

Meet the editor

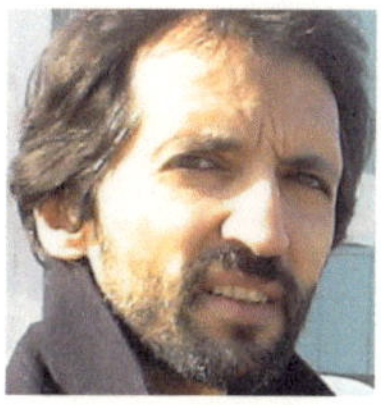

Dr. Mohammad Hosein Kalantar Motamedi is currently Professor at the Trauma Research Center, Baqiyatallah University of Medical Sciences and at the Azad University of Medical Sciences, Tehran, Iran. He has had 33 International Conference Presentations, has published 11 textbooks, supervised 52 doctorate theses and has published 105 papers indexed in PUBMED and SCOPUS. He is an Associate Editor for the Biomed Central "BMC Oral Health" Journal and Associate Editor for BMC Research Notes Journal. He is also listed in the Marquis Book "Who's Who in the World" (1999-2011) and also in the Marquis Book "Who's Who in Healthcare and Medicine" (2002-2011).

Contents

Preface XI

Part 1 Immunology 1

Chapter 1 **Immunopathogenesis of Sarcoidosis 3**
Giorgos A. Margaritopoulos, Foteini N. Economidou, Nikos M. Siafakas and Katerina M. Antoniou

Chapter 2 **Immunopathogenesis and Presumable Antigen Pathway of Sarcoidosis: A Comprehensive Approach 21**
Atsushi Kurata

Part 2 Diagnosis 35

Chapter 3 **Basic Diagnostic Approaches in Sarcoidosis 37**
Louis Gerolemou and Peter R. Smith

Chapter 4 **Diagnosis of Pulmonary Sarcoidosis 47**
Tiberiu Shulimzon and Matthew Koslow

Chapter 5 **Imaging in Sarcoidosis 71**
M. Reza Rajebi, Nicole A. Zimmerman, Roozbeh Sharif, Ernest M. Scalzetti, Stuart A. Groskin and Rolf A. Grage

Chapter 6 **Bronchoalveolar Lavage and Sampling in Pulmonary Sarcoidosis 101**
Edvardas Danila

Part 3 Management 123

Chapter 7 **Updated Guidelines for the Treatment of Pulmonary Sarcoidosis 125**
Luis Jara-Palomares, Candela Caballero-Eraso, Alicia Díaz-Baquero and Jose Antonio Rodríguez-Portal

Chapter 8 **Prognostic Factors in Sarcoidosis 137**
Wojciech J. Piotrowski

Chapter 9 **Lung Transplantation for Pulmonary Sarcoidosis 163**
Dominic T. Keating

Part 4 Extrapulmonary Sarcoidosis 189

Chapter 10 **Clinical Features of Skin 191**
Dilek Biyik Ozkaya

Chapter 11 **Acquired Ichthyosiform Erythrodermia Sarcoidosis 199**
Hui-Jun Ma

Chapter 12 **Orofacial Sarcoidosis and Granulomatosis 203**
Mohammad Hosein Kalantar Motamedi, Mohammad Ghasem Shams and Taghi Azizi

Chapter 13 **Diagnostic and Therapeutic Management of Cardiac Sarcoidosis -Application of High Resolution Electrocardiography 217**
Kenji Yodogawa

Chapter 14 **Neurological Sarcoidosis 223**
J. Chad Hoyle and Herbert B. Newton

Chapter 15 **Spinal Cord Sarcoidosis Accompanied with Compressive Cervical Myelopathy 239**
Yoshihito Sakai, Yukihiro Matsuyama and Shiro Imagama

Part 5 Sarcoid-Like Reactions 251

Chapter 16 **Sarcoid-Like Reactions 253**
Shweta Nag

Chapter 17 **Granulomatosis and Cancer 269**
Michel Pavic and Florian Pasquet

Preface

Sarcoidosis is a type of inflammation that occurs in various locations of the body for no known reason. Normally, when foreign substances or organisms enter the body, the immune system retaliates by activating an immune response. Inflammation is a normal part of this immune response that subsides once the antigen is gone. In sarcoidosis, the inflammation persists, and immune cells form abnormal tissue called granulomas. Although the disease can affect any organ, it is most likely to occur in the lungs i.e. the skin, eyes, liver, or lymph nodes. The etiology of sarcoidosis is not known; research suggests that it may be due to an extreme immune response or sensitivity to certain substances and seems to have a genetic component as well. When sarcoidosis occurs in the lungs, it can lead to wheezing, coughing, shortness of breath, and chest pain. Other possible symptoms that affect other body systems include night sweats, fever, weight loss, and seizures. Some cases of sarcoidosis resolve spontaneously , while others may last indefinitely. Treatment of sarcoidosis is designed to reduce inflammation and usually includes corticosteroids and immunosuppression therapy.

As a contemporary comprehensive book relating to sarcoidosis focusing on the aforementioned issues was lacking, INTECH took the opportunity to seek out top researchers on the subject worldwide in order to collate data and publish a diagnostic and management update on this mysterious disease. To this end more than 30 contemporary scientists worldwide were consulted. Based on their specific area of expertise and recently published research indexed in PUBMED, each contributed generously to a section of this book. This book has 5 basic sections : Immunology, Diagnosis, Management, Extrapulmonary Sarcoidosis and Sarcoid-like Reactions. It includes 17 chapters which cover the topics of: Immunopathogenesis and antigen pathway of sarcoidosis, Diagnostic Approaches in Sarcoidosis, Imaging in Sarcoidosis, Bronchoalveolar lavage and sampling, Treatment update in pulmonary sarcoidosis, Prognostic Factors in Sarcoidosis, Lung Transplantation, Extrapulmonary Sarcoidosis (skin, face, mouth, heart, brain, spine) and Sarcoid-like reactions.

For me, it was indeed both an honor and a privilege to work with these noble researchers. Anyone who has authored a book knows how hard a task it is to compile,complete, edit and publish it. This indeed was a great undertaking on behalf of INTECH and the international authors and collaborators. I hereby express my gratitude and sincere appreciation to each and every one of them for their unyielding and relentless efforts in this arduous task. I would like to also thank INTECH open access publisher, Ms. Ana Nikolic Head of Editorial Consultants and the Publishing Managers Mr. Niksa Mandic and Ms. Martina Blecic for their kind help throughout the past 12 months without which this undertaking would not have been possible.

Mohammad Hosein Kalantar Motamedi
Professor, Trauma Research Center,
Baqiyatallah University of Medical Sciences, Tehran,
IR Iran

Part 1

Immunology

1

Immunopathogenesis of Sarcoidosis

Giorgos A. Margaritopoulos[1], Foteini N. Economidou[2],
Nikos M. Siafakas[2] and Katerina M. Antoniou[2]
[1]Royal Brompton Hospital, London UK,
[2]Thoracic Medicine Department, University Hospital of Heraklion Crete,
Greece

1. Introduction

Sarcoidosis is a multisystemic disease in which inflammatory cells gather and form nodules known as non caseating epithelioid granulomas. The most commonly affected organs are the lungs, the eyes and the skin whereas all the organs can be potentially affected. The disease can develop when genetically susceptible individuals are exposed to environmental agents with antigenic properties. These can be either exogenous agents (infections, antigenic structures) or endogenous agents produced by damaged cells. Usually the immune system is able to eliminate the granulomas over a few years but if this is not the case, a progression to fibrosis and permanent organ damage is observed.
It is commonly accepted that the pathogenesis of the disease is mediated by an interplay of cells of both innate and adaptive immunity as well as by their products. Interestingly, the pathogenetic process is compartmentalized and there is an exuberant immune response occurring in the affected tissues such as increase of lymphocytes in the bronchoalveolar lavage fluid in contrast to the peripheral blood lymphocytopenia and cutaneous anergy to tuberculin and other skin tests (Daniele& Rowlands, 1976; Hunninghake,1979,1981; Siltzbach et al,1974; Winterbauer et al,1993; Yeager et al 1977). The role of the immune cells and cytokines involved in the pathogenesis of sarcoidosis will be discussed in this chapter.

2. Innate and adaptive immune system

Lungs, which represent a frequent site of infections, are constantly exposed to either microorganisms and their by-products or to antigenic structures. Innate immunity represents the first line of host defence against these threats and is able to withhold the majority of them. A vast number of cells such as neutrophil granulocytes, macrophages, dentritic cells and natural killer cells as well as receptors such as toll-like receptors (TLRs), nucleotide-binding oligomerization domain-containing protein (NOD)-like receptors are part of the innate immune system. Should it fail to eradicate the infection or the antigenic structures, a second line of host defence, namely adaptive immune system, is being activated. T-cells, B-cells, antigen presenting cells (APCs) are part of it.

2.1 Receptors

Toll-like Receptors (TLRs) are pattern-recognition receptors that play a key role in the innate immunity and their role in the pathogenesis of sarcoidosis has been investigated in many studies. TLRs localize to various cellular compartments depending on the nature of the ligands they recognize. Thus, TLRs involved in recognition of lipid and protein ligands are expressed on the plasma membrane (TLR-1, TLR-2, TLR-4, TLR-5 and TLR-6), whereas TLRs that detect viral nucleic acids are localized in endolysosomal cellular compartments (TLR-3, TLR-7, TLR-8, TLR-9). TLRs recognize various conserved pathogen associated molecular patterns (PAMPs) such as viral derived RNA (TLR3-, TLR-7, TLR-8), and DNA (TLR-9), as well as endogenous ligands (TLR-2, TLR-4) called damage association molecular patterns (DAMPs) released following tissue damage, cell death, oxidative stress and decomposition of extracellular matrix (ECM) [Bianchi,2007;Tsan&Gao,2004; Wagner,2006]. Serum amyloid-A has been found to play an important role in the innate immune response in chronic sarcoidosis by inducing the release of TNFa via TLR-2 and nuclear factor kB activation (Chen, 2010). Once TLRs bind to products of various PAMPs and DAMPs, intracellular signaling pathways are being activated and pro-inflammatory chemokines and cytokines are released (Bianchi,2007). TLR-9 has been observed to be overexpressed in the BAL of patients with sarcoidosis compared to normal controls (Margaritopoulos et al,2010). A higher expression of TLR-2 and TLR-4 has been demonstrated in peripheral blood monocytes [Wiken,2009], and linkage analysis has indicated that an unidentified polymorphism of TLR-4 is associated with sarcoidosis [Schurmann et al,2008].

2.2 Neutrophil granulocytes

These cells can detect invading microorganisms through the presence of TLRs and eliminate them through the process of phagocytosis. They are amongst the first cells migrating to the site of infection. They have been identified in granulomas of human lungs affected by tuberculosis and demonstrated to be essential for the initiation of pulmonary granuloma formation in M. Tuberculosis-affected C57BL/6 mice (Seiler et al,2003;D'Souza,1997). Various inflammatory cells such as monocytes and macrophages as well as alveolar epithelial cells type II and fibroblasts produce chemokines such as Interleukin-8 (IL-8) and epithelial neutrophil activating protein (ENA)-78 which can attract neutrophils (Pechkovsky et al,2000;Larsen et al,1989;) which in turn produce IL-1, Tumor necrosis factor-α (TNF-α), IL-12 and CXCR3 ligands resulting in an amplification of the inflammatory response in sarcoidosis. On the other hand, these cells produce reactive oxygen species and proteases which can cause damage to the lung. In accordance with this, the presence of high percentage of BAL neutrophils is associated with disease progression, radiographic evidence of fibrosis and to a more likely IPF-like outcome (Tutor-Ureta et al,2006; Ziegenhagen et al,2003;Borzi et al,1993).

2.3 Alveolar macrophages

Alveolar macrohages (AMs) are part of both innate and adaptive immune system. These cells along with their ancestor cells namely monocytes play an important role in the pathogenesis of sarcoidosis. This is highlighted by various events such as macrophagic alveolitis which is a common finding in sarcoidosis, early migration of monocytes from capillaries to alveolar interstitium (Soler&Basset,1976), and formation of macrophages aggregates and their differentiation into epithelioid and multinucleated giant cells which form the core of granuloma. Moreover, activated AMs produce TNF and other cytokines which promote the formation of granuloma in sarcoidosis (Müller-Quernheim et al,1992; Ziegenhagen& Müller-Quernheim,2003).

Infections have been implicated in the pathogenesis of sarcoidosis. Both AMs and monocytes express CD14 which is a membrane-bound lipopolisaccharide (LPS) receptor. It has no intracellular tail and in order to initiate cell activation acts in synergy with TLR-4 which is in close vicinity. When this complex is activated leads to release of NF-kB dependent cytokines such as IL-1,-6,-8 and TNF-α. Intracellular bacteria such as mycobacteria and propionibacteria have been identified as possible causative agents since DNA has been found in sarcoid tissue (Saboor et al,1992;Abe et al,1984). These bacteria are detected by intracellular PRRs such as NOD-1, 2 and TLR-9.

Activation of PRRs leads to the release of cytokines. TNF-α is a proinflammatory cytokine actively produced by sarcoid alveolar macrophages (Fehrenbach et al,2003). It has an important role in lung injury and in the regulation of fibroblast via induction of IL-6. Chronic overexpression of TNF-α and IFN-γ is crucial for the persistence and progression of inflammation and tissue damage in sarcoidosis (Agostini et al,1996). The release of TNF-α is compartmentalized since it has been observed that it is increased in the cultures of BAL cells whereas it is not in peripheral blood cells of the same patient (Müller-Quernheim et al,1992). This suggests that the trigger for the release of this cytokine should be within the lungs and recently is has been proposed that serum amyloid A induces TNF-α release through activation of the innate immune system via TLR-2 (Chen,2010).

Both IL-12, produced by alveolar macrophages, lymphocytes and NK cells and IL-18, produced by alveolar macrophages and dendritic cells are cytokines which have been found up-regulated in the BAL fluid of sarcoid patients, whereas serum levels of IL-12 was decreased in patients group in accordance to TNF- behaviour (Lammas et al,2002;Antoniou et al,2006). These cytokines are involved in Th1 immune response inducing the Th0 to Th1 shift, and when acting in synergy induce production of IFN-γ from Th1 cells (Shigehara et al, 2001). Other cytokines produced by activated AMs are IL-1, IL-6, and IL-15 which favor T-cell proliferation as well as sarcoid fibroblast proliferation and collagen production.

AMs can also act as antigen presenting cells and take part in the adaptive immune response. In sarcoidosis, they develop an increased antigen presenting capacity compared to controls and furthermore, this happens only in AMs from patients with active sarcoidosis and non in AMs from patients with inactive disease (Lem et al,1985;Venet et al,1985;Ina et al,1990;Zissel et al,1997). When in contact with the antigen, the process of phagocytosis begins. T cells recognize the antigen through a T cell receptor, when it is presented within the binding groove of the major histocompatibility complex (MHC) molecule. What follows is a subsequent expansion of antigen specific CD4+ T-cells. It has been observed that the number of MHC II molecules is increased in the surface of AMs of patients with active sarcoidosis, something that has been also related to increased antigen–presenting capacity and moreover that some HLA-DR subtypes are associated with the clinical course of sarcoidosis (Rossi et al,1986;Berlin et al,1997;Martinetti et al,2002; Schürmann et al,2002). Several co-stimulatory molecules expressed on AMs and involved in the interaction between AMs and T-cells are found increased in patients with sarcoidosis. These include CD154 (ligand for CD40), CD72 (ligand for CD5), CD80 and CD86 (ligand for CD28), CD153 (ligand for CD30L) (Wahlström et al,1999;Hoshino et al,1995;Nicod&Isler,1997;Kaneko et al,1999;Agostini et al,1999;Zissel,1999). Adhesion molecules such as CD54 and CD11a-c are also expressed highly in epithelioid cells forming sarcoid granulomas (Zissel,1997).

AMs can be activated by different stimuli and produce different types of cytokines and costimulatory molecules with different actions. Activation by LPS or IFN-γ leads to inflammatory response and production of proinflammatory cytokines and increased expression of CD16, CD32 and CD64. On the other hand, activation by IL-4, IL-10 and IL-13 leads to a fibrotic response and production of CCL17, CCL18, CCL22, IL-1Rα (Prasse,2006).

2.4 Dendritic cells

Dendritic cells (DCs) are antigen presenting cells and have the ability to induce primary immune response in T cells (Banchereau et al,2000). Two subtypes have been identified, the CD11c+ subtype which belongs to the myeloid lineage and the CD11- subtype which belongs to the lymphoid lineage (Ito et al,1999;Siegal et al,1999). The CD11+ myeloid subset has been found to be able to polarize naïve CD4+T cells towards IFN-γ producing - Th1 cells, depending on IL-12 production whereas the CD11c- plasmacytoid subset drives IL-4 producing-Th2 cells upon IL-13 exposure (Rissoan et al,1999). Pulmonary DCs are functionally immature whereas in case of inflammation express high surface amounts of MHC class II and costimulatory molecules and mature into functional APCs (Banchereau&Steinman,1998;Sallusto et al,1998). They also express CCR7 in their surface and under the influence of its ligands such as CCL19 and CCL21 they migrate into the T-cell areas of regional lymphnodes replaced by peripheral blood precursors (Jang et al,2006;Legge&Braciale,2003). Therefore, lymphadenopathy seen in sarcoidosis can be the consequence of the accumulation of DCs in hilar lymphnodes. DCs are components of granuloma observed in sarcoidosis and studies have shown a premature and rapid involvement of these cells at the sites of inflammation and in the formation of granuloma (Iyonaga et al,2002;Ota et al,2004;Chiu et al,2004).

2.5 T-cells

The presence and accumulation of T-cells is critical for the granuloma formation and this is supported by the fact that T-cell depleted mice are incapable of granuloma formation. Lung T-cells from patients with pulmonary sarcoidosis express markers of activation such as IL-2R, CD69 and CD26 (Semenzato et al,1984; Wahlström et al,1999). IL-2R is found to be related with disease severity (Ziegenhagen et al,1997). These activated T-cells are predominantly CD4+, produce mainly IFN-γ and IL-2 and thus belong to the Th1-cell subtype (Pinkston et al,1983;Robinson et al,1985). They represent the immunological hallmark of the disease. Even though in tissues affected by sarcoidosis has been observed that the ratio CD4/CD8 is extremely high, CD8+ cells are capable of releasing IFN-γ and IL-2 as well, adding to the overall Th-1 associated cytokine release in sarcoidisis (Prasse et al,2000). On the contrary, marker cytokines of Th2 cells such as IL-4, IL-5, IL-10, IL-13 are not elevated in sarcoid body fluids or cell culture supernatants of sarcoid T-cells.

T-cell activation occurs when antigens are internalised by APCs, digested into small fragments and loaded into the peptide binding groove of MHC molecules. The variable portions of the T-cell receptors (TCR) are then able to bind to MHC-antigen complex and are clonally expanded (Moller,1998). The cell surface TCR number is then down-regulated and serves as a marker of recent engagement (DuBois et al,1992). Moreover, activation of T-cells requires binding of costimulatory molecules on the cell surface to the appropriate ligand on the APC. The most important molecule expressed by T-cells is CD28 which interacts with CD80 and CD86 on APCs to effectively stimulate T-cells (Pathak et al, 2007).

Both Th1 and Th2 lymphocytes produce cytokines which are responsible for driving the development of granulomatous reactions in the sarcoid lung. IL-2 is released by pulmonary T-cells and acts as a local growth factor for lung T-cells in sarcoidosis (Moller et,1996). Addition of IL-2 in AMs leads to their activation and production of granulocyte-macrophage-colony stimulating factor (GM-CSF). Binding sites for IL-2 have also been observed in human lung fibroblasts and the addition of this cytokine leads to an increased expression of the gene coding for monocyte chemoattractant protein-1 which is involved in fibrosis. IFN-γ, which is expressed by Th1-cells infiltrating the sarcoid tissue, favours the development of the hypersensitivity reaction and on the other hand can inhibit the development of fibrosis. It also regulates the expression of costimulatory molecules such as CD80 and CD86 on accessory cells (Agostini et al,1999). It also induces the release of ELR-chemokines such as CXCL9, CXCL10, CXCL11 and CXCL16 by AMs and alveolar epithelial cells type II (Sugiyama et al,2006;Agostini et al,2005;Takeuchi et al,2006,Morgan et al,2005). Th1-cells expressing receptors for these chemokines such as CXCR3 and CXCR6 are then recruited in the inflamed tissues. IL-4 is released by Th-2 cells and acting in synergy with IL-2 stimulates the growth of T-cells. It has been related to the development of pulmonary fibrosis in sarcoidosis (Gurrieri et al,2005;Wallace&Howie,1999;Tsoutsou et al,2006). IL-10 is released by Th2-cells as well as by CD4+CD25+T regulatory cells (Freeman et al,2005). IL-13 is considered a major inducer of fibrosis and is released by Th0 and Th2-cells. Together with TNFα, induces the release of TGF-β1 in AMs through a process that involves the IL-13rα receptor. Blockade of this receptor signaling results to a decreased production of TGF-β1 and collagen deposition in bleomycin-induced lung fibrosis (Fichtner-Feigl et al 2008).

3. Granuloma

Granuloma is a feature of many chronic interstitial lung diseases, e.g. sarcoidosis, hypersensitivity pneumonitis, berylliosis and histiocytosis X. Granulomas are highly organized structures created by macrophages, epithelioid cells, giant cells, and T cells. It is generally accepted that initiation of granuloma formation requires T cell activation. In contrast, diminished T cell response inhibits granuloma formation. This is shown by Taflin et al who demonstrate that functional regulatory T cells diminish in vitro granuloma formation (Taflin et al,2009). In addition, TNF released by alveolar macrophages is also required for the induction and maintenance of granuloma, as sarcoid patients with macrophage aggregates in their lung parenchyma, which may be regarded as granulomas in status nascendi, disclosed higher levels of TNF release than patients with differentiated granulomas (Fehrenbach et al,2003). In contrast, blockade of TNF in granuloma inducing conditions inhibits granuloma formation (Smith et al,1997).Thus the development of granuloma requires the finetuned interplay of a variety of cell types and cytokines.

An initial event triggering granuloma formation in diseases of known origin is the deposition of antigenic substances in the lung, as observed in tuberculosis and hypersensitivity pneumonitis. In berylliosis the triggering event seems to be the binding of beryllium to HLA molecules on the surface of the immune cells (Newman,1993). The immune system, however, recognizes peptides in the context of self on the surface of antigen-presenting cells and the sole binding of beryllium may not be a sufficiently stimulating event. Therefore, other triggers such as an altered cleavage of self-antigens, caused by a beryllium-induced shift of the specificity of restriction proteases, and subsequent presentation of these new peptides in the context of the MHC, are conceivable.

In experimental models such a metal-induced presentation of new self-antigens recognized as nonself by the immune system has been identified as a cause of autoimmunity (Kubicka-Muranyi et al,1995,1996). In sarcoidosis, however, the initiating agent is not known, but it may be found in the membrane of alveolar macrophages, as demonstrated by a granulomatous skin reaction elicited by membrane fragments of sarcoid alveolar macrophages (Holter et al,1992).

Many structurally different agents are known to stimulate the formation of immune granulomas and they share some characteristics. Firstly, in the case of infectious agents their habitat is the macrophage or, owing to their particulate nature, they have the propensity to be phagocytosed by macrophages. Secondly, they have the capability to persist within tissues or macrophages, either because the micro-organisms involved are resistant to intracellular killing or because the materials resist enzymatic degradation. Thirdly, without a specific T-cell response immune granuloma cannot be generated and therefore, the inducing agents have to be immunogenic. The unknown aetiological sarcoidosis-inducing agent should fulfil these three criteria.

One of the major impediments to studying sarcoidosis is the lack of a widely accepted animal model. In many murine models, granulomas are induced by injection of tail vein with antigens, a route of antigen exposure that does not employ the airway (as is thought to be important in sarcoidosis). Infection model studies with organisms that produce granulomatous inflammation typically study the course of infection that can be either self-limited or fatal. Thus, models often focus on the acute phase of inflammation and granuloma formation, a time frame that is incompatible with chronic persistent sarcoidosis. Nevertheless, recent findings suggest certain cytokines and antigenic exposures may be more applicable to sarcoid research.

Sequential analysis of the cellular components of the sarcoid granulomas has demonstrated their dynamic nature. An influx, local multiplication and cell death of immune cells can be observed, most probably governed by inflammatory signals. In immune granulomas, as in sarcoidosis, these signals are likely to be cytokines and cell-cell interactions of lymphocytes, macrophages and their derivatives, and fibroblasts (Kunkel et al,1989). Blocking CD80 and CD86, molecules mediating the accessory signals of macrophages in T-cell activation (Zissel et al,1997), by monoclonal antibodies suppressed helminth-induced granuloma formation and cytokine release of T-cells, highlighting the interdependence of these processes in granuloma formation (Subramanian et al,1997).

After phagocytosis of the inducing agent the macrophage releases a number of cytokines which mediate migration of activated lymphocytes and monocytes out of the bloodstream into sites of inflammation. Osteopontin, also known as early T-lymphocyte activation protein 1 (Eta-1),is a cytokine produced by macrophages and other cells which promotes macrophage and T-cell chemotaxis (O'Regan et al,1999). Osteopontin deficient mice are prone to disseminated bacille Calmette-Guérin (BCG) infection, presumably because of inadequate local control by poorly formed granulomas (Nau et al,1999). Eta-1 was released in high quantities by macrophages immediately after the phagocytosis of M. tuberculosis, but only in minute amounts when phagocytosing inert particles. Normal lung and granulation tissue did not stain positive for Eta-1 but it was identified by immunohistochemistry in macrophages, lymphocytes and the extracellular matrix of pathological tissue sections of patients with tuberculosis or silicosis (Nau et al,1997). Finally, osteopontin-deficient mice recruit fewer macrophages and epithelioid cells in a Schistosoma hypersensitivity pulmonary granuloma model (O'Regan et al,2001). Yamagami et al used Mycobacterium tuberculosis surface glycolipids (cord factor) to induce both foreign body and hypersensitivity type granulomas in mice (Yamagami et al,2001). Mice were first immunized with heat killed M. tuberculosis before intravenous injection of glycolipid cord factor preparations. Immunized mice developed more severe inflammatory lesions suggesting an immune component (in addition to a foreign body type) to granuloma formation (Yamagami et al,2001). Although both aforementioned models developed immunemediated granulomatous inflammation, both used an intravenous injection and/or a sensitization step as a means of forming pulmonary granulomas.

Other animal models use a variety of knockout mice and antigenic stimuli to elicit pulmonary granulomas. In the study of sarcoidosis, the most common pathogen challenges are with Propionibacterium and Mycobacterium (Seiler et al,2003;Co et al,2004;Kunkel et al,1998;Nishiwaki et al,2004;Perez et al,2003;Minami et al,2003). Finally, some early animal models exposed mice to Kveim reagent or homogenates of sarcoid tissue in an attempt to create a "sarcoid mouse." Belcher and Reid followed mice after footpad injection with sarcoid homogenates for up to 1 year (Belcher&Reid,1975). At autopsy, granulomas were observed equally in animals that received sarcoid tissue homogenates and control animals (Belcher&Reid,1975). However, Mitchell et al showed mice inoculated with sarcoid tissue homogenates manifest granulomas in many organs and tissues for up to 15 months (Mitchell et al,1976). Studies using Kveim reagent in an animal model are appealing, in theory, as the granulomatous inflammation would likely mirror that of sarcoidosis.

Granuloma formation in sarcoidosis requires interplay between APCs, antigen, and T-cells . This immune response will occur in a genetically susceptible individual (ie, BTNL2), and severity will depend on disease-modifying genes (ie, HLA, TNF). During the initiation phase of granuloma formation, macrophages undergo "frustrated phagocytosis" when in contact with the inciting antigen. The antigen in sarcoidosis is believed to be processed in a classic MHC-II restricted pathway (taken up by phagocytosis and degraded in the endosome/lysosome compartment) with subsequent expansion of antigen-specific CD4+ T-cells. Activation of these macrophages recruits mononuclear cells, predominantly monocytes, and CD4+ T-cells. These cells accumulate at the site of inflammation in an attempt to wall off the antigen or pathogen. Next, inflammatory cells are recruited to the granuloma by chemokines TNF-α, IL-1, IN-γ and others that regulate trafficking to the site of inflammation. Animal studies of immune and foreign-body granulomas suggest that IL-1 is important in the early recruitment stages of granuloma formation, while TNF-α may take part in later maintenance or effector functions (Chensue et al,1989). This view is supported by the observation that depletion of TNF-α led to a rapid regression of fully developed immune granulomas and suppressed the accumulation of mRNA in macrophages surrounding the granuloma. The latter indicates that TNF-α enhances its own synthesis and release, thus favouring further macrophage accumulation and differentiation leading to bacterial elimination (Kindler et al,1989). The requirement of IFN-γ for granuloma formation is demonstrated by the absence of granulomas in IFN-γ gene knockout mice, which do not respond with a granulomatous reaction after exposure to thermophilic bacteria (Gudmundsson&Hunninghake,1997).

During the effector phase of granuloma formation, specific cells are recruited to the site of inflammation. In the case of sarcoidosis, CD4 T-cells predominate. However, if the granuloma is skewed by the initial antigenic burden, eosinophils and neutrophils can be aggressively recruited to the site of inflammation, as is the case with some infection models of granulomatous inflammation. Whether granulomatous inflammation resolves, persists, or leads to fibrosis will depend on a delicate balance of inflammatory cells, regulatory cells, apoptosis, and TH1/TH2 cytokine responses.

The role of T-cells in the development and maintenance of granuloma can be studied in infectious diseases and their animal models. Experimental infection of susceptible mice with Leishmani major results in a disseminated, lethal disease and the infected animals respond with CD4+ Th2 cells secreting IL4, IL-5, IL-6 and IL-10, promoting a humoral and suppressing a cellular immune response. In marked contrast, CD4+ IL-2, IFN-γ and TNF-β-releasing Th1 cells are observed in resistant strains which respond with a strong cellular immune reaction. Evidence from human leishmaniosis suggests that the Th1 or Th2 polarized response determines whether subclinical or progressive disease develops (Kemp et al,1996). Using mycobacterial and schistosomal antigens Type 1 (IFN-γ and TNF-β dominant) and Type 2 (IL-4 and IL-5 dominant) granulomatous responses can be elicited in normal mice. Knockout of the IFN-γ gene converts the Type 1 response to a response with decreased TNF-β and increased secretion of IL-4, IL-5 and other Type 2 cytokines and eosinophilic infiltration. IL-4 gene knockout exacerbates Type 1 response with compartmentalization of the expected exaggerated IFN-γ release to the lymph nodes and a decrease in IFN-γ transcripts in the lung. Most interestingly, IL-4 gene knockout did not convert Type 2 to Type 1 granulomas (Chensue et al,1997). Along this line a Type 1 cytokine pattern has to be expected in tuberculous and sarcoid granulomas. Bergeron et al analysed the presence of mRNA of 16 cytokines in granulomatous lymph node tissue of patients with tuberculosis and sarcoidosis and found a Type 1 response in sarcoidosis and Type 0 response (less polarized to Type 1) in tuberculosis (Lammas et al,2002). In addition, they demonstrated that distinct histological features were associated with characteristic cytokine patterns, e.g. neutrophilic infiltration heralded the presence of IL-8 transcripts (Bergeron et al, 1997).

4. Fibrosis

In 60% of patients with sarcoidosis, the course of the disease is self-limiting with spontaneous resolution of the granuloma, whereas patients with progressive sarcoidosis show massive development of granulomas and do not recover even if strong immunosuppressive therapy is used. The uncontrolled development of granulomas results in fibrosis. The immune cells composing the granuloma secrete cytokines that attract, stimulate and deactivate fibroblasts, which seems to be dependent on immunological cytokines such as interferon (Subramanian et al,1997;Smith et al,1995,Rolfe,1991). Extracellular matrix is found also in the outer rim of and within the granuloma, indicating that the granuloma is the starting point of fibrosis in sarcoidosis (Limper et al,1994;Marshall et al,1996).

Although the reversible phases of initial alveolar injury in the sarcoid process are mediated by Th1 lymphocytes, the fibrotic changes that follow the sarcoid Th1 immune response are modulated by macrophages, neutrophils, eosinophils and mast cells, which, via overproduction of the superoxide anion, oxygen radicals and proteases, can cause local injury, disruption of the epithelial basement membrane, alteration of epithelial permeability and consequent derangement of the normal architecture of lung parenchyma (Bjemer et al,1987;Inoue et al,1996;Agostini&Semenzato,1998). By releasing a number of molecules, including transforming growth factor (TGF)-b and the family of TGF-related cytokines, platelet-derived growth factor and insulin-like growth factor I, sarcoid macrophages may mediate fibrosis. These growth factors for fibroblasts and epithelial cells and their receptors are abundantly expressed in fibrotic lung. They cooperate with the TGF family in promoting fibroblast growth and deposition of collagen fibrils. Furthermore, macrophage-derived cytokines which are overexpressed at sites of granuloma formation (including IL-1, IL-6, IFN-c, TNF-a and GM-CSF) and immunoglobulin G immune complexes may upregulate the expression of the inducible form of nitric oxide synthase and nitric oxide production in granuloma cells, thus contributing to the injury and consequent reparative processes (Ishioka et al,1996;Homma et al,1995;Bost et al,1994;Facchetti et al,1999).

Prasse and his colleagues recently demonstrated also, increased release of the profibrotic chemokine CCL18 (a chemokine released by M2 macrophages), by alveolar macrophages from patients with fibrotic sarcoidosis (Prasse et al,2006). The induction of M2 alveolar macrophages in chronic sarcoidosis might emerge due to different mechanisms. First, the activation of alveolar macrophages might be induced in a total lack of T cell activation, possibly because there is no relevant T cell antigen or the T cells are anergic. Engagement of the innate PRRs would induce macrophage activation, which would be boosted by chemokines such as CCL2 released by alveolar epithelial cells type II (Pechkovsky et al,2005). This scenario is rather unlikely because the limited activation of the alveolar macrophages would not result in sufficient granuloma formation. In addition, the involvement of T cells in sarcoid granuloma has been demonstrated (Bergeron et al,1997). Thus, it is more likely that after granuloma formation the T cell activation is downregulated or shifts from a Th1- to a Th2-dominated phenotype. Downregulation of T cell activation but persistent macrophage activation again might result in a shift from classical to alternative activation as already described. A shift from a Th1 T cell activation pattern to a Th0/Th2 pattern can be seen in tuberculosis, but in sarcoidosis IL-4 and Il-10 producing T cells are also present and the contribution of their cytokine release might increase during a downregulation of the Th1 response (Somoskovi et al,1999;Baumer et al,1997;Mollers et al,2001). This shift fosters M2 activation because IL-4 and IL-10 are the main inducers of CCL18 and downregulate M1-related cytokine release (Zissel et al,1996). Besides CCL18, the profibrotic cytokine TGF-b is also found in close proximity to the granuloma, inducing extracellular matrix deposition and downregulating M1-related cytokine release (Zissel et al,1996). CCL18 release is amplified by extracellular matrix, Th2 cytokines, and contact to fibroblasts initiating a vicious cycle and accelerating pulmonary fibrosis.

The recruitment of fibroblasts and the subsequent increased production of matrix macromolecules are crucial to the fibrotic process. The migration of fibroblasts and epithelial cells from the interstitium to the alveolar spaces and adhesive interactions of fibroblasts with the surrounding interstitial matrix are the major factors contributing to the development of fibrosis. The migratory process of fibroblasts reflects the local release of a variety of molecules which can act as chemoattractant factors for fibroblasts, such as chemokines, products of coagulation and the fibrinolytic cascade, as well as matrix proteins (collagen peptides, laminin, fibronectin and elastin-derived peptides) (Marshall et al,1996;Shigehara et al,1998;Probst-Cousin et al,1997;Roman et al,1995). Most of these are actively produced in sarcoid lung. Molecules secreted by sarcoid inflammatory cells are also able to prime fibroblasts to enter the G1 phase of the growth cycle, and thus to proliferate.

A way of estimating the status of fibroblasts is to monitoring the turn-over of cellular matrix in the process of fibrosis. Several parameters have been thoroughly evaluated to serve as markers for pulmonary fibrosis (type III procollagen peptide, collagenase, hyaluronan, and fibrinogen and its degradation products) (Bjemer et al,1991;Mornex et al,1994;Pohl et al,1992;O'Connor et al,1989;Perez et al,1993;Schaberg et al,1994). The problem encountered with this concept is that none of the named markers can differentiate between pathological fibrosis and normal tissue turnover in inflammation, as demonstrated by the fact that some markers correlate with parameters of alveolitis (Perez et al,1993), although conflicting results have been obtained in longitudinal studies (Pohl et al,1992;O'Connor et al,1989).

5. References

Abe C, Iwai K, Mikami R, Hosoda Y. (1984). Frequent isolation of Propionibacterium acnes from sarcoidosis lymph nodes. *ZentralblBakteriolMikrobiolHyg A*, 256:541-547.

Agostini C, Zambello R, Sancetta R, Cerutti A, Milani A, Tassinari C, et al.(1996). Expression of tumor necrosis factor-receptor superfamily members by lung T lymphocytes in interstitial lung disease. *Am J Respir Crit Care Med*, 153:1359-1367.

Agostini C, Semenzato G.(1998). Cytokines in sarcoidosis.*SeminRespir Infect*,13: 184–196.

Agostini C, Trentin L, Perin A, Facco M, Siviero M, Piazza F, et al.(1999). Regulation of alveolar macrophage-T cell interactions during Th1-type sarcoid inflammatory process. *Am J Physiol*, 277:L240-250.

Agostini C, Cabrelle A, Calabrese F, Bortoli M, Scquizzato E, Carraro S, et al.(2005). Role for CXCR6 and its ligand CXCL16 in the pathogenesis of T-cell alveolitis in sarcoidosis. *Am J RespirCrit Care Med*,172:1290-1298.

Antoniou KM, Tzouvelekis A, Alexandrakis MG, Tsiligianni I, Tzanakis N, Sfiridaki K, et al. (2006). Upregulation of Th1 cytokine profile (IL-12, IL-18) in bronchoalveolar lavage fluid in patients with pulmonary sarcoidosis. *J Interferon Cytokine Res*, 26:400-405.

Banchereau J, Steinman RM. (1998). Dendritic cells and the control of immunity. *Nature*, 392:245-52.

Banchereau J, Briere F, Caux C, Davoust J, Lebecque S, Liu YJ, et al.(2000). Immunobiology of dendritic cells. *Annu Rev Immunol*, 18:767-811.

Baumer I, Zissel G, Schlaak M, Mu¨ller-Quernheim J. (1997). Th1/Th2 cell distribution in pulmonary sarcoidosis. *Am J Respir Cell MolBiol*, 16:171–177.

Belcher RW, Reid JD. (1975). Sarcoid granulomas in CBA/J mice.Histologic response after inoculation with sarcoid and nonsarcoid tissue homogenates. *Arch Pathol*, 99:283-285.

Bergeron A, Bonay M, Kambouchner M, et al. (1997). Cytokine patterns in tuberculous and sarcoid granulomas: correlations with histopathologic features of the granulomatous response. *J Immunol*, 159: 303–443.

Berlin M, Fogdell-Hahn A, Olerup O, Eklund A, Grunewald J. (1997). HLA-DR predicts the prognosis in Scandinavian patients with pulmonary sarcoidosis. *Am J RespirCrit Care Med*, 156:1601-1605.

Bianchi ME. (2007). DAMPs, PAMPs and alarmins: all we need to know about danger. *J Leukoc Biol*, 81:1-5.

Bjermer L, Engstrom-Laurent A, Thunell M, Hallgren R. (1987). The mast cell and signs of pulmonary fibroblast activation in sarcoidosis. *Int Arch Allergy ApplImmunol*, 82: 298–301.

Bjermer L, Eklund A, Blaschke E.(1991). Bronchoalveolar lavage fibronectin in patients with sarcoidosis: correlation to hyaluronan and disease activity. *EurRespir J*, 4:965–971.

Borzì RM, Grigolo B, Meliconi R, Fasano L, Sturani C, Fabbri M, et al.(1993). Elevated serum superoxide dismutase levels correlate with disease severity and neutrophil degranulation in idiopathic pulmonary fibrosis. *ClinSci (Lond)*, 85:353-359.

Bost TW, Riches DW, Schumacher B, et al. (1994). Alveolar macrophages from patients with beryllium disease and sarcoidosis express increased levels of mRNA for tumor necrosis factor-a and interleukin-6 but not interleukin-1b. *Am J Respir Cell MolBiol*, 10: 506–513.

Chen ES, Song Z, Willett MH, Heine S, Yung RC, Liu MC et al. (2010). Serum amyloid A regulates granulomatous inflammation in sarcoidosis through Toll-like receptor-2. *Am J RespirCrit Care Med*, 181:360-373.

Chensue SW, Otterness IG, Higashi GI, ShmyrForsch C, Kunkel SL. (1989). Monokine production by hypersensitivity (Shistosomamansoni egg) and foreign body (Sephadex bead)-type granuloma macrophages. Evidence for sequential production of IL-1 and tumor necrosis factor.*J Immunol*, 142: 1281–1286.

Chensue SW, Warmington K, Ruth JH, Lukacs N, Kunkel SL.(1997). Mycobacterial and schistosomal antigen-elicited granuloma formation in IFN-gamma and IL-4 knockout mice: analysis of local and regional cytokine and chemokine networks. *J Immunol*, 159: 356–573.

Chiu BC, Freeman CM, Stolberg VR, Hu JS, Komuniecki E, Chensue SW.(2004). The innate pulmonary granuloma: characterization and demonstration of dendritic cell recruitment and function. *Am J Pathol*,164:1021-1030.

Co DO, Hogan LH, Il-Kim S, Sandor M. (2004). T cell contributions to the different phases of granuloma formation. *Immunol Lett*, 92:135-142.

Daniele RP, Rowlands DT Jr. (1976) Lymphocyte subpopulations in sarcoidosis: correlation with disease aetivity and duration. *Ann Intern Med*, 85:593-600.

D'Souza CD, Cooper AM, Frank AA, Mazzaccaro RJ, Bloom BR, Orme IM. (1997). An anti-inflammatory role for gamma delta T lymphocytes in acquired immunity to Mycobacterium tuberculosis. *J Immunol*, 158:1217-1221.

Du Bois RM, Kirby M, Balbi B, Saltini C, Crystal RG. (1992). T-lymphocytes that accumulate in the lung in sarcoidosis have evidence of recent stimulation of the T-cell antigen receptor. *Am Rev Respir Dis*, 145:1205-1211.

Facchetti F, Vermi W, Fiorentini S, et al. (1999). Expression of inducible nitric oxide synthase in human granulomas and histiocytic reactions. *Am J Pathol*, 154: 145–152.

Fehrenbach H, Zissel G, Goldmann T, Tschernig T, Vollmer E, Pabst R, et al. (2003). Alveolar macrophages are the main source for tumour necrosis factor-alpha in patients with sarcoidosis. *Eur Respir J*, 21:421-428.

Fichtner-Feigl S, Young CA, Kitani A, Geissler EK, Schlitt HJ, Strober W. (2008). IL-13 signaling via IL-13R alpha2 induces major downstream fibrogenic factors mediating fibrosis in chronic TNBS colitis. *Gastroenterology*, 135:2003-2013

Freeman CM, Chiu BC, Stolberg VR, Hu J, Zeibecoglou K, Lukacs NW, et al. (2005). CCR8 is expressed by antigen-elicited, IL-10-producing CD4+CD25+ T cells, which regulate Th2-mediated granuloma formation in mice. *J Immunol*, 174:1962-1970.

Gudmundsson G, Hunninghake GW. (1997). Interferon-γ is necessary for the expression of hypersensitivity pneumonitis. *J Clin Invest*, 99: 2386–2390.

Gurrieri C, Bortoli M, Brunetta E, Piazza F, Agostini C. (2005) Cytokines, chemokines and other biomolecular markers in sarcoidosis. *SarcoidosisVasc Diffuse Lung Dis*, 22Suppl 1:S9-14

Holter J, Park H, Sjoerdsma K, Kataria Y. (1992). Nonviable autologous bronchoalveolar lavage cell preparations induce intradermal epithelioid cell granulomas in sarcoidosis patients. *Am Rev Respir Dis*, 145: 864–871.

Homma S, Nagaoka I, Abe H, et al. (1995). Localization of platelet-derived growth factor and insulin-like growth factor I in the fibrotic lung. *Am J Respir Crit Care Med*, 152: 2084–2089.

Hoshino T, Itoh K, Gouhara R, Yamada A, Tanaka Y, Ichikawa Y, et al. (1995). Spontaneous production of various cytokines except IL-4 from CD4+ T cells in the affected organs of sarcoidosis patients. *ClinExpImmunol*, 102:399-405.

Hunninghake GW, Crystal RG. (1981). Pulmonary sarcoidosis: a disorder mediated by excess helper T-lymphocyte activity at sites of disease activity. *N Engl J Med*, 305:429-434.

Hunninghake GW, Fulmer JD, Young RC Jr, Gadek JE, Crystal RG. (1979) Localization of the immune response in sarcoidosis. *Am Rev Respir Dis*, 120:49-57.

Ina Y, Takada K, Yamamoto M, Morishita M, Miyachi A. (1990). Antigen-presenting capacity in patients with sarcoidosis. *Chest*, 98:911-916.

Inoue Y, King TE Jr, Tinkle SS, Dockstader K, Newman LS. (1996). Human mast cell basic fibroblast growth factor in pulmonary fibrotic disorders. *Am J Pathol*, 149: 2037–2054.

Ishioka S, Saito T, Hiyama K, et al. (1996). Increased expression of tumor necrosis factor-a, interleukin-6, platelet-derived growth factor-B and granulocyte-macrophage colony-stimulating factor Mrna in cells of bronchoalveolar lavage fluids from patients with sarcoidosis.*SarcoidosisVasc Diffuse Lung Dis*, 13: 139–145.

Ito T, Inaba M, Inaba K, Toki J, Sogo S, Iguchi T, et al.(1999). A CD1a+/CD11c+ subset of human blood dendritic cells is a direct precursor of Langerhans cells. *J Immunol*, 163:1409-1419.

Iyonaga K, McCarthy KM, Schneeberger EE. (2002). Dendritic cells and the regulation of a granulomatous immune response in the lung. *Am J Respir Cell Mol Biol*, 26:671-679.

Jang MH, Sougawa N, Tanaka T, Hirata T, Hiroi T, Tohya K, et al. (2006). CCR7 is critically important for migration of dendritic cells in intestinal lamina propria to mesenteric lymph nodes. *J Immunol*, 176:803-810.

Kaneko Y, Kuwano K, Kunitake R, Kawasaki M, Hagimoto N, Miyazaki H et al. (1999). Immunohistochemical localization of B7 costimulating molecules and major histocompatibility complex class II antigen in pulmonary sarcoidosis. *Respiration*, 66:343-348.

Kemp M, Theander TG, Kharazmi A. (1996). The contrasting roles of CD4+ T cells in the intracellular infections in humans: leishmaniasis as an example. *Immunol Today,* 17: 13–16.

Kindler V, Sappino A, Grau G, Piguet P, Vassalli P. (1989). The inducing role of tumor necrosis factor in the development of bactericidal granulomas during BCG infection.*Cell*,56: 731–740.

Kubicka-Mulanyi M, Kremer J, Rottmann N, et al. (1996). Murine systemic autoimmune disease induced by mercuric chloride: T helper cells reacting to self proteins. *Int Arch Allergy Immunol,* 109: 11–20.

Kubicka-Muranyi M, Griem P, Lübben B, Rottmann N, Lührmann R, Gleichmann E. (1995). Mercuric-chloride-induced autoimmunity in mice involves up-regulated presentation by spleen cells of altered and unaltered nucleolarself antigen. *Int Arch Allergy Immunol,* 108: 1–10.

Kunkel SL, Chensue SW, Strieter RM, Lynch JP, Remick DG.(1989). Cellular and molecular aspects of granulomatous inflammation. *Am J Respir Cell MolBiol,* 1: 439–447.

Kunkel SL, Lukacs NW, Strieter RM, Chensue SW. (1998). Animal models of granulomatous inflammation. *SeminRespir Infect,* 13:221-228.

Lammas DA, De Heer E, Edgar JD, Novelli V, Ben-Smith A, Baretto R, et al. (2002). Heterogeneity in the granulomatous response to mycobacterial infection in patients with defined genetic mutations in the interleukin 12-dependent interferon-gamma production pathway. *Int J ExpPathol*,83:1-20.

Larsen CG, Anderson AO, Oppenheim JJ, Matsushima K. (1989). Production of interleukin-8 by human dermal fibroblasts and keratinocytes in response to interleukin-1 or tumour necrosis factor. *Immunology,* 68:31-36.

Legge KL, Braciale TJ. (2003). Accelerated migration of respiratory dendritic cells to the regional lymph nodes is limited to the early phase of pulmonary infection. *Immunity,* 18:265-277.

Lem VM, Lipscomb MF, Weissler JC, Nunez G, Ball EJ, Stastny P, et al. (1985). Bronchoalveolar cells from sarcoid patients demonstrate enhanced antigen presentation. *J Immunol,* 135:1766-1771.

Limper AH, Colby TV, Sanders MS, Asakura S, Roche PC, DeRemee RA. (1994). Immunohistochemical localization of transforming growth factor-b 1 in the nonnecrotizing granulomas of pulmonary sarcoidosis. *Am J Respir Crit Care Med,* 149:197–204.

Margaritopoulos GA, Antoniou KM, Karagiannis K, Samara KD, Lasithiotaki I, Vassalou E, et al. (2010). Investigation of Toll-like receptors in the pathogenesis of fibrotic and granulomatous disorders: a bronchoalveolar lavage study. *Fibrogenesis Tissue Repair,* 11;3:20.

Marshall BG, Wangoo A, Cook HT, Shaw RJ. (1996). Increased inflammatory cytokines and new collagen formation in cutaneous tuberculosis and sarcoidosis. *Thorax,* 51:1253–1261.

Martinetti M, Luisetti M, Cuccia M. (2002). HLA and sarcoidosis: new pathogenetic insights. *SarcoidosisVasc Diffuse Lung Dis,* 19:83-95.

Minami J, Eishi Y, Ishige Y, et al. (2003). Pulmonary granulomas caused experimentally in mice by a recombinant trigger-factor protein of Propionibacterium acnes. *J Med Dent Sci*, 50:265-274.

Mitchell DN, Rees RJ, Goswami KK. (1976). Transmissible agents from human sarcoid and Crohn's disease tissues. *Lancet*, 2:761-765.

Moller DR, Forman JD, Liu MC, Noble PW, Greenlee BM, Vyas P, et al. (1996). Enhanced expression of IL-12 associated with Th1 cytokine profiles in active pulmonary sarcoidosis. *J Immunol*, 156:4952-4960.

Moller DR. (1998). Involvement of T cells and alterations in T cell receptors in sarcoidosis. *SeminRespir Infect*, 13:174-183.

Mollers M, Aries SP, Dro¨mann D, Mascher B, Braun J, Dalhoff K. (2001). Intracellular cytokine repertoire in different T cell subsets from patients with sarcoidosis. *Thorax*, 56:487–493.

Morgan AJ, Guillen C, Symon FA, Huynh TT, Berry MA, Entwisle JJ, et al. (2005). Expression of CXCR6 and its ligand CXCL16 in the lung in health and disease. *Clin Exp Allergy*, 35:1572-1580

Mornex JF, Leroux C, Greenland T, Ecochard D. (1994). From granuloma to fibrosis in interstitial lung disease: molecular and cellular interactions. *Eur Respir J*, 7: 779–785.

Müller-Quernheim J, Pfeifer S, Männel D, Strausz J, Ferlinz R. (1992). Lung-restricted activation of the alveolar macrophage/monocyte system in pulmonary sarcoidosis. *Am Rev Respir Dis*, 145:187-192.

Nau GJ, Guilfoile P, Chupp GL, et al. (1997). A chemoattractant cytokine associated with granulomas in tuberculosis and silicosis. *ProcNatlAcadSci USA*, 94: 6414–6419.

Nau GJ, Liaw L, Chupp GL, Berman JS, Hogan BL, Young RA. (1999). Attenuated host resistance against Mycobacterium bovis BCG infection in mice lacking osteopontin. *Infect Immun*,67:4223-4230.

Newman LS. (1993). To Be2+ or not to Be2+: immunogenetics and occupational exposure (Comment). *Science*, 262: 197–198.

Nicod LP, Isler P. (1997). Alveolar macrophages in sarcoidosiscoexpress high levels of CD86 (B7.2), CD40, and CD30L. *Am J Respir Cell Mol Biol*, 17:91-96.

Nishiwaki T, Yoneyama H, Eishi Y, et al. (2004). Indigenous pulmonary Propionibacterium acnes primes the host in the development of sarcoid-like pulmonary granulomatosis in mice. *Am J Pathol*,165:631-639.

O'Connor CM, Ward K, van Breda A, McIlgorm A, Fitz-Gerald MX. (1989). Type 3 procollagen peptide in bronchoalveolar lavage fluid.Poor indicator of course and prognosis in sarcoidosis. Chest, 96: 339–344.

O'Regan AW, Chupp GL, Lowry JA, Goetschkes M, Mulligan N, Berman JS. (1999). Osteopontin is associated with T cells in sarcoid granulomas and has T cell adhesive and cytokine-like properties in vitro. *J Immunol*, 162:1024-1031.

O'Regan AW, Hayden JM, Body S, et al. (2001). Abnormal pulmonary granuloma formation in osteopontin-deficient mice. *Am J Respir Crit Care Med*, 164:2243-2247.

Ota M, Amakawa R, Uehira K, Ito T, Yagi Y, Oshiro A, et al. (2004). Involvement of dendritic cells in sarcoidosis. *Thorax*, 59:408-413.

Pathak SK, Basu S, Basu KK, Banerjee A, Pathak S, Bhattacharyya A et al. (2007). Direct extracellular interaction between the early secreted antigen ESAT-6 of

Mycobacterium tuberculosis and TLR2 inhibits TLR signaling in macrophages. *Nat Immunol*, 8:610-618.

Pechkovsky DV, Zissel G, Ziegenhagen MW, Einhaus M, Taube C, Rabe KF et al. (2000). Effect of proinflammatory cytokines on interleukin-8 mRNA expression and protein production by isolated human alveolar epithelial cells type II in primary culture. *Eur Cytokine Netw*, 11:618-625.

Pechkovsky DV, Goldmann T, Ludwig C, et al. (2005). CCR2 and CXCR3 agonistic chemokines are differently expressed and regulated in human alveolar epithelial cells type II. *Respir Res*, 6:75.

Perez RL, Duncan A, Hunter RL, Staton GL. Elevated D dimer in the lungs and blood of patients with sarcoidosis. Chest 1993; 103: 1100–1106.

Perez RL, Rivera-Marrero CA, Roman J. (2003). Pulmonary granulomatous inflammation: from sarcoidosis to tuberculosis. *Semin Respir Infect*,18:23-32.

Pinkston P, Bitterman PB, Crystal RG. (1983). Spontaneous release of interleukin-2 by lung T lymphocytes in active pulmonary sarcoidosis. *N Engl J Med*, 308:793-800.

Pohl WR, Thompson AB, Köhn H, et al.(1992). Serum procollagen III peptide levels in subjects with sarcoidosis. A 5-year follow-up study. *Am Rev Respir Dis*, 145:412–417.

Prasse A, Georges CG, Biller H, Hamm H, Matthys H, LuttmannW,et al. (2000). Th1 cytokine pattern in sarcoidosis is expressed by bronchoalveolar CD4+ and CD8+ T cells. *Clin Exp Immunol*, 122:241-248.

Prasse A, Pechkovsky DV, Toews GB, Jungraithmayr W, Kollert F, Goldmann T, et al. (2006). A vicious circle of alveolar macrophages and fibroblasts perpetuates pulmonary fibrosis via CCL18. *Am J Respir Crit Care Med*, 173:781-792.

Probst-Cousin S, Poremba C, Rickert CH, Bocker W, Gullotta F. (1997). Factor XIIIa expression in granulomatous lesions due to sarcoidosis or mycobacterial infection. *Pathol Res Pract*, 193:741–745.

Rissoan MC, Soumelis V, Kadowaki N, Grouard G, Briere F, de Waal Malefyt R, et al. (1999). Reciprocal control of T helper cell and dendritic cell differentiation. *Science*, 283:1183-1186.

Robinson BW, McLemore TL, Crystal RG. (1985). Gamma interferon is spontaneously released by alveolar macrophages and lung T lymphocytes in patients with pulmonary sarcoidosis. *J Clin Invest*, 75:1488-1495.

Rolfe MW, Kunkel SL, Standiford TJ, et al. (1991). Pulmonary fibroblast expression of interleukin-8: a model for alveolar macrophage-derived cytokine networking. *Am J Respir Cell Mol Biol*, 5: 493–501.

Roman J, Jeon YJ, Gal A, Perez RL. (1995). Distribution of extracellular matrices, matrix receptors, and transforming growth factor-b1 in human and experimental lung granulomatous inflammation. *Am J Med Sci*, 309: 124–133.

Rossi GA, Zocchi E, Sacco O, Balbi B, Ravazzoni C, Damiani G. (1986). Alveolar macrophage stimulation of T-cell proliferation in autologous mixed lymphocyte reactions. Role of HLA-DR antigens. *Am Rev Respir Dis*, 133:78-82.

Saboor SA, Johnson NM, McFadden J. (1992). Detection of mycobacterial DNA in sarcoidosis and tuberculosis with polymerase chain reaction. *Lancet*, 339:1012-1015.

Sallusto F, Schaerli P, Loetscher P, Schaniel C, Lenig D, Mackay CR, et al. (1998). Rapid and coordinated switch in chemokine receptor expression during dendritic cell maturation. *Eur J Immunol*, 28:2760-2769

Schaberg T, Orzechowski K, Oesterling C, Lode H, Schuppan D. (1994). Simultaneous measurement of collagen type-VI-related antigen and procollagen type-N-propeptide levels in bronchoalveolar lavage. *Eur Respir J*, 7: 1221–1226.

Schürmann M, Bein G, Kirsten D, Schlaak M, Müller-Quernheim J, Schwinger E. (1998). HLA-DQB1 and HLA-DPB1 genotypes in familial sarcoidosis. *Respir Med*, 92:649-652.

Schürmann M, Kwiatkowski R, Albrecht M, Fischer A, Hampe J, Müller-Quernheim J, Schwinger E, Schreiber S. (2008). Study of Toll-like receptor gene loci in sarcoidosis. *Clin Exp Immunol*, 152:423-431.

Seiler P, Aichele P, Bandermann S, Hauser AE, Lu B, Gerard NP et al. (2003). Early granuloma formation after aerosol Mycobacterium tuberculosis infection is regulated by neutrophils via CXCR3-signaling chemokines. Eur J Immunol, 33:2676-2686.

Semenzato G, Agostini C, Trentin L, Zambello R, Chilosi M, Cipriani et al. (1984). Evidence of cells bearing interleukin-2 receptor at sites of disease activity in sarcoid patients. *Clin Exp Immunol*, 57:331-337.

Shigehara K, Shijubo N, Hirasawa M, Abe S, Uede T. (1998). Immunolocalization of extracellular matrix proteins and integrins in sarcoid lymph nodes. *Virchows Arch*, 433: 55–61.

Shigehara K, Shijubo N, Ohmichi M, Takahashi R, Kon S, Okamura H, et al. (2001). IL-12 and IL-18 are increased and stimulate IFN-gamma production in sarcoid lungs. *J Immunol*, 166:642-649.

Siegal FP, Kadowaki N, Shodell M, Fitzgerald-Bocarsly PA, Shah K, Ho S, et al. The nature of the principal type 1 interferon-producing cells in human blood.Science. 1999 Jun;284:1835-7.

Siltzbach LE, James DG, Neville E, Turiaf J, Battesti JP, Sharma OP, et al. (1974). Course and prognosis of sarcoidosis around the world. *Am J Med*, 57:847-852.

Smith D, Hansch H, Bancroft G, Ehlers S. (1997). T-cell-independent granuloma formation in response to Mycobacterium avium: role of tumour necrosis factor-alpha and interferon-gamma. *Immunology*, 92:413–421.

Smith RE, Strieter RM, Zhang K, Phan SH, Standiford TJ, Lukacs NW.A role for C-C chemokines in fibrotic lung disease.J LeukocBiol 1995; 57: 782–787.

Soler P, Basset F. (1976). Morphology and distribution of the cells of a sarcoid granuloma: ultrastructural study of serial sections. *Ann N Y Acad Sci*, 278:147-160.

Somoskovi A, Zissel G, Zipfel PF, et al. (1999). Different cytokine patterns correlate with the extension of disease in pulmonary tuberculosis. *Eur Cytokine Netw*, 10:135–142.

Subramanian G, Kazura JW, Pearlman E, Jia X, Malhtra I, King CL. (1997). B7-2 requirement for helminth-induced granuloma formation and CD4 Type 2 T helper cell cytokine expression. *J Immunol*, 158: 5914–5920.

Sugiyama K, Mukae H, Ishii H, Kakugawa T, Ishimoto H, Nakayama S, et al. (2006). Elevated levels of interferon gamma-inducible protein-10 and epithelial neutrophil-activating peptide-78 in patients with pulmonary sarcoidosis. *Respirology*, 11:708-714.

Taflin C, Miyara M, Nochy D, et al. (2009). FoxP3þ regulatory T cells suppress early stages of granuloma formation but have little impact on sarcoidosis lesions. *Am J Pathol,* 174:497–508.

Takeuchi M, Oh-I K, Suzuki J, Hattori T, Takeuchi A, Okunuki Y et al. (2006). Elevated serum levels of CXCL9/monokine induced by interferon-gamma and CXCL10/interferon-gamma-inducible protein-10 in ocular sarcoidosis. *Invest Ophthalmol Vis Sci,* 47:1063-1068.

Tsan MF, Gao B. (2004). Endogenous ligands of Toll-like receptors. *J Leukoc Biol,* 76:514-519.

Tsoutsou PG, Gourgoulianis KI, Petinaki E, Germenis A, Tsoutsou AG, Mpaka M, et al. (2006). Cytokine levels in the sera of patients with idiopathic pulmonary fibrosis. *Respir Med,* 100:938-945.

Tutor-Ureta P, Citores MJ, Castejón R, Mellor-Pita S, Yebra-Bango M, Romero Y et al. (2006). Prognostic value of neutrophils and NK cells in bronchoalveolar lavage of sarcoidosis. *Cytometry B Clin Cytom,* 70:416-422.

Venet A, Hance AJ, Saltini C, Robinson BW, Crystal RG. (1985). Enhanced alveolar macrophage-mediated antigen-induced T-lymphocyte proliferation in sarcoidosis. *J Clin Invest,* 75:293-301.

Wagner H. (2006). Endogenous TLR ligands and autoimmunity. *Adv Immunol,* 91:159-173.

Wahlström J, Berlin M, Sköld CM, Wigzell H, Eklund A, Grunewald J. (1999). Phenotypic analysis of lymphocytes and monocytes/macrophages in peripheral blood and bronchoalveolar lavage fluid from patients with pulmonary sarcoidosis. *Thorax,* 54:339-346.

Wallace WA, Howie SE. (1999). Immunoreactive interleukin 4 and interferon-gamma expression by type II alveolar epithelial cells in interstitial lung disease. *J Pathol,* 187:475-480.

Wikén M, Grunewald J, Eklund A, Wahlström J. (2009). Higher monocyte expression of TLR2 and TLR4, and enhanced pro-inflammatory synergy of TLR2 with NOD2 stimulation in sarcoidosis. *J Clin Immunol,* 29:78-89.

Winterbauer RH, Lammert J, Selland M, Wu R, Corley D, Springmeyer SC. (1993). Bronchoalveolar lavage cell populations in the diagnosis of sarcoidosis. *Chest,* 104:352-361.

Yamagami H, Matsumoto T, Fujiwara N, et al. (2001). Trehalose 6,6'-dimycolate (cord factor) of Mycobacterium tuberculosis induces foreign-body- and hypersensitivity-type granulomas in mice. *Infect Immun,* 69:810-815.

Yeager H Jr, Williams MC, Beekman JF, Bayly TC, Beaman BL. (1977). Sarcoidosis: analysis of cells obtained by bronchial lavage. *Am Rev Respir Dis,* 116:951-954.

Ziegenhagen MW, Benner UK, Zissel G, Zabel P, Schlaak M, Müller-Quernheim J. (1997). Sarcoidosis: TNF-alpha release from alveolar macrophages and serum level of sIL-2R are prognostic markers. *Am J Respir Crit Care Med,* 156:1586-1592.

Ziegenhagen MW, Müller-Quernheim J. (2003). The cytokine network in sarcoidosis and its clinical relevance. *J Intern Med,* 253:18-30.

Zissel G, Schlaak J, Schlaak M, Mu¨ller-Quernheim J. (1996). Regulation of cytokine release by alveolar macrophages treated with interleukin-4, interleukin-10, or transforming growth factor beta. *Eur Cytokine Netw,* 7:59–66.

Zissel G, Ernst M, Schlaak M, Müller-Quernheim J. (1997). Accessory function of alveolar macrophages from patients with sarcoidosis and other granulomatous and nongranulomatous lung diseases. *J Investig Med*, 45:75-86.

Zissel G, Ernst M, Schlaak M, Müller-Quernheim J. (1999). Pharmacological modulation of the IFNgamma-induced accessory function of alveolar macrophages and peripheral blood monocytes. *Inflamm Res*, 48:662-668.

2

Immunopathogenesis and Presumable Antigen Pathway of Sarcoidosis: A Comprehensive Approach

Atsushi Kurata
Department of Molecular Pathology,
Tokyo Medical University,
Japan

1. Introduction

Sarcoidosis is a multisystemic disorder of unknown etiology. Formation of non-caseating epithelioid cell granulomas in the involved organs is the main feature. Sarcoidal granulomas may involve any organ, but generally clinical sarcoidosis manifests intrathoracic lymph node enlargement, pulmonary involvement, skin or ocular signs and symptoms, or some combination of these findings. Epidemiologically, sarcoidosis affects people of all racial and ethnic groups, although the incidence of sarcoidosis varies widely throughout the world and is most common in women and in people of Scandinavian or African-American descent. Sarcoidosis may occur at any age, but is usually seen in adults under the age of 50 (Dempsey et al., 2009; Iannuzzi et al., 2007; Fernandez-Faith & McDonnell, 2007).

Sarcoidosis has long been characterized by many unknown variables: antigen, genetic susceptibility, and factors influencing severity (Noor & Knox, 2007). Clinically, non-specific systemic symptoms such as fatigue, night sweats, and weight loss are common in sarcoidosis patients. Tuberculin skin test is classically negative in patients with sarcoidosis, since activated T-lymphocytes are sequestered at the site of sarcoidal granulomas, leading to peripheral depletion (Dempsey et al, 2009). However, a negative result of the tuberculin test is not specific to sarcoidosis. The Kveim-Siltzbach test, in which cutaneous injection of homogenate of human sarcoid tissue extract and subsequent biopsy are performed, is currently less often used because of many constraints and lower sensitivity. Sarcoidal granulomas produce angiotensin I-converting enzyme (ACE), whose levels are elevated in 60% of patients with sarcoidosis, but the importance of using serum ACE levels in diagnosing sarcoidosis remains controversial (Iannuzzi et al., 2007).

Currently, the diagnosis of sarcoidosis is based on three different features: (1) a typical clinico-radiological presentation, (2) the histological evidence of non-caseating granuloma, and (3) exclusion of other possible diseases causing granuloma (Ma et al., 2007). The typical clinico-radiological presentation includes the presence of bilateral hilar adenopathy in chest radiograph of an asymptomatic patient, Löfgren syndrome (combination of erythema nodosum, bilateral hilar adenopathy in chest radiograph, and arthritis), and a gallium-67 uptake in the parotid and lacrimal glands (Panda sign) as well as in the right paratracheal and bilateral hilar (Lambda sign). Diagnostic criteria of sarcoidosis have been thus

established; however, in practice, its diagnosis is made arbitrarily because complete exclusion of other granulomatous disorders is impossible (Baughman et al., 2010).
In order to understand and explore the solutions of the problems thus far mentioned, in this chapter, comprehensive approaches from pathological and immunological aspects of sarcoidosis, including the comparison with other granulomatous disorders, are presented.
In general, granulomas form as a result of the persistent presence of a nondegradable product or of delayed type hypersensitivity (Kobayashi et al., 2001). The former includes silica, tuberculosis, Toxoplasma gondii, and foreign bodies, while the latter includes sarcoidosis, Crohn's disease, and (tumor-related) sarcoid reactions. It is understood that granuloma-formation is observed in virtually all the hosts in the former, while it is found in limited hosts in the latter. Administration of beryllium oxide or zirconium lactate into subcutaneous tissue usually causes formation of foreign body granulomas, while it may result in hypersensitivity granuloma in a small percentage of individuals (Maceira et al., 1984). Furthermore, most delayed-type hypersensitivity reactions, including contact dermatitis, tuberculin reaction, and tumor immunity, do not form granulomas (Fig. 1).

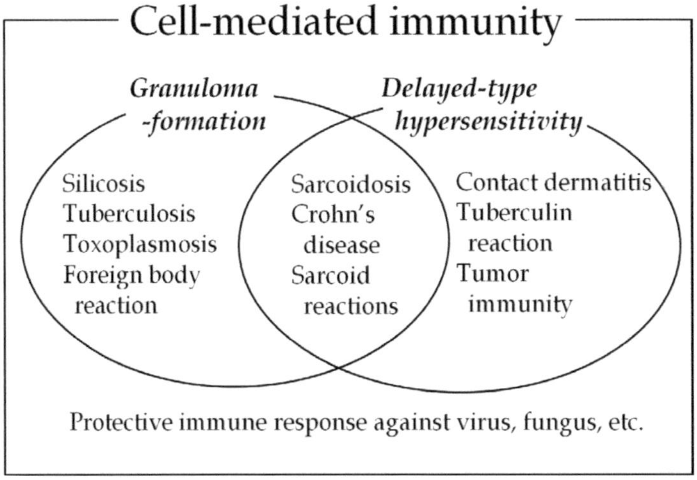

Fig. 1. Sarcoidosis and associated immunoreactions

2. Histology of sarcoidal granulomas and differential diagnosis of granulomatous disorders

Sarcoid lesions vary according to the different stages of the disease. In the earliest stage in the lung, mild alveolitis without granuloma formation is seen. However, characteristic non-necrotizing epithelioid cell granulomas usually occur thereafter. The granulomas have a compact appearance with sharp circumscription from the surrounding lung (Fig. 2a). The granulomas are mainly composed of epithelioid cells, tightly-assembled macrophages with spindle features that are microscopically reminiscent of epithelial cells, and are occasionally surrounded by a rim of lymphocytes. Multinucleated giant cells may be intermingled, which are formed by the fusion of epithelioid macrophages (Ma et al., 2007). Cutaneous manifestations have been classified into nonspecific lesions without granuloma formation such as erythema nodosum and specific lesions with presence of the granulomas (Fig. 2b), similar to the respiratory counterparts (Fernandez-Faith & McDonnell, 2007).

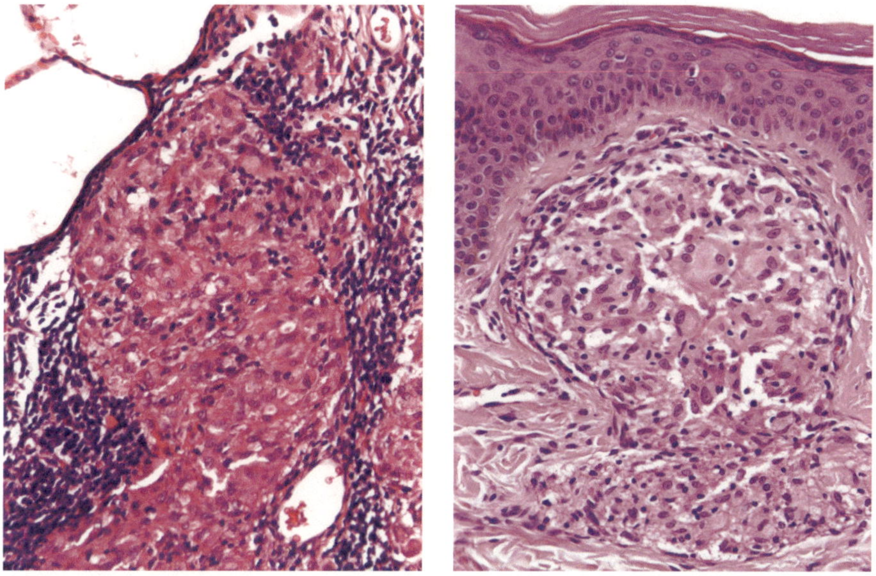

(a) (b)

Fig. 2. Typical sarcoidal granulomas in the lung and skin. (a) Non-necrotizing epithelioid cell granulomas in the lung with surrounding lymphocytes. Original magnification: x200. (b) Dermal sarcoidal granulomas formed beneath the epidermis, accompanied by intermingled giant cells. Original magnification: x200.

The subsequent outcome of granulomas seems to be common in different organs of varying etiologies. That is, cellular and discrete granulomas in the early stages of the disease may resolve with little consequence, or become more fibrotic as the disease advances (Fig. 3); eventually they may appear as confluent hyalinized nodules (Iannuzzi et al., 2007; Ma et al., 2007).

Several characteristic histological features have been proposed that are useful in the differential diagnosis of various granulomatous disorders. It is well known that tuberculous granulomas are accompanied by caseous necrosis, and Crohn's disease is usually manifested as small-sized granulomas (Fig. 4a). Toxoplasmic lymphadenopathy is characterized by the presence of microgranulomas without multinucleated giant cells (Fig. 4b) (Eapen et al., 2006).

However, specific features of sarcoidal granulomas have not been identified. Although asteroid and Schaumann's bodies may appear in sarcoidal granuolomas (Fig. 5a) (Ma et al., 2007), these may be found in other granulomatous disorders as well (Fernandez-Faith & McDonnell, 2007). Therefore, diagnostic problems occasionally arise. For example, there are difficulties in differentiation of sarcoidosis vs. foreign body granuloma if polarizable foreign body particles are detected in sarcoidal granuloma (Fig. 5b) (Marcoval et al., 2001), and of sarcoidosis vs. sarcoid reactions, which occur in approximately 4% of carcinomas (Brincker, 1986), if a patient with cancer is accompanied by granulomas in lymph nodes or other organs such as the spleen (Marruchella, 2009; Kurata et al., 2010b).

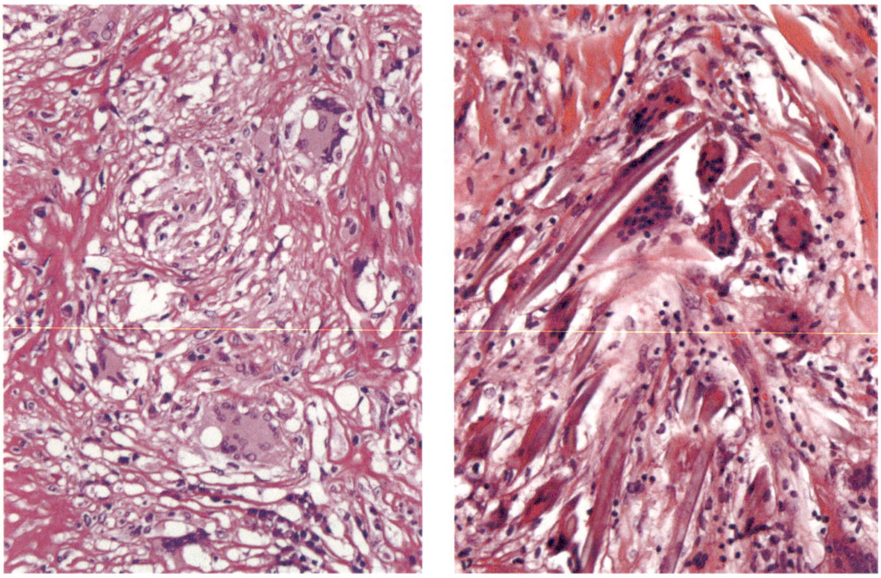

(a) (b)

Fig. 3. Examples of old granulomas accompanied by fibrosis in cases other than sarcoidosis. (a) Old granulomas divided by hyaline in the lymph node sarcoid reactions. Original magnification: x200. (b) A thread granuloma, representative foreign body reaction, is tightly packed by fibrotic capsule. Original magnification: x200.

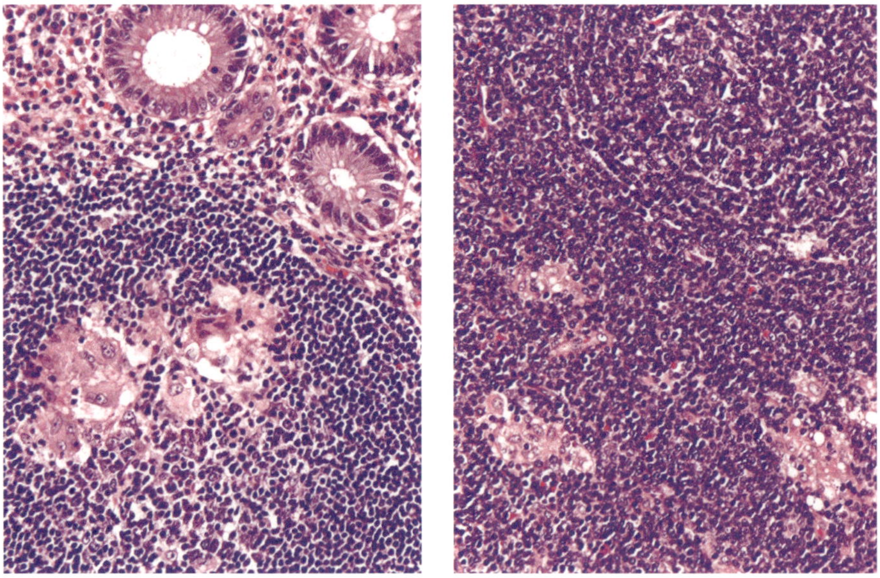

(a) (b)

Fig. 4. Examples of small granulomas in cases other than sarcoidosis. (a) Small-sized granulomas in the intestinal mucosa in Crohn's disease. Original magnification: x200. (b) Scattered microgranulomas in Toxoplasmic lymphadenitis. Original magnification: x200.

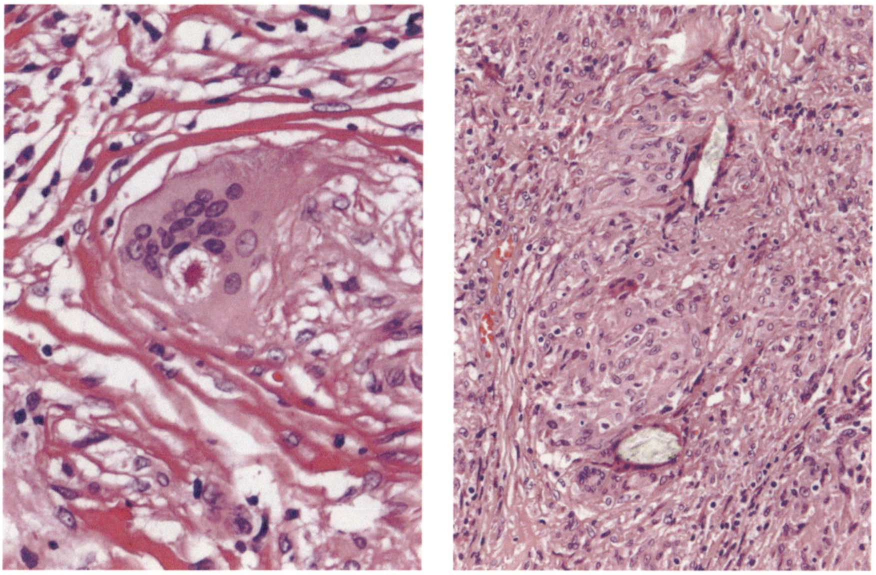

(a) (b)

Fig. 5. Examples of inclusions and foreign bodies in sarcoidal granulomas. (a) Asteroid body (arrow), a star-shaped spiculated structure, within multinucleated giant cells of sarcoidal granuloma. Original magnification: x400. (b) Foreign body particles identified in sarcoidal granulomas of the skin. Original magnification: x200.

3. Immunohistochemical characteristics of cells constituting granulomas

Granulomas are usually accompanied by $CD4^+$ T-lymphocytes in the center and $CD8^+$ T-lymphocytes in the periphery (Fig. 6), but B-lymphocytes are rarely observable within granulomas (Kurata et al., 2005; Ma et al., 2007; Noor & Knox, 2007). These observations are compatible with the below-mentioned postulation that granulomas are caused by cell-mediated immunity, and that $CD4^+$ T-lymphocytes are primary cells that recruit other T-lymphocytes and macrophages.

Epithelioid cells and giant cells as well as other macrophages including alveolar macrophages in the lung and sinus histiocytes in the lymph nodes are immunohistochemically positive for CD68, a marker for pan-macrophages. In contrast, macrophages within granulomas are selectively positive for ACE by immunohistochemistry in both sarcoidosis and sarcoid reactions (Fig. 7a), and probably in other granulomas. ACE is selectively expressed in macrophages with particular differentiation including those with epithelioid formation.

The macrophages constituting these granulomas originate from blood monocytes, not from resident tissue macrophages. This was verified by presence of a large amount of mononuclear cells within and around granulomas, regardless of the developmental stage, that were immunohistochemically labeled by myeloid-related protein 8 and 14 (S100A8 and S100A9, respectively), which are only expressed in freshly recruited macrophages (Fig. 7b) (Kurata et al., 2005). Besides T-lymphocytes and macrophages, below-mentioned dendritic cells (DCs) are interspersed within granulomas (Noor & Knox, 2007).

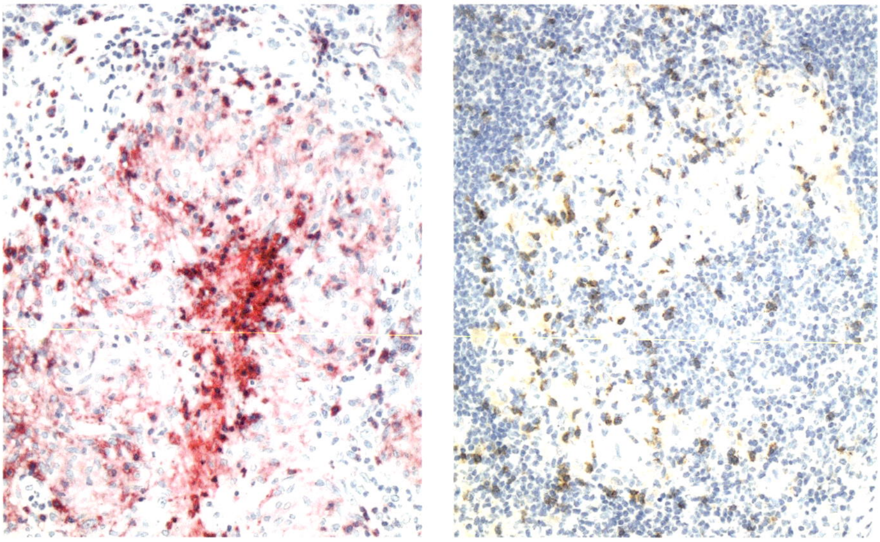

(a) (b)

Fig. 6. Immunohistochemitry of lymphocytes in lymph node sarcoid reactions. (a) $CD4^+$ T-lymphocytes are abundantly seen especially in the center of the granuloma. Positive signal is red. Original magnification: x200. (b) $CD8^+$ T-lymphocytes are scattered especially in the periphery of the granuloma. Positive signal is brown. Original magnification: x200.

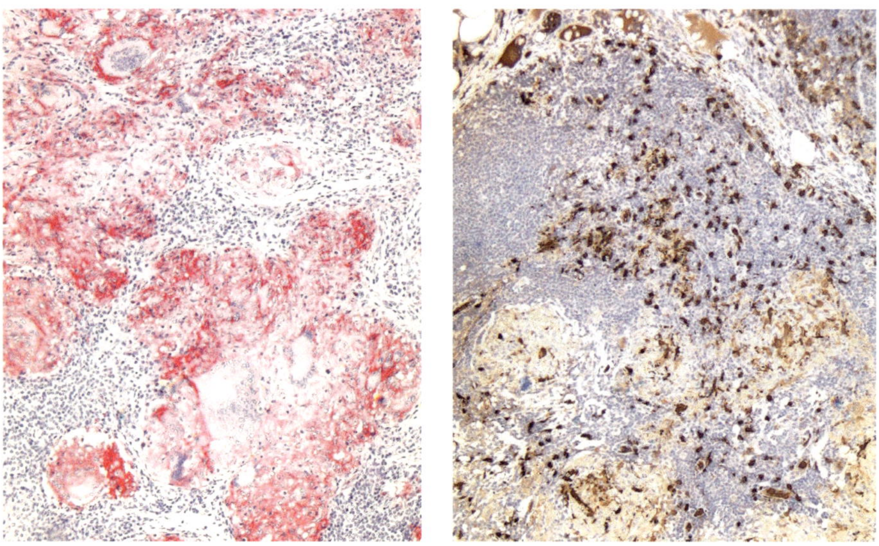

(a) (b)

Fig. 7. Immunohistochemitry of macrophages in lymph node sarcoid reactions. (a) Angiotensin I-converting enzyme is selectively expressed in macrophages observed in granulomas. Positive signal is red. Original magnification: x100. (b) Myeloid-related protein 8-positive cells indicating freshly recruited macrophages are abundantly seen in and around the granulomas. Positive signal is brown. Original magnification: x100.

4. Pathogenesis of granulomatous disorders

It is generally believed that sarcoidosis occurs in genetically susceptible hosts exposed to specific but unknown environmental agents (Dempsey et al., 2009). Pathogenesis of sarcoidosis is thought to be similar to other granulomatous diseases of known cause, such as chronic beryllium disease. That is, the exogenous antigens are phagocytosed and processed by antigen presenting cells, followed by antigen presentation through human leukocyte antigen (HLA) class II molecules to naïve CD4+ T-lymphocytes. The immune reaction begets polarization of the T-lymphocytes to a T-helper 1 phenotype (Th1), followed by cellular recruitment and differentiation leading to formation of the sarcoidal granuloma through the secretion of interferon-γ and interleukin-2 (Baughman et al., 2010; Iannuzzi et al., 2007). However, this sequence is identical to delayed-type hypersensitivity in general such as a tuberculin reaction except for the formation of granulomas (Kobayashi et al., 2001). Therefore, the causative factors specific to granuloma formation are obscure (Fig. 8). Although tumor necrosis factor alpha (TNF-α), macrophage inflammatory protein 1 (MIP-1), monocyte chemotactic protein 1 (MCP-1), and granulocyte macrophage colony-stimulating factor (GM-CSF) may be involved in the formation of granulomas (Baughman et al., 2010; Iannuzzi et al., 2007), their decisive roles in the formation of granulomas in comparison with cell-mediated immunity in general have not been proved. Furthermore, although TNF antagonists are effective in treating some patients with sarcoidosis (Baughman et al., 2010), paradoxical occurrence of sarcoid-like granulomas has been reported in patients treated with TNF blockers (Daïen et al., 2009).

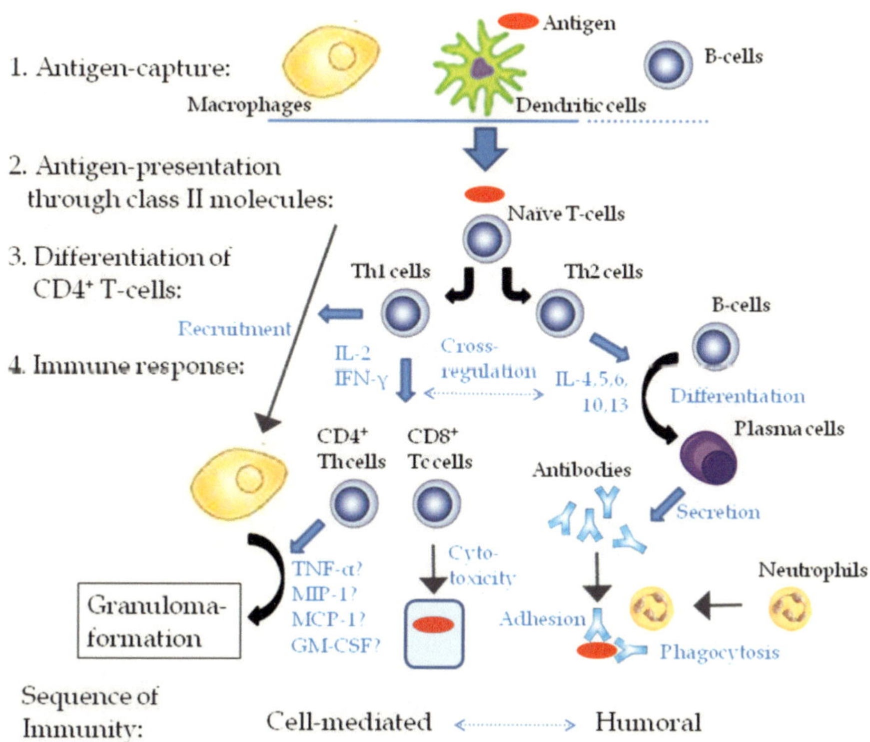

Fig. 8. Paradigm of immunoreactions of Th1 and Th2.

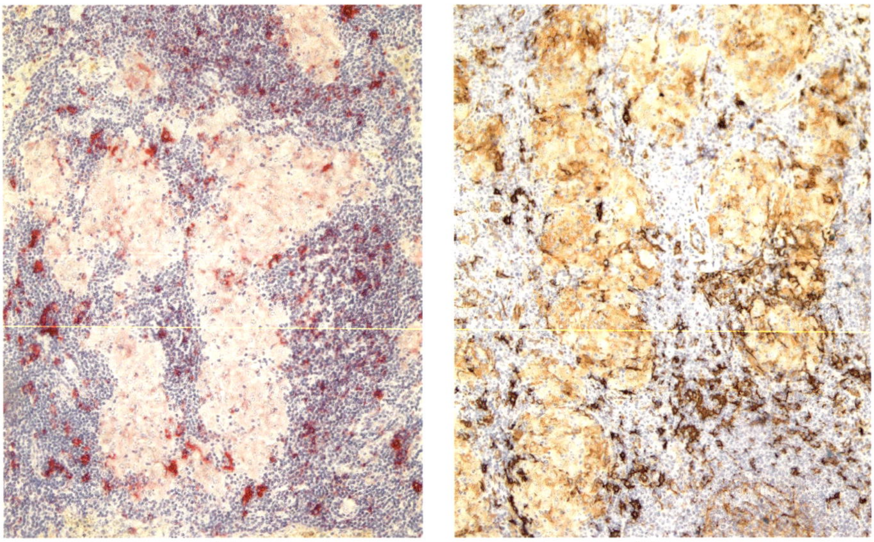

(a) (b)

Fig. 9. Immunohistochemitry for antigen-presenting cells in lymph node sarcoid reactions. (a) HLA-DR+ antigen-presenting cells in the vicinity and inside the granulomas. Positive signal is red. Original magnification: x100. (b) Fascin+ mature dendritic cells in the vicinity and inside the granulomas. Positive signal is brown. Original magnification: x100.

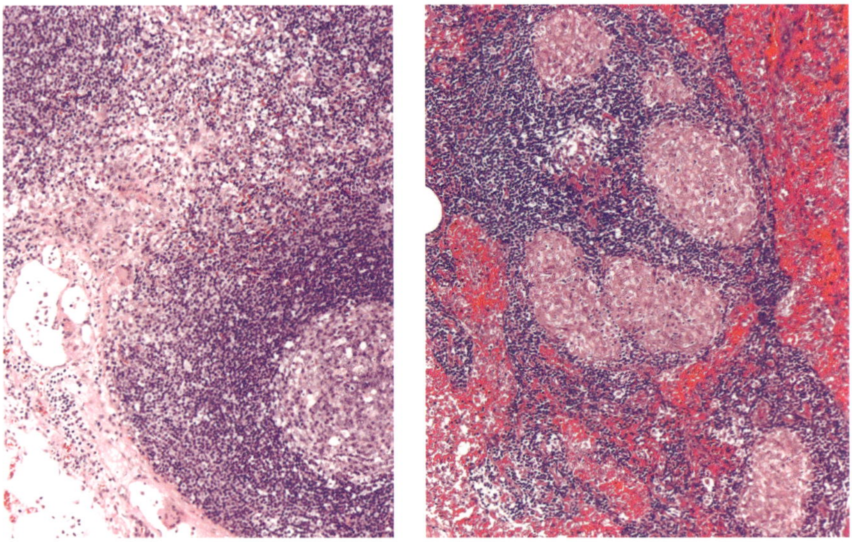

(a) (b)

Fig. 10. Pathogenesis of granulomas of lymph nodes exemplified by sarcoid reactions. (a) Solitary granuloma being formed between sinus and T-zone. Original magnification: x100. (b) Multiple granulomas in the T-zone around the lymph follicles. Original magnification: x100.

Emergence of HLA-DR+ antigen-presenting cells in the vicinity and inside the granulomas has been shown in sarcoidosis (Ota et al., 2004) and in lymph node sarcoid reactions (Kurata et al., 2005) (Fig. 9a). These cells grossly corresponded to mature DCs, which are representative antigen presenting cells, as verified by expression of below-mentioned fascin and CD83 (Fig. 9b). Further, cell-to-cell contact between T-lymphocytes and HLA-DR$^+$ mature DCs in sarcoidal granulomas has been demonstrated by immunohistochemical double staining (Ota et al., 2004).

Although granulomas in the lymph nodes are usually of the large confluent type in systemic sarcoidosis, some of those in sarcoid reactions are solitary or of multiple types. Solitary type is formed between sinus and T-zone (Fig. 10a), while multiple type occurs exclusively in the sinus or T-zone (Fig. 10b). These data are consistent with the contribution of T-cell-mediated immunity in granuloma formation. However, we have not yet identified any specific feature(s) that can differentiate sarcoid reactions from sarcoidosis by immunohistochemical analysis of lymphocytes, DCs, and macrophages (Kurata et al., 2005).

5. Maturation of dendritic cells above granulomas and with relation to lymphatic vessels in cutaneous sarcoidosis

As mentioned earlier, DCs play central roles in antigen presentation. CD1a$^+$ immature DCs, a subpopulation of which is also known as Langerhans cells, are capable of antigen uptake and processing, but unable to present antigens to naïve T-lymphocytes. Immature DCs, after the capture of antigens, generally begin to mature en route through the lymphatic vessels. After maturation, they can express antigen molecules to naïve T-lymphocytes in the lymph nodes. In contrast, some DCs that are activated in the peripheral tissues stay at the site of activation, where they mature and may contribute to the initiation of local inflammation (Wilson & Villadangos, 2004; Kurata et al., 2010b).

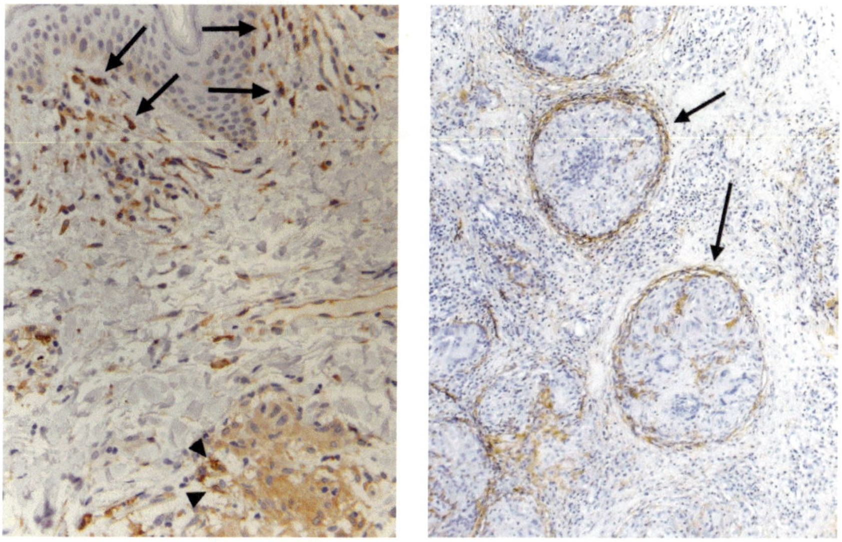

(a) (b)

Fig. 11. Immunohistochemistry of cutaneous sarcoidosis (a) Mature fascin$^+$ DCs proliferate in the upper dermis (arrows) and appear in dermal granulomas (arrowheads). Blood vessel endothelial cells are also positive for fascin. Original magnification: x100. (b) Granulomas in deeper dermis encircled by D2-40$^+$ lymphatic vessel endothelial cells (arrows). Original magnification: x100.

In cutaneous sarcoidosis, it was previously reported that Langerhans cells in the epidermis overlying the dermal granuloma increase in number compared with those in the epidermis of age-, sex-, and race-matched controls (Martin et al., 1986). We have recently identified that mature DCs, which are immunohistochemically positive for fascin and CD83, proliferate in the upper dermis overlying the dermal granulomas (Fig. 11a), compared with other granulomatous skin disorders or various skin diseases. In addition, dermal granulomas, especially those located in the deeper dermis, were occasionally encircled by D2-40$^+$ lymphatic vessel endothelial cells (Fig. 11b), whereas no dermal granuloma was encircled by fascin$^+$ blood vessel endothelial cells (Kurata et al., 2010a). We have re-checked the granulomas in all 11 specimens of cutaneous sarcoidosis used in the above-mentioned research for CD31, a more specific marker for blood vessel endothelial cells, and confirmed that no granuloma was encircled by blood vessels. Therefore, cutaneous sarcoidosis has common pathogenesis with Crohn's disease in that granulomas appear to be in and around the lymphatic vessels (Van Kruiningen & Colombel, 2008). These data suggest that the antigen pathway of cutaneous sarcoidosis is from epidermis through dermis to lymphatic vessels, and not from other organs such as lungs through the vascular pathway.

6. Presumable antigen pathway and proposed antigen of sarcoidosis

The hypothesis that the antigen enters through the skin in cutaneous sarcoidosis is in accordance with the observations that cutaneous sarcoidosis is usually seen at the onset of systemic sarcoidosis (Fernandez-Faith & McDonnell, 2007). However, cutaneous manifestation in sarcoidosis occurs in only about 20-35% of patients (Fernandez-Faith & McDonnell, 2007). It is conceivable that antigen enters not from the skin, e.g. through the respiratory tracts, in the other 65-80% of patients. Alternatively, it is also possible to speculate that the initial skin lesions are overlooked in a considerable number of sarcoidosis patients. The supposed antigen pathways are shown in Fig. 12. Granulomas may be formed at arbitrary sites in the course of these pathways. However, bilateral pulmonary hilar lymph nodes may be the most important sentinels against the antigens. Although we have not investigated ocular sarcoidosis, local entry of the antigen in ocular sarcoidosis ("ocular pathway") is also possible.

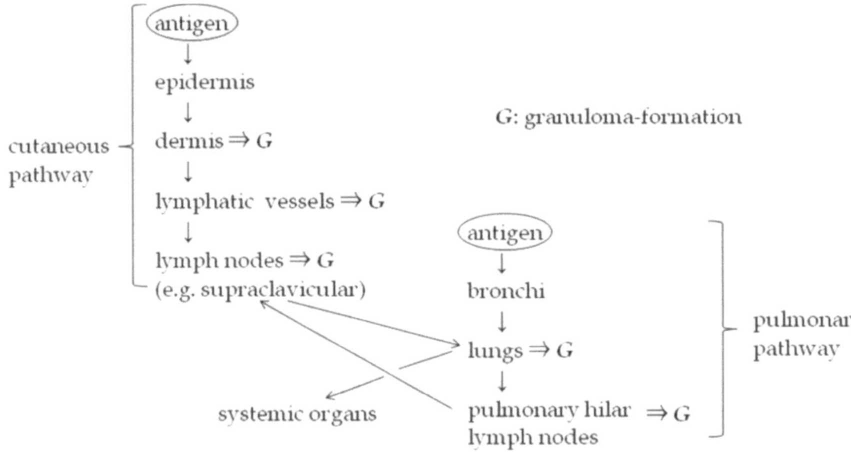

Fig. 12. Presumable antigen pathway of sarcoidosis

The common antigen of sarcoidosis patients remains unknown. Mycobacterium species are suspected in Western countries, and Propionibacterium (P.) species are suspected in Japan. It has been reported that *P. acnes* DNA are highly detected in lymph nodes of Japanese and European patients with sarcoidosis (Eishi et al., 2002). Therefore, *P. acnes* is a likely candidate as the antigen of sarcoidosis. Since *P. acnes* is indigenous to the skin, the "cutaneous pathway" may bring this antigen to systemic organs. Further studies are necessary to investigate the specificity of *P. acnes* in causing sarcoidosis, e.g. if *P. acnes* is more often detected in cutaneous granulomas in sarcoidosis than in other granulomatous skin diseases.

Alternatively, since the association with various environmental exposures has been reported in sarcoidosis patients, it has been proposed that "the development of sarcoidosis is probably the end result of immune responses to various ubiquitous environmental triggers" (Iannuzzi et al., 2007). Combining this proposal and the "cutaneous pathway" theory, it is postulated that environmental antigens may often enter through the skin. In this hypothesis, cutaneous sarcoidosis is likely to be the granuloma-forming variant of contact dermatitis, along the same line as sarcoid reactions being the granuloma-forming variant of tumor immunity (Fig. 1). The fact that *P. acnes* is highly detected in sarcoidosis lesions may not indicate that *P. acnes* is a causative agent, rather, it may be the supporting evidence that other antigens enter through the skin along with *P. acnes* that is indigenous to the skin. To confirm this possibility, further experimental research is necessary, such as testing the skin reaction by topical application of various environmental factors to the sarcoidosis patients' skin in order to identify the antigen.

7. Further hypothesis on susceptibility to sarcoidosis

As mentioned earlier, sarcoidosis is thought to occur in genetically susceptible hosts exposed to specific but unknown environmental antigens. Genetic susceptibility due to particular immunity profiles including expression of specific HLA-molecules and T-cell receptors has been proposed, since the pathogenesis of sarcoidosis seems to involve the interplay between antigens, HLA class II molecules, and T-cell receptors (Baughman et al., 2010). For example, HLA class II antigens encoded by HLA-DRB1 and DQB1 alleles have been reported to be associated with sarcoidosis (Rossman et al., 2003; Iannuzzi et al., 2003). However, no single gene appears to be responsible for sarcoidosis; rather, the susceptibility is likely to be based on more than one gene (Ma et al., 2007).

Alternatively, it is also conceivable that environmental factors may affect the susceptibility. For example, the prevalence of allergic diseases such as wheeze, atopic dermatitis, and rhinitis in children has increased throughout the world in the past 50 years (Yura et al., 2011). This phenomenon cannot be explained only by genetic susceptibility, since the prevalence of susceptible genes has not been changed during these 50 years. Interestingly, it has been reported that infants who received Diptheria-Pertussis-Tetanus (DPT) vaccination subsequently show significantly higher incidence of bronchial asthma, allergic rhinitis, and atopic dermatitis, compared with those who did not receive it in a remote island in Japan (Yoneyama et al., 2000). This may be explained by the hypothesis that those who received DPT vaccination escaped from natural immunoreaction against these intracellular pathogens, thus the paucity of defense against intracellular pathogens brings about a Th1-less and Th2-dominant constitution, leading to increased susceptibility to allergic pathogens that are associated with humoral immunity because Th1 and Th2 cytokines suppress each other (Kobayashi et al., 2001) (Fig. 13).

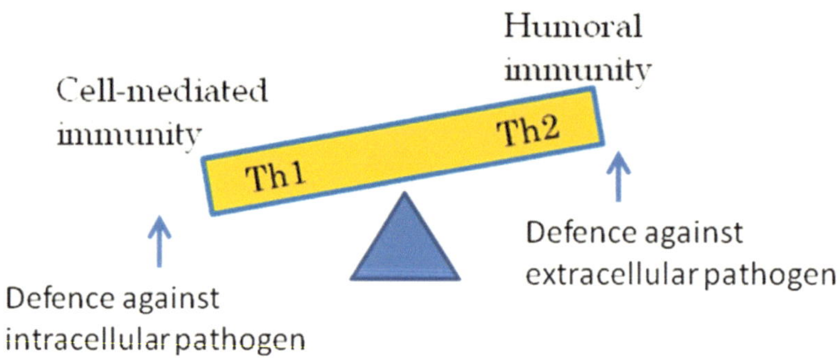

Fig. 13. The interrelation between Th1 and Th2 immunophenotypes.

Contrary to the atopic predisposition, sarcoidosis patients may tend to have a Th1-dominant constitution. This is partially verified by the fact that the incidence of atopic diseases including asthma and allergic rhinitis in sarcoidosis patients is much lower than the usual atopy prevalence (Kokturk et al., 2005). Although highly speculative, Scandinavian people are more often exposed than other Europeans to intracellular pathogens such as viruses that prefer a colder environment, whereas Americans of African descent live in an environment where more viruses are found than their natural environment. These external factors may promote the susceptibility of Scandinavian and African-American hosts to sarcoidosis.

8. Conclusion

Sarcoidosis is an elusive disorder that has long been characterized by many unknown factors. Although its hallmark feature is formation of non-necrotizing epithelioid cell granulomas in the involved organs, exclusion of other granulomatous disorders is necessary in its diagnosis, and a unique histological feature is lacking. However, due to the recent advances in the fields of immunology and immunohistochemistry, the characteristics of sarcoidosis have gradually emerged. It is obvious that sarcoidal granuloma is formed through antigen presentation by DCs and sequential Th1 immunoreactions. Th1-associated cytokines recruit blood monocytes, leading to granuloma formation, although the critical cytokines are still under discussion. Immunohistochemical characteristics of cells constituting granulomas seem to be common between sarcoidosis and other granulomatous disorders including the expression of ACE and the contribution of mature DCs. Although causative antigens are still unknown, the local antigen pathway in cutaneous sarcoidosis has been proposed, since DCs mature above dermal granulomas and dermal granulomas are often associated with local lymphatic vessels. Environmental factors in addition to genetic susceptibility may be associated with not only the onset of but also the predisposition to sarcoidosis.

9. References

Baughman, R.P., Culver, D.A. & Judson, M.A. (2011) A Concise Review of Pulmonary Sarcoidosis, *Am J Respir Crit Care Med* 183(5):573-81.

Brincker, H. (1986) Sarcoid reactions in malignant tumours, *Cancer Treat Rev* Vol. 13(3):147-56.

Daïen, C.I., Monnier, A., Claudepierre, P., Constantin, A., Eschard, J.P., Houvenagel, E., Samimi, M., Pavy, S., Pertuiset, E., Toussirot, E., Combe, B., Morel, J. & Club Rhumatismes et Inflammation (CRI) (2009) Sarcoid-like granulomatosis in patients treated with tumor necrosis factor blockers: 10 cases, *Rheumatology (Oxford)* Vol. 48(8):883-6.

Dempsey, O.J., Paterson, E.W., Kerr, K.M. & Denison, A.R. (2009) Sarcoidosis, *BMJ* Vol. 339:620-5. URL: www.bmj.com

Eapen, M., Mathew, C.F. & Aravindan, K.P. (2005) Evidence based criteria for the histopathological diagnosis of toxoplasmic lymphadenopathy, *J Clin Pathol* Vol. 58(11):1143-6.

Eishi, Y., Suga, M., Ishige, I., Kobayashi, D., Yamada, T., Takemura, T., Takizawa, T., Koike, M., Kudoh, S., Costabel, U., Guzman, J., Rizzato, G., Gambacorta, M., du Bois, R., Nicholson, A.G., Sharma, O.P. & Ando, M. (2002) Quantitative analysis of mycobacterial and propionibacterial DNA in lymph nodes of Japanese and European patients with sarcoidosis, *J Clin Microbiol* Vol. 40(1):198-204.

Fernandez-Faith, E. & McDonnell, J. (2007) Cutaneous sarcoidosis:differential diagnosis, *Clin Dermatol* Vol. 25(3):276-87.

Iannuzzi, M.C., Maliarik, M.J., Poisson, L.M. & Rybicki, B.A. (2003) Sarcoidosis susceptibility and resistance HLA-DQB1 alleles in African Americans. *Am J Respir Crit Care Med* Vol. 167(9):1225-31.

Iannuzzi, M.C., Rybicki, B.A. & Teirstein, A.S. (2007) Sarcoidosis, *N Engl J Med* Vol. 357(21):2153-65.

Kobayashi, K., Kaneda, K. & Kasama, T. (2001) Immunopathogenesis of delayed-type hypersensitivity, *Microsc Res Tech* Vol. 53(4):241-5.

Kokturk, N., Han, E.R. & Turktas, H. (2005) Atopic status in patients with sarcoidosis, *Allergy Asthma Proc* Vol. 26(2):121-4.

Kurata, A., Terado, Y., Schulz, A., Fujioka, Y. & Franke, F.E. (2005) Inflammatory cells in the formation of tumor-related sarcoid reactions, *Hum Pathol* Vol. 36(5):546-54.

Kurata, A., Terado, Y., Izumi, M., Fujioka, Y. & Franke, F.E. (2010a) Where does the antigen of cutaneous sarcoidosis come from?, *J Cutan Pathol* Vol. 37(2):211-21.

Kurata, A., Takayama, N., Terado, Y., Hirano, K., Yokoyama, K. & Fujioka, Y. (2010b) Sarcoidal granulomas in the spleen associated with multiple carcinomas, *Sarcoidosis Vasc Diffuse Lung Dis* Vol. 27(2):153-9.

Ma, Y., Gal, A. & Koss, M.N. (2007) The pathology of pulmonary sarcoidosis: update, *Semin Diagn Pathol* Vol. 24(3):150-61.

Maceira, J.M., Fukuyama, K., Epstein, W.L. & Rowden, G. (1984) Immunohistochemical demonstration of S-100 protein antigen-containing cells in beryllium-induced, zirconium-induced and sarcoidosis granulomas, *Am J Clin Pathol* Vol. 81(5):563-8.

Marcoval, J., Mañá, J., Moreno, A., Gallego, I., Fortuño, Y. & Peyrí, J. (2001) Foreign bodies in granulomatous cutaneous lesions of patients with systemic sarcoidosis, *Arch Dermatol* Vol. 137(4):427-30.

Marruchella, A. (2009) Sarcoidosis or sarcoid reaction?, *Chest* Vol. 136(3):943-4.

Martin, A.G., Kleinhenz, M.E. & Elmets, C.A. (1986) Immunohistologic identificationof antigen-presenting cells in cutaneous sarcoidosis, *J Invest Dermatol* Vol. 86(6):625-9.

Noor, A. & Knox, K.S. (2007) Immunopathogenesis of sarcoidosis, *Clin Dermatol* Vol. 25(3):250-8.

Ota, M., Amakawa, R., Uehira, K., Ito, T., Yagi, Y., Oshiro, A., Date Y, Oyaizu H, Shigeki T, Ozaki Y, Yamaguchi K, Uemura Y, Yonezu S, Fukuhara S. (2004) Involvement of dendritic cells in sarcoidosis. *Thorax* Vol. 59(5):408-13.

Rossman, M.D., Thompson, B., Frederick, M., Maliarik, M., Iannuzzi, M.C., Rybicki, B.A., Pandey, J.P., Newman, L.S., Magira, E., Beznik-Cizman, B., Monos, D. & ACCESS Group (2003) HLA-DRB1*1101: a significant risk factor for sarcoidosis in blacks and whites, *Am J Hum Genet* Vol. 73(4):720-35.

Van Kruiningen, H.J. & Colombel, J.F. (2008) The forgotten role of lymphangitis in Crohn's disease, *Gut* Vol. 57(1):1-4

Wilson, N.S. & Villadangos, J.A. (2004) Lymphoid organ dendritic cells: beyond the Langerhans cells paradigm, *Immunol Cell Biol* Vol. 82(1):91-8.

Yoneyama, H., Suzuki, M., Fujii, K., Odajima, Y (2000) The effect of DPT and BCG vaccinations on atopic disorders, *Arerugi* (*Japanese Journal of Allergology*: Japanese with English abstract) Vol. 49(7):585-92.

Yura, A., Kouda, K., Iki, M. & Shimizu, T. (2011) Trends of allergic symptoms in school children: large-scale long-term consecutive cross-sectional studies in Osaka Prefecture, Japan, *Pediatr Allergy Immunol* 2011: Doi: 10.1111/j.1399-3038.2011.01159.x.

Part 2

Diagnosis

3

Basic Diagnostic Approaches in Sarcoidosis

Louis Gerolemou and Peter R. Smith
Division of Pulmonary Medicine,
SUNY Downstate Medical Center,
University Hospital of Brooklyn at long Island College Hospital,
Brooklyn, NY USA

1. Introduction

Sarcoidosis was first described by a British dermatologist, Jonathan Hutchison in 1869. Since then it has been seen in almost every part of the world and continues to engender considerable interest and concern amongst scientists and medical providers alike because 1) the cause is unknown, 2) it may involve any organ system in the body, 3) the course and prognosis vary from spontaneous resolution to progressive disability and death, and 4) there is no truly satisfactory treatment. Just as there are many unknowns about the illness in general, its diagnosis remains problematic despite extensive study and voluminous reporting in the scientific literature. Our objective in this chapter is to provide an overview of current knowledge on the diagnostic approach in sarcoidosis.

2. Definition

Sarcoidosis is a granulomatous disease of unknown etiology with protean manifestations that affects people throughout the world (1).

3. Diagnostic criteria

In many respects, sarcoidosis is a diagnosis of exclusion. Although it has been asserted that the method of diagnosis has been established (1), a more recent expert view is that the diagnosis is never completely secure (2). There is no single diagnostic test. It is often suspected when a chest radiograph performed for non-specific symptoms such as dyspnea or chest pain shows the characteristic findings of bilateral hilar adenopathy with or without diffuse lung infiltrates. In other cases, especially when thoracic manifestations are atypical or absent, the diagnosis remains obscure. Thus, the diagnostic approach may be straight forward, but in some situations will be complex and involve multiple diagnostic modalities.
The diagnosis of sarcoidosis is based on the following criteria: 1) a compatible clinical and/or radiographic picture 2) histological evidence of non-caseating granulomas and 3) exclusion of other conditions with similar histology. An algorithm for approaching the diagnosis which reflects currently available data is shown in figure 1. The diagnostic evaluation should also evaluate the extent and severity of organ involvement, and assess disease stability and the need for treatment with corticosteroids (1).

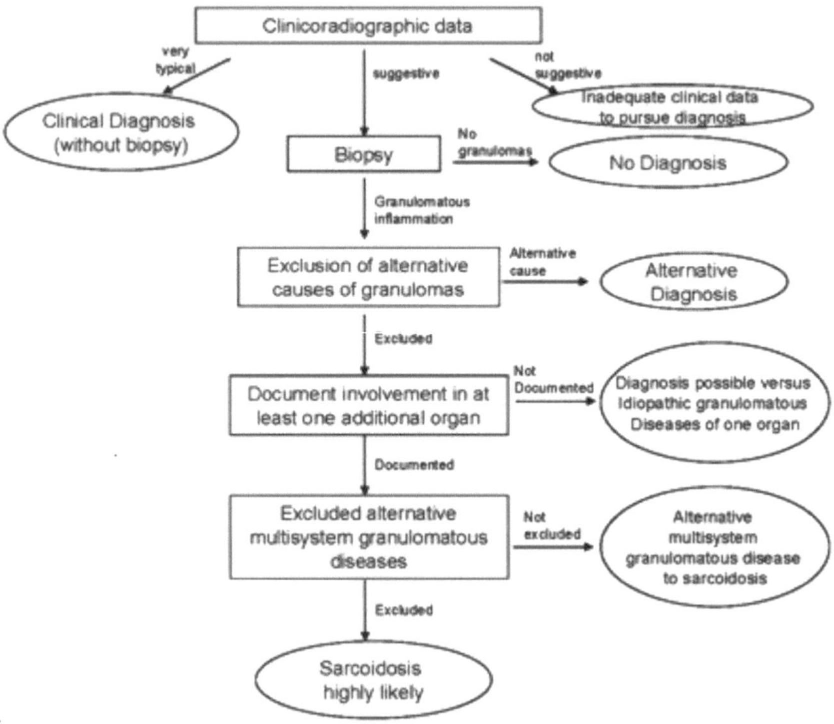

Fig. 1. An approach to the diagnosis of sarcoidosis*

4. Initial evaluation

Key data from the medical history, physical findings, and routine laboratory and radiographic studies figure prominently in the diagnostic approach to sarcoidosis. Nonspecific constitutional manifestations such as fever, fatigue, malaise, and weight loss occur in up to one third of patients with sarcoidosis (3). Sarcoidosis can involve virtually every organ system and the review of systems can provide important diagnostic clues. Factors associated with a higher clinical likelihood of sarcoidosis include African American or Northern European descent, nonsmokers, and a family history of sarcoidosis (4-7). A detailed occupational history should include prior exposure to beryllium, risk factors for hypersensitivity pneumonitis, and exposure to tuberculosis or fungal pathogens all of which can mimic sarcoidosis (1).

The physical examination should be performed with similar attention to detail. Respiratory findings may include wheezing or rales. Frequently encountered extra-thoracic manifestations include peripheral lymphadenopathy, liver or splenic enlargement, ocular involvement, parotitis, facial nerve palsy, and a variety of cutaneous lesions including direct involvement by sarcoidosis and non-specific lesions especially erythema nodosum (8).

Initial laboratory studies should include a complete blood count and comprehensive metabolic panel with particular attention to liver function and calcium levels. A tuberculin skin test and (where appropriate) fungal skin tests and serologies should be done. A variety

* Reprinted with permission. Judson MA. The diagnosis of sarcoidosis. Clinics in Chest Medicine 2008; 29:415-427. Copyright Elsevier.

of electrocardiographic abnormailities may indicate cardiac sarcoidosis including conduction defects, atrial and ventricular extrasystoles and arryhythmias. Pulmonary function tests are crucial for quantification of pulmonary impairment, and to provide a baseline for assessment of future stability or progression. Restrictive and/or obstructive ventilatory defects and diffusion impairment are common.

Compatible radiographic imaging is one of the diagnostic criteria for sarcoidosis. The most common abnormalities on plain chest radiographs are bilateral, symmetric hilar adenopathy with or without lung infiltrates. The classification system developed by Scadding 50 years ago remains in use today (9). In stage I hilar and mediastinal lymphadenopathy alone are present. Stage II is defined by adenopathy plus pulmonary infiltrates, stage III by pulmonary infiltrates alone and stage IV includes radiographic evidence of pulmonary fibrosis (Figs. 2a-2d). More recently stage 0 has been added when the chest roentgenogram shows none of these abnormalities. The classification has prognostic value as originally described by Scadding with a 90% likelihood of resolution in 2 years with stage 1, compared to about 30% with stage 3.

Although the radiologic staging does tend to correlate with physiologic impairment, its value in managing individual patients is limited (2).

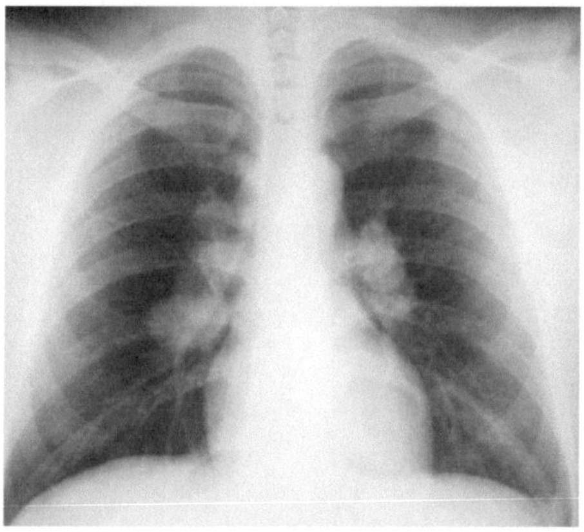

(a) Stage I

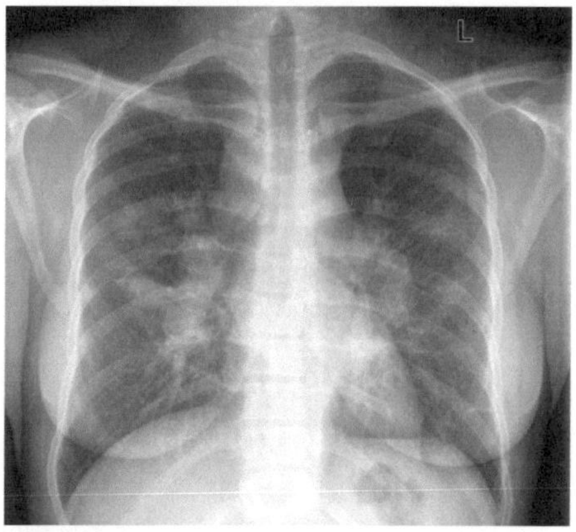

(b) Stage II

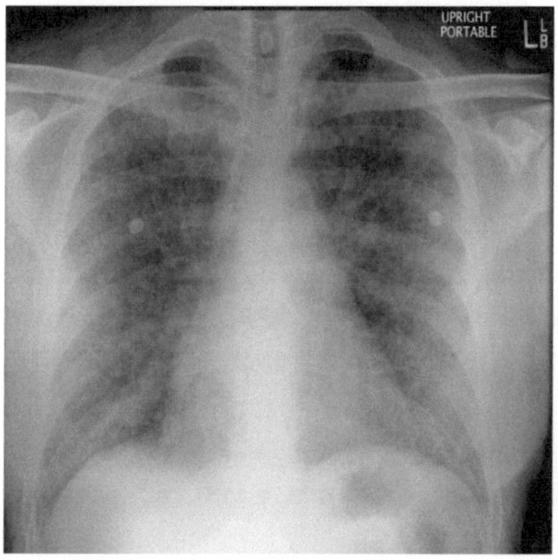

(c) Stage III

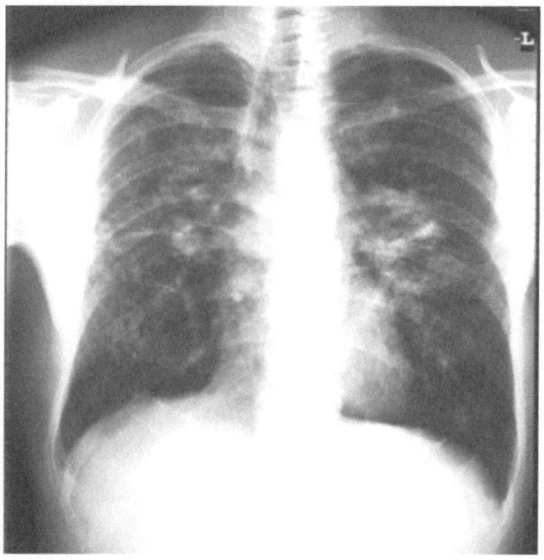

(d) Stage IV

Fig. 2. Chest radiographs showing sarcoidosis stages I-IV.

Computed tomographic scans (CT scans) especially using high resolution technique (HRCT), provide much greater detail than routine chest radiographs. Common patterns in sarcoidosis include widespread pulmonary nodules, infiltrates with a bronchovascular and subpleural distribution (fig.3a), thickened intralobular septa, and as shown in figure 3b, architectural distortion, and conglomerate masses (10).

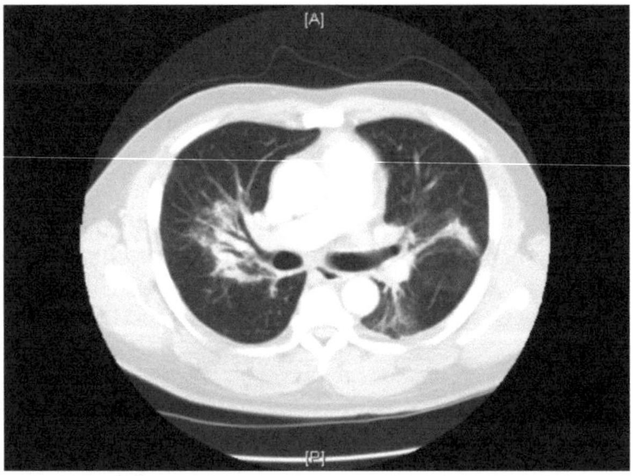

(a)

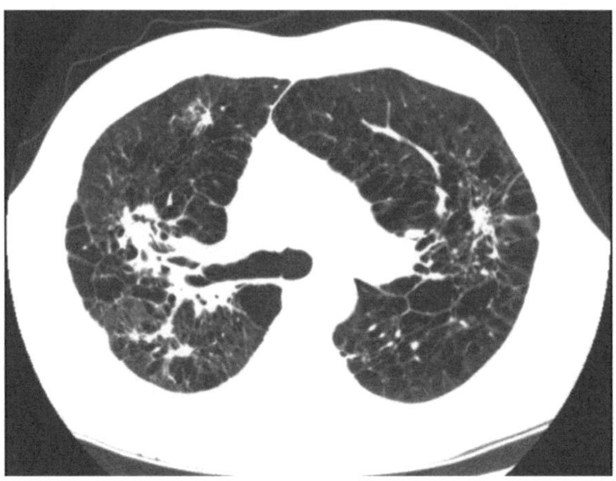

(b)

Fig. 3. (a) CT scan showing bronchovascular distribution of pulmonary infiltrates in stage III sarcoidosis.

Intrathoracic adenopathy is also more often detected on CT (11). It is unclear, however, that CT scanning adds critical diagnostic information beyond that of plain chest radiographs in the initial evaluation of most patients with suspected sarcoidosis. Whatever additional information is derived must be balanced against the added expense and radiation exposure associated with CT scans.

Gallium-67 scanning may be of value in the initial diagnostic evaluation. Parotid and lacrimal gland uptake (positive Panda sign) plus bilateral hilar and right paratracheal lymph node uptake (positive Lambda sign) strongly support the diagnosis (11) (Figs 4a,b). Like CT scans, the additional cost and radiation exposure with gallium scanning are not warranted in most cases. Angiotensin-converting enzyme (ACE) is produced in epithelioid cells within sarcoid granulomas. Elevated levels of ACE were once felt to be diagnostic of sarcoidosis (12). More recent data indicate that ACE levels are neither sufficiently sensitive nor specific to confirm a diagnosis of sarcoidosis although they may have some value as supportive evidence for or against the diagnosis (2).

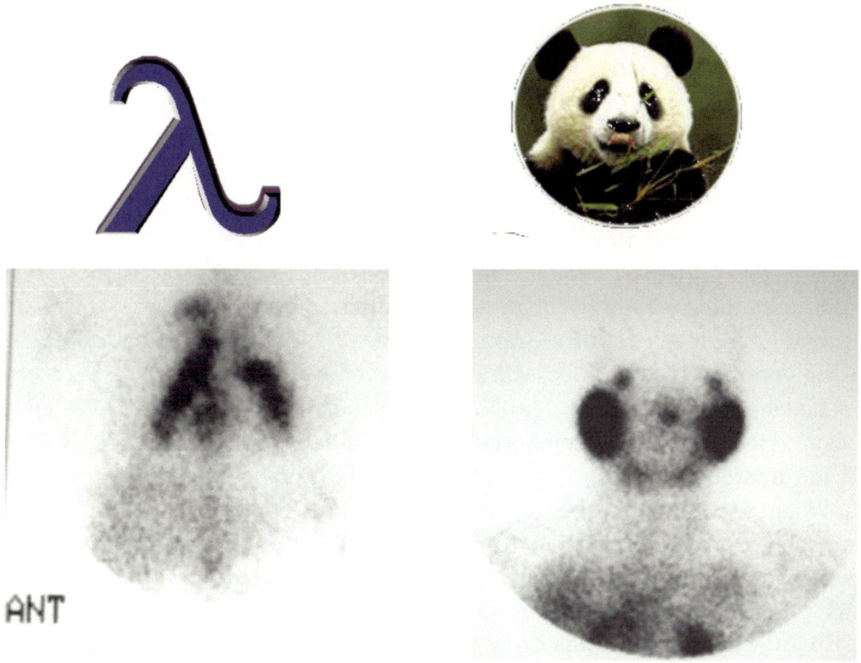

(a) (b)

Fig. 4. (a) Gallium scan showing (a) Lamda sign; (b) Panda sign.

5. Diagnosis without biopsy

There are 4 circumstances where the diagnosis of sarcoidosis may be confidently made without biopsy because the combined clinical and radiographic findings are highly specific (2, 11). These situations are as follows: 1) asymptomatic patients with bilateral hilar adenopathy on chest x-ray, 2) Lofgren's syndrome which consists of bilateral hilar adenopathy, erythema nodosum, and often fever and arthritis, 3) Heerfordt syndrome which includes uveitis, parotiditis and fever, and 4) when a gallium-67 scan shows Panda and Lambda signs as previously described.

6. Invasive diagnostic modalities and appropriate biopsy sites

Most patients with suspected sarcoidosis require histologic confirmation for diagnosis. Since sarcoidosis is a multi-system disorder, evidence of granulomatous inflammation in at least 2 organs is required to distinguish it from granulomatous disorders of individual organs such as granulomatous hepatitis and idiopathic panuveitis (2, 11). However, biopsy confirmation from one organ is deemed sufficient if compatible clinical, laboratory, or radiologic findings are consistent with the diagnosis in at least one additional organ and alternative diagnoses have been excluded (2, 11). Positive biopsy material from more than one organ system may be necessary when sarcoidosis presents in an atypical fashion (11).

The choice of biopsy site should be guided by what is least invasive and most likely to yield diagnostic material. Enlarged peripheral lymph nodes, skin involvement, and conjunctival nodules permit minimally invasive procedures. The Kveim test developed more than 50 years ago (13), involves a subcutaneous injection of material from a human spleen involved with sarcoidosis. A positive test is defined by the appearance of a nodular lesion at the site after 4-6 weeks which on biopsy shows non-caseating granulomas. The Kveim test has been reported to be fairly specific, but the sensitivity is low (11). It is not in general use because both sensitivity and specificity vary with the splenic material used, and it is not approved by the Food and Drug Administration in the United States (11)..

Since over 90% of patients present with intra-thoracic involvement, bronchoscopy is often the diagnostic procedure of choice. Flexible fiberoptic bronchoscopy provides multiple options for obtaining diagnostic material. Lung parenchyma can be sampled by transbronchial lung biopsy (TBLB). Granulomas may be identified via endobronchial biopsy (EBB) in the central airways. Mediastinal and hilar lymph nodes may be accessed with transbronchial needle aspiration (TBNA). Bronchalveolar lavage (BAL) yields liquid material from one or more lung segments that can be helpful diagnostically. It also provides substrate for microbiologic studies to exclude conditions which figure strongly in the differential diagnosis, such as tuberculosis and fungal infections.

The diagnostic yield of TBLB ranges from 60% to 97% depending on the radiographic stage of the disease and the number of biopsies performed (14). In radiographic stage I where the pulmonary parenchyma appears normal on plain radiograph, the yield is approximately 50% (15, 16). Even when the lungs do not show abnormalities on HRCT, TBLB may still be diagnostic (17). The number of biopsies required to maximize diagnostic yield plateaus at 4-5 specimens (18).

Endobronchial involvement is frequent in sarcoidosis. In the presence of abnormalities of the bronchial mucosa including nodularity, hypervascularity and bronchial stenosis, EBB has been reported to be diagnostic in over 90% of cases (19). Even when the mucosa appears normal, a positive biopsy may be obtained in about 30% of cases (19, 20). Moreover, the addition of EBB to TBLB increases overall diagnostic yield (19, 20). EBB should probably be considered in all patients undergoing bronchoscopy for suspected sarcoidosis since it adds minimally in terms of risk and procedure time.

Bronchoalveolar lavage (BAL) can be of value in the diagnosis of sarcoidosis. Analysis of BAL fluid typically shows a normal or modestly increased cell count, a lymphocyte predominance in over 90% of patients, a normal percentages of neutrophils and eosinophils, and absence of foamy alveolar macrophages and plasma cells (10, 21). These findings are helpful in distinguishing sarcoidosis from several conditions with similar clinical and radiologic features, specifically, extrinsic allergic alveolitis, nonspecific interstitial pneumonia, and idiopathic pulmonary fibrosis. Examination of lymphocyte populations (CD4/CD8 ratio) may also be diagnostically helpful. Several studies have shown that a CD4/CD8 ratio of greater than 3.5 has a specificity of 93-96%, although the sensitivity is low (53-59%) (22-25).In inactive sarcoidosis, the ratio is usually normal. In patients with only extrathoracic manifestations, BAL may still show findings typical of sarcoidosis even when thoracic imaging studies are normal (26).

Endobronchial ultrasound (EBUS) is a new approach to obtain histologic confirmation of intrathoracic sarcoidosis. Formerly, transbronchial needle aspiration (TBNA) using anatomical landmarks and fluoroscopy to guide the site of needle insertion in the airway was the standard bronchoscopic technique for sampling mediastinal lymph nodes in suspected sarcoidosis and other conditions particularly bronchogenic carcinoma. The ability to visualize lymph nodes via EBUS has resulted in diagnostic yields in sarcoidosis approaching 85% in experienced hands (27, 28). In one study, the diagnosis was confirmed in 96% of patients using EBUS compared to 73% using TBNA without EBUS despite the use of smaller gauge needles (19g for TBNA alone vs 22g with EBUS) (29). Furthermore, EBUS has the added ability to biopsy smaller nodes not easily accessible by blind TBNA or mediastinoscopy. Procedure times and amount of sedation needed tend to be modestly higher with EBUS compared to blind TBNA. The frequency of complications is low for both techniques and roughly similar (29). Combining endoscopic (esophageal) ultrasound (EUS) with EBUS has the added advantage of accessing additional lymph node stations in the mediastinum and has proven to be an invaluable tool in lung cancer staging. In the evaluation of sarcoidosis it remains unclear if the combined modality (EBUS plus EUS) results in improved diagnostic yield (29).

When less invasive modalities are inconclusive in suspected sarcoidosis, confirmation using one of several surgical options may be necessary. Mediastinoscopy remains the "gold standard" to evaluate abnormal mediastinal lymph nodes. For mediastinal lymph adenopathy of diverse etiologies, mediastinoscopy is diagnostic in 82-97% of reported cases (30). The high yield reflects the generous volume of biopsy material obtainable with this technique. However, significant morbidity ranges from 1.4-2.3% (31). Other disadvantages include higher cost compared to less invasive procedures, the need for general anesthesia, and the cosmetic effects of a neck scar. Video-assisted thoracoscopic surgery (VATS) or open thoracotomy provide the ultimate approach for biopsy of lung parenchyma and/or mediastinal and hilar lymph nodes in sarcoidosis.

7. Additional diagnostic modalities

Occasionally, the clinical presentation suggests the diagnosis of sarcoidosis but no readily available biopsy site is identified, or only a single organ system is involved. Under such vexing clinical scenarios additional studies may be warranted to help identify occult sites of disease for diagnostic biopsy or to help identify the presence of granulomatous inflammation in relatively inaccessible organs (ie.. heart and brain). Traditionally gallium scanning was used in this regard, however newer modalities including F-18 fluorodeoxyglucose positron emission tomography (PET) and gadolinium enhanced magnetic resonance imaging (MRI) may have improved diagnostic sensitivity (32). FDG PET scanning has been shown to be sensitive for evaluating areas of active granulomatous inflammation in sarcoidosis. When interpreting PET scans caution is appropriate as positive scans can also be seen in patients with other granulomatous diseases, infections, and neoplasms. It has recently been proposed that combining a more specific tracer L- (3-18F) - alpha - methytyrosine scan with an FDG PET scan can help differentiate neoplasm from sarcoidosis (33). PET scanning has also been shown to have a specific pattern in cardiac sarcoidosis.

Like PET scanning, the use of MRI in suspected sarcoidosis has been shown to have value in the identification of occult disease especially cardiac and central nervous system involvement (34). Recent studies suggest that PET scanning may be more sensitive than MRI for detection of cardiac sarcoidosis. However, MRI appears to have a higher specificity (35), and unlike PET, MRI does not expose patients to ionizing radiation.

8. Conclusions

The diagnostic approach in sarcoidosis can be relatively straight forward, but not infrequently it is arduous and complex. The multi-system nature of the condition, its protean manifestations, and unknown causation, all contribute to its elusive diagnostic nature. The routine clinical tools and diagnostic modalities discussed in this chapter provide an approach that will usually succeed. However, a degree of skepticism and ample consideration of alternative diagnoses are warranted.

9. References

[1] Hunninghake GW, Costabel U, Ando M, et al. American Thoracic Society/European Respiratory Society/ World Association of Sarcoidosis and Other Granulomatous Disorders: Statement on Sarcoidosis. SarcoidosisVasc Diffuse Lung Dis 1999; 16: 149-173.

[2] Baughman RP, Culver DA, Judson MA.A concise review of pulmonary sarcoidoisis. Am Rev Respir Crit Care Med. 2011;183:573-581.

[3] Drent M, Wirnsberger RM, De Vries J. Association of fatigue with an acute phase response in sarcoidosis. Eur Respir J 1999; 13: 718-722.

[4] Milman N, Selroos O. Pulmonary Sarcoidosis in the Nordic Countries 1950-1982. Epidemiology and Clinical Picture. Sarcoidosis 1990; 7: 50-7.

[5] Rybicki BA, Major M, Popovich J, et al. Racial differences in sarcoidosis incidence: a 5 year study in a health maintenance organization. Am J Epidemiology 1997; 145:234-41.

[6] RyabickiVA, Iannuzzi MC, Frederick MM, et al. Familial aggregation of sarcoidosis. A case control etiologic study of sarcoidosis (ACCESS). Am J Respir Crit Care Med 2001; 164:2085-91.

[7] Newman LS, Rose CS, Bresnitz EA, et al. A case control etiologic study of sarcoidosis: environmental and occupational risk factors. Am J Respir Crit Care Med 2004; 170:1324-30.

[8] Baughman RP, TeirsteinAS, Judson MA, et al. Clinical characteristics of patients in a case control study of sarcoidosis. Am J Resp Crit Care Med 2001; 164:1885-9.

[9] Scadding JG. Prognosis of intrathoracicsarcoidosis in England. BMJ 1961;4:1165-1172.

[10] Costabel U, Guzman J, Drent M. Diagnostic approach to sarcoidosis. Eur Respir Mon, 2005; 32:259-264.

[11] Judson, MA. The Diagnosis of Sarcoidosis. Clin Chest Med 2008; 29:415-427.

[12] Lieberman J, Nosal A, Schleissner A, Sastre-Foken A. Serum angiotensin converting enzyme for diagnosis and therapeutic evaluation of sarcoidosis. Am Rev Respir Dis 1979;120:329-335.

[13] Siltzbach LE. The Kveim test in sarcoidosis.A study of 750 patients. JAMA 1961;178:476-482.

[14] Lynch JP 3rd, Kazerooni EA, Gay SE. Pulmonary sarcoidosis. Clin Chest Med. 1997;18:7557-85.

[15] Koonitz CH, Joyner LR, Nelson RA. Transbronchial lung biopsy via the fiberoptic bronchoscope in sarcoidosis. Ann Intern Med. 1976;85:64-66.

[16] Poe RH, Israel RH, Utell MJ, Hall WJ. Probability of a positive transbronchial lung biopsy result in sarcoidosis. Arch Intern Med. 1979;139:761-763

[17] Smith PR. Personal observations

[18] Gilman MJ, Wang KP. Transbronchial lung biopsy in sarcoidosis. An approach to determine the optimal number of biopsies. Am Rev Respir Dis 1980; 122:721-4.

[19] Armstrong JR, Radke JR, Kvale PA, Eichenhorn MS, Popovich J Jr. Endoscopic findings in sarcoidosis. Characteristics and correlations with radiographic staging and bronchial mucosal biopsy yield. Ann Otol Rhinol Laryngol. 1981;90 :339-43.

[20] Shorr AF, Torrington KG, Hnatiuk OW. Endobronchial biopsy for sarcoidosis: A prospective study. Chest 2001; 120:109-114.

[21] Drent M, Mansour K, Linssen C. Bronchoalveolar lavage in Sarcoidosis. Semin Resp Crit Care Med 2007;28:486-495.

[22] Costabel U, Zaiss A, Wagner DJ, et al. Value of bronchoalveolar lavage lymphocyte subpopulations for the diagnosis of sarcoidosis. In: Grassi C, Rizzato G, Pozzi E, eds. Sarcoidosis and other granulomatous disorders. Amsterdam: Elsevier, 1988; 429-432.

[23] Winterbauer RH, Lammert J, Selland M, Wu R, Corley D, Springmeyer SC. Bronchoalveolar lavage cell populations in the diagnosis of sarcoidosis. Chest 1993;104:352-361.

[24] Thomeer M, Demedts M. Predictive value of CD4/CD8 ratio in bronchoalveolar lavage in the diagnosis of sarcoidosis [abstract]. Sarcoidosis Vasc Diffuse Lung Dis. 1997;14(suppl 1):36

[25] Korosec P, Rijavec M, Silar M, Kern I, Kosnik M, Osolnik K. Deficiency of pulmonary Valpha24 Vbeta11 natural killer T cells in corticosteroid-naïve sarcoidosis patients. Respir Med. 2010;104:571-577.

[26] Costabel U, Bonella F, Ohshimo S, Guzman J. Diagnostic modalities in sarcoidosis: BAL, EBUS, and PET. SeminRespirCrit Care Med. 2010;31:404- 8

[27] Garwood S, Judson MA, Siverstri G, et al. Endobronchial Ultrasound for the diagnosis of pulmonary sarcoidosis. Chest 2007; 132:1298-304.

[28] Wong, M, Yasufuku K, Nakajima T, et al. Endobronchial Ultrasound: New insight for the diagnosis of sarcoidosis. Eur Respir J 2007; 29:1182-6.

[29] Tremblay, A, Stather DR, Maccachern P, Khalil M, Field SK. A Randomized controlled trial of standard versus endobronchial ultrasonography guided transbronchial needle aspiration in patients with suspected sarcoidosis. Chest 2009; 136:340-346.

[30] Gossot D, Toledo L, Frisch S, et al. Mediastinoscopy versus thoracoscopy for mediastinal biopsy: Results of a prospective randomized study. Chest 1996; 110: 1328-1331

[31] Reich JM, Brouns MC, OConnor EA et al. Mediastinoscopy in patients with presumptive stage I sarcoidosis: A risk/benefit, cost/benefit analysis. Chest 1998; 113:147-152.

[32] Teirstein AS, Machac J, Almeida O, Lu P, Padilla M, Iannuzzi M. Results of 188 whole body fluorodeoxyglucose positron emission tomography scans in 137 patients with sarcoidosis. Chest 2007; 132:1949-1953.

[33] Kaira K, Oriuchi N, Otani Y, et al.. Diagnostic usefulness of fluorine -18- alpha methyltyrosine positron emission tomography in combination with 18 Fluorodeoxyglucose in sarcoidosis patients. Chest 2007; 131:1019-1027

[34] Nunes H, Brillet PY, Valcyre D, Brauner MW, Wells AU. Imaging in sarcoidosis. Semin Respir Crit Care Med 2007; 28:102-120.

[35] Tadamura E, Yamamuro M, Kubo S, et al., Images in cardiovascular medicine. Multimodality imaging of cardiac sarcoidosis before and after steroid therapy. Circulation 2006; 113:771-773.

4

Diagnosis of Pulmonary Sarcoidosis

Tiberiu Shulimzon and Matthew Koslow
The Pulmonary Institute, The Chaim Sheba Medical Center, affiliated to the Sackler's School of Medicine, Tel Aviv University, Israel

"Absolute certainty in diagnosis is unattainable, no matter how much information we gather, how many observations we make, or how many tests we perform. Our task is not to attain certainty, but rather to reduce the level of diagnostic uncertainty enough to make optimal therapeutic decision"
J.P. Kassirer, The New England Journal of Medicine, 1989

1. Introduction

1.1 Imaging

As previously described, the majority of patients with sarcoidosis are asymptomatic. The main reason patients seek medical attention is an abnormal imaging study. By far the most common situation is a chest radiography that was performed for an alternative diagnosis or as a routine procedure before anesthesia or surgery.

In recent years the increased use of computed tomography (CT) in various screening programs for malignancy (colon, lung) or in cardiology has led to an explosion of "lung abnormalities," many of which are eventually attributed to sarcoidosis. For example, 25% of solitary pulmonary nodules (SPN) on chest CT were attributable to "nonspecific granulomas" after tissue biopsy (Albert and Russell 2009).

The recent report of the National Lung Screening Trial in USA favors a CT scan program for reducing the all cause mortality attributable to lung cancer (The National Lung Screening Trial Research Team 2011). This recommendation is expected to dramatically increase the number of chest CT examinations performed for screening purposes. It is likely that many of the abnormalities found in the lung parenchyma will undergo biopsy and be diagnosed as granulomatous sarcoid-like lesions. A practical approach to their management is needed.

From a historical perspective, the suspicion of sarcoidosis is typically initiated by abnormal imaging. In fact, the pragmatic "Statement on Sarcoidosis" dedicates a subchapter to this issue in the "patient without histology" (Hunninghake et al. 1999). The authors claim that clinical and/or radiological features alone may be diagnostic for patients with stage I disease (98% reliability) or stage II (89% reliability), but less accurate for stage III (52% reliability). In a review of 100 patients with bilateral hilar lymphadenopathy, sarcoidosis was diagnosed if symptoms were limited to uveitis or erythema nodosum or in asymptomatic patients with a negative physical examination (74% of all patients). In these patients, the authors conclude that biopsy confirmation is not necessary.

1.2 The chest radiograph

The classical staging system for sarcoidosis progression was described more than 50 years ago by Scadding. In a modified version it includes:

- stage 0 : no adenopathy or infiltrate
- stage I : hilar and mediastinal adenopathy alone
- stage II : adenopathy and pulmonary infiltrates
- stage III : pulmonary infiltrates alone
- stage IV : pulmonary fibrosis (Scadding 1961)

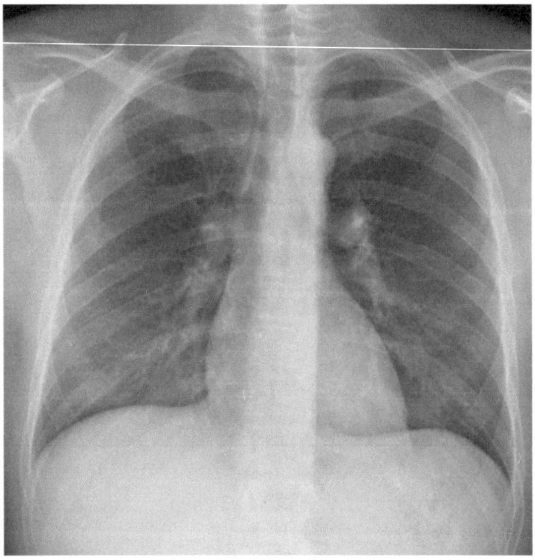

Fig. 1. Stage I sarcoidosis on chest radiography

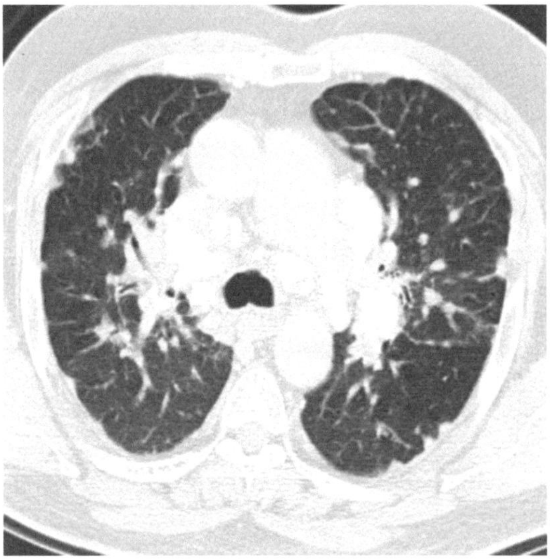

Fig. 2. Stage II parenchymal change on Chest CT

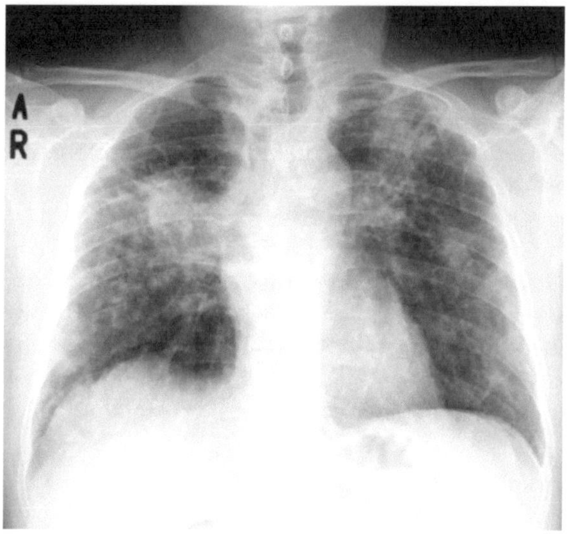

Fig. 3. Stage III sarcoidosis on chest radiography

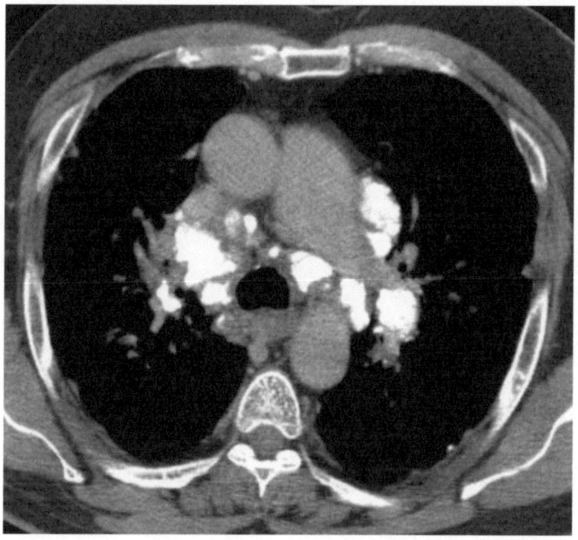

Fig. 4. Lymph node calcifications in sarcoidosis on Chest CT(contributed by Dr. Judith Rosenman, The Radiology Department, The Chaim Sheba Medical Center, Tel Aviv, Israel)

The Scadding staging system has important prognostic significance. Scadding noticed that stage I patients have more than 90% resolution of their radiographic findings within 2 years, while those with stage III disease demonstrate resolution in less than 1/3 of cases.
However, the chest radiograph does not correlate well with sarcoidosis symptoms (e.g. dyspnea) or functional parameters such as spirometry nor the six-minute walk test (Yeager et al. 2005; Judson et al. 2008; Baughman, Sparkman, and Lower 2007). Furthermore, there is poor interobserver reliability among various specialists according to a recent study of chest roentgenograms in sarcoidosis patients during a trial of infliximab (Baughman et al. 2009).

The characteristic histology of sarcoidosis is the granuloma formation. Granulomas may be seen along the lymphatics of the bronchovascular bundle, interlobular septa, major fissures and subpleural areas. These are the anatomic areas that deserve attention on regular chest X rays. The majority of patients present with stage I disease in which the differential diagnosis includes lymphoma, infectious diseases (fungal, mycobacterial) or occupational diseases (beryliosis) and support the need for biopsy confirmation.
Specific situations may preclude the need for biopsy based on radiologic and clinical findings alone. Examples include the Lofgren syndrome (bilateral hilar adenopathy, erythema nodosum, fever and arthritis), the Heerfodt syndrome (uveitis, fever and parotiditis) and the presence of isolated bilateral hilar adenopathy on the chest radiography in a asymptomatic patient. Furthermore, the Gallium 67 scan may demonstrate the typical "Panda sign" (Heerfodt syndrome) or "Lambda sign" (Lofgren syndrome) providing further support for these diagnoses and avoiding the need for histological diagnosis.

1.3 Computed Tomography (CT) scanning

With recent advances in computed tomography technology, especially the high resolution multi-slice CT scan (HRCT), the diagnostic imaging of sarcoidosis has improved. Nishino et al. describes the broad spectrum of pulmonary sarcoidosis and clues for the HRCT interpretation (Nishino et al. 2010). Disease manifestations are classified as parenchymal, airway involvement, mediastinal and hilar adenopathy and complications.

1.3.1 Parenchymal change

Nodules are the main feature of this type of interstitial lung disease. They are small (1-3 mm), peripheral in distribution and typically involve the bronchovascular bundle and interlobar septa. In our practice we use involvement of the major and minor fissures as a typical feature of pulmonary sarcoidosis. Nodules typically involve the upper lobes and lead to distortion of lung parenchyma. Less frequently, pulmonary sarcoidosis may manifest as multifocal opacities of various sizes (cm) described as "the sarcoid galaxy sign" (Nakatsu et al. 2002).
Fibrotic changes are not specific for sarcoidosis, and may represent the end stage of various interstitial lung diseases. While a honeycomb pattern is not common in fibrotic sarcoidosis (Abehsera et al. 2000), we believe fibrotic changes should discourage a decision for histological diagnosis since therapy at this stage is unlikely to affect disease evolution.
Another supportive sign of pulmonary sarcoidosis is the air trapping at end expiration on CT. In a comparative study of sarcoidosis patients with and without a history of smoking, the air-trapping sign was present in the majority of cases (Terasaki et al. 2005).

1.3.2 Airway involvement

A minority of patients with lung sarcoidosis may present with airway involvement. The small airways- lobar and subsegmental bronchi- are most commonly affected while, less frequently, disease of the large airways may manifest as tracheomalacia (Lenique et al. 1995).

1.3.3 Mediastinal and hilar lymphadenopathy

This is the main radiologic feature of sarcoidosis. Symmetric hilar adenopathy is the most typical followed by disease in the subcarina and paratracheal lymph nodes stations. Calcification and necrosis are rare features in sarcoidosis (Figure 4).

1.3.4 Complications

Hawtin et al describes sarcoidosis as the "great pretender (Hawtin et al. 2010). " Atypical features of sarcoidosis may lead to an incorrect diagnosis and treatment. Challenging examples include:

- Aspergillosis/aspergilloma may complicate sarcoidosis
- Cavity formation may appear in large nodules due to ischaemic necrosis. Mycetoma may also complicate it (Rohatgi and Schwab 1980).
- Pleural disease including effusion occur in only 2% of cases. Chylothorax and pneumothorax were described in case reports (Huggins et al. 2006).
- Large vessel (venous/arterial) involvement is the result of external compression while necrotising angiitis on small vessels raises the possibility of other vasculitides (like Wegener's disease)
- Lymphangitis on lung imaging raises the possibility of malignancy. The typical interlobular septal thickening is less marked in sarcoidosis than in lymphangitic carcinomatosis (Shadid and ter Maaten 2002).
- Cystic air spaces may be described in stage IV disease. They have a central distribution (in contrast to the peripheral honeycomb pattern of usual interstitial pneumonitis, UIP) and predominate in the upper lobes (Morello, Ali, and Cesani 1998).
- Diffuse mediastinal infiltration with compression of adjacent structures (Devaraj et al. 2007).
- Pulmonary veno-occlusive disease (POVD) is described in the absence of lung fibrosis (Nunes et al. 2006). Features include a high occurrence of ground glass attenuation in patients with pulmonary non-fibrotic sarcoidosis and pulmonary hypertension (sarcoid vasculopathy).
- "Vanishing lung disease" may mimic severe bullous emphysema mainly of the upper lobes (Judson 1998).

Radiologic changes provide a target for various examinations including tissue biopsy, bronchoalveolar lavage (BAL) for cytology or bacteriology investigation etc. However, the radiographic changes are not always sufficient to provide a target with significant yield. Metabolic activity at the site of the targeted lesions is essential for diagnosis and two modalities may be used for this purpose: Gallium isotope scanning or a PET examination.

1.4 Nuclear medicine

Gallium 67 scanning is one of the oldest radionuclide imaging techniques used for sarcoidosis diagnosis. This isotope is taken up in lesions having an inflammatory or infectious cause producing an increased blood flow. Its sensitivity ranges from 60 to 90% and appears as two distinct patterns:

- the "lambda pattern": bilateral symmetrical uptake in the parahilar and infrahilar lymph nodes and right parahilar lymph node
- the "panda pattern": symmetrical uptake in the parotid, lacrimal and salivary glands

The presence of both patterns is regarded as highly specific for sarcoidosis (Nunes et al. 2007).

The uptake of Gallium 67 may be noticed in other organs including the liver and spleen, but this abnormal uptake has low sensitivity and specificity. The usefulness of Gallium 67 as a marker of disease activity is controversial (Mana 2002). Gallium 67 scanning is a time-consuming procedure requiring up to 48-72 hours for completion and diagnosis. It is also an expensive diagnostic tool requiring isotope availability (Sulavik et al. 1990).

The [18F]-fluorodeoxyglucose-positron emission tomography (FDG-PET) is a non-invasive imaging technique widely used in oncology for the evaluation of active metabolic malignancy. Since inflammatory cells, such as neutrophils, activated macrophages and lymphocytes, also have increased FDG uptake FDG-PET is useful for both the diagnosis and/or therapeutic response in sarcoidosis.

FDG uptake in sarcoidosis was described in the early '90 s but considered neither sufficiently sensitive in uptake intensity nor specific since the pattern is also seen in lymphoma and diffuse metastatic disease (Lewis and Salama 1994). Moreover, PET-CT scans are not universally available and are expensive. The identification of potential biopsy sites is the main indication we recommend the use of either PET-CT or Gallium 67 scanning (depending on institution availability).

In a small retrospective study, Braun et al. compared the clinical utility of FDG-PET/CT and Gallium 67 scanning in biopsy-proven sarcoidosis. FDG-PET was able to provide a complete morpho-functional mapping of the inflammatory active areas and follow therapy response in patients with sarcoidosis (Braun et al. 2008). In a larger study, PET-CT helped direct the biopsy procedure and diagnose disease in difficult to reach areas such as the heart (Hollister et al. 2005). Cardiac sarcoidosis has a specific pattern and, represents, one of the main indications for PET-CT imaging in sarcoidosis. It may also be performed in patients with pacemakers. In one series, up to 40% of sarcoidosis patients had cardiac involvement based on MRI or PET-CT scanning. However, these were asymptomatic patients and the need for specific therapy was controversial (Mehta et al. 2008).

The need for differentiating malignant lesions from inflammatory/sarcoid lesions led to the use of different tracers. In a recent study from Japan, the fluorine 18 alpha methyl tyrosine tracer was used in positron emission tomography and was able to differentiate malignancy (high uptake) from sarcoidosis (negative uptake) (Kaira et al. 2007).

In conclusion, imaging is a key component in the evaluation of suspected sarcoidosis. The "classical" findings on chest radiographs and CT scans suggest the diagnosis while nuclear imaging techniques help target sites for biopsy and assess disease activity. However, results should be regarded with caution when considering therapeutic decisions because the natural history of disease is extremely variable and prognostic factors for progression of disease are lacking. Therefore, atypical radiographic presentation will usually require histological diagnosis and correlation with other diagnostic methods help decrease diagnostic uncertainty (see further in this chapter).

2. Pulmonary Function Tests (PFT)

As more than 90% of patients with sarcoidosis present with lung involvement, it is reasonable that pulmonary function tests (PFT), both static and at exercise, are affected. As mentioned in previous sections for other diagnostic tests, these PFT changes are not specific. We use PFT for two main purposes:

- establish the disease severity
- establish the disease activity and response to therapy

A pattern of both restrictive and obstructive defects has been described. In the ACCESS study, 14-20% of the enrolled patients had a restrictive pattern and up to 13.6% had a forced vital capacity (FVC) of less than 70% on spirometry (Baughman et al. 2001). The obstructive pattern was often described in the African American population (Sharma and Johnson 1988). We have also noticed this mixed pattern in one of our patients of African Israeli origin.

The explanation of the obstructive pattern may be related to the endobronchial involvement by sarcoidosis or to airways hyperreactivity. This last phenomenon was described in up to 80% of patients with sarcoidosis, depending on the study design and patient selection (Shorr, Torrington, and Hnatiuk 2001). Symptoms of hyperreactive airways may bring the patient to medical attention but a clear connection between symptoms and PFT, especially spirometric measurements, was not established. A fixed obstructive pattern on PFT was associated with doubling the risk for mortality.

According to The Statement of Sarcoidosis, abberations of pulmonary function tests are found in up to 20% of patients with stage I disease and up to 70% of patients with stages II, III and IV disease (Hunninghake et al. 1999).

Diffusion capacity (DLCO) measurement is characteristic for evaluation of any interstitial lung disease. As a sensitive parameter, DLCO is a marker of gas exchange impairment due to both air and vascular lung architecture disturbances. DLCO measurements are the preferred diagnostic tool to predict gas exchange disturbances during moderate exercise in patients with sarcoidosis.

In a retrospective cohort study of patients listed for lung transplantation, the single independent prognostic factor for survival was right heart ventricle hemodynamics (Arcasoy et al. 2001). This is a consequence of pulmonary hypertension and altered gas exchange as showed by other studies (Judson 1998). Therefore, gas exchange impairment as a consequence of vascular bed involvement and pulmonary hypertension may be a more sensitive parameter for sarcoidosis severity and activity. In fact, some authors suggest the DLCO measurement is the most sensitive of the pulmonary function tests in stages II-IV disease (Huang et al. 1979). Conversely, others believe that measuring diffusion capacity is not a sensitive indicator of pulmonary pathology in sarcoidosis since lung volume can be altered independently of DLCO abnormalities. It is established that gas exchange at a given degree of volume restriction differs in sarcoidosis compared with idiopatic pulmonary fibrosis (Dunn et al. 1988).

What about exercise testing? A retrospective study of 48 patients with biopsy-proven sarcoidosis suggests that changes in gas exchange with exercise may be the most sensitive physiologic measurement to assess the extent of disease in early radiographic stages of sarcoidosis (Medinger, Khouri, and Rohatgi 2001).

The 6-minute walk test is easy to perform and proved to be useful in disability assessment and prognosis in lung diseases. In a prospective study, 142 patients performed the 6-minute walk distance test and were monitored for the lowest oxygen saturation. The 6-minute walk distance was reduced in most patients but mainly in those with pulmonary hypertension. The only independent predictors of the 6-minute walk distance were the Saint George Quality of Life Questionaire (SGRQ) , the forced vital capacity (FVC) and the lowest oxygen saturation (Baughman, Sparkman, and Lower 2007).

The distance-saturation product is a new parameter defined as the product of the 6-minute walk distance and the lowest oxygen saturation during the test. This parameter was found to be well correlated with a number of factors contributing to reduced test performance. These factors are: forced expiratory volume in 1 second (FEV1), partial pressure of oxygen PAO2, Borg dyspnea score, gender and pulmonary hypertension. This specific parameter was also associated with the degree of fibrosis documented by computed tomography (CT) and a positive response to therapy (Alhamad et al. 2010).

Dyspnea is the most common presentation in early to moderate advanced sarcoidosis. Up to half of patients have disease involvement of the skeletal muscles. Maximal respiratory

muscle force generation has been shown to be a more reliable index of functional work capacity than the standard static lung function tests (Kabitz et al. 2006).
When measuring the impairment of the inspiratory muscle strength with volitional tests (PE max, PI max), results may be misleading since these tests are highly dependent on patient motivation and cooperation. The use of non-volitional tests for this purpose may be more reliable. One of these non-volitional tests is the measurement of the twitch-mouth pressure during bilateral anterior magnetic phrenic nerve stimulation (Winterbauer and Hutchinson 1980).
So what are the most sensitive tests for evaluating sarcoidosis severity and/or disease activity? They include the static PFT based on lung volumes and diffusion capacity measurements, the exercise tests, hemodynamic evaluation and perhaps the respiratory muscle impairment serial measurements. About 30 years ago, Winterbauer and Hutchinson formulated some guidelines which we believe are still relevant in today's clinical practice:

- Pulmonary function tests data should be corelated with clinical (symptomatic) and radiological information
- There are no known PFT criteria that allow the clinician to predict the natural course of lung parenchymal sarcoidosis or response to therapy
- The best parameters to use for clinical follow up are the vital capacity (VC) and the diffusion capacity (DLCO), through sequential measurements (comparing an individual with himself through time).

The vital capacity and diffusion capacity share a common direction of change on sequential testing in 2/3 of patients with parenchymal sarcoidosis. The remaining 1/3 show a change in only one of the measured functions (Bradley et al. 2008)
As with all forms of interstitial lung disease, there has never been a formal evaluation of the diagnostic accuracy of exercise testing. In clinical practice, a normal study is useful to exclude significant interstitial lung disease in a symptomatic patient with normal rest PFT and chest radiography. The role of exercise testing in grading disease severity and prognosis is uncertain (Bradley et al. 2008).
We prefer the 6-minute walking distance test as a tool for clinical follow up and prognostic assessment along with hemodynamic evaluation of the pulmonary vascular bed (pulmonary hypertension). These measurements combined with sequential vital capacity and diffusion capacity measurements comprise a fair use of the pulmonary function tests in the diagnostic approach to sarcoidosis.

3. Biomarkers in sarcoidosis

Biomarkers are largely used in medicine for the diagnosis and follow up of a therapeutic response. Two recently published reviews (Manolio 2003; Tzouvelekis et al. 2005) describe the properties of an "ideal" serum biomarker :

- increase in the presence of disease (high sensitivity)
- normal levels in the absence of the disease (high specificity)
- add information on the risk and progression of disease
- correlate with disease activity
- correlate with disease extent/burden
- reproducible (a low coefficient of variation)
- easy/inexpensive determination

Such an ideal serum biomarker is difficult to find in most of the systemic diseases and sarcoidosis is not an exception. Sarcoidosis is a systemic inflammatory disease and so most of the biomarkers are serum markers of disease activity. They include various cytokines, enzymes, soluble cytokine receptors and various proteins.

Following the widespread use of flexible bronchoscopy and the technique of the bronchoalveolar lavage (BAL), a score of immunologic studies were performed on cell populations obtained from the respiratory epithelium. They include both bronchial and alveolar cell origin.

In two separate studies, Ziegenhagen et al. described the TNF alpha, released by the macrophages, and the serum level of sIL-2R as reliable biomarkers reflecting sarcoidosis severity and prognosis (Ziegenhagen et al. 2003).

In a well-designed retrospective study, the clinical usefulness of various serologic markers of inflammation were studied in 185 sarcoidosis patients followed in a dedicated sarcoidosis center for 4 years (Rothkrantz-Kos et al. 2003). Disease severity was assessed by ROC curves and logistic regression analyses. The disease severity was also compared to the lung function tests results. The sIL-2R had the largest area under the curve (AUC) in the untreated patients. The same parameter had the highest sensitivity, specificity, positive and negative predictive values among all the evaluated markers.

So what is the sIL-2R marker? In sarcoidosis, activated alveolar macrophages produce interleukin 1 and 6 (IL-1 and IL-6). The cytokines stimulate the production of SAA (serum amyloid A) and IL-2. The IL-2 production leads to T cell activation which express the IL-2 receptor on their surface IL-2R and release a soluble form of it in serum (s IL-2R). The s IL-2R marker was found to be increased in active disease (Muller-Quernheim 1998).

Another biomarker is derived from the lung epithelium specific proteins. The pneumoprotein KL-6 (Krebs von den Lungen) was initially described as a marker of sarcoidosis by Kobayashi et al. Increased serum levels of KL-6 indicated alveolitis activity and disease severity (Kobayashi and Kitamura 1996).

In a recent retrospective study from Japan, 43 patients with pulmonary sarcoidosis were observed. The initial serum IL-2R, lysozime and KL-6 levels reflected lymphocytic alveolitis. The initial serum KL-6 level was also associated with increased parenchymal infiltration (Miyoshi et al. 2010). This was also demonstrated by a strong correlation between the serum IL-2R and KL-6 markers levels and the bronchoalveolar lavage (BAL) fluid number of total lymphocytes and CD4.

By far the most studied and controversial serum marker for sarcoidosis is the angiotensin converting enzyme (ACE). Elevated levels were found in up to 60% of the patients with active sarcoidosis (Sharma and Alam 1995). This is an exopeptidase playing a central role in the control of blood pressure through conversion of the decapeptide angiotensin I to the octapeptide angiotensin II and through bradykinin inactivation. Most of the angiotensin I–angiotensin II conversion occurs through a single lung passage. ACE activity takes place on the luminal surface of the pulmonary endothelium but also on non-pulmonary vascular bed (Ng and Vane 1967).

In his pioneer study from 1975, J. Lieberman measured the serum ACE level in 200 patients with chronic lung disease and 200 controls (Lieberman 1975). While the serum ACE level was reduced in patients with COPD, CF, tuberculosis and lung cancer, the ACE level was significantly higher in sarcoidosis (greater than 2 standard deviation above the mean) for 15 of 17 patients with the disease. In sarcoidosis patients treated with steroids the level was normal. He concluded that an assay of serum ACE is useful for confirming sarcoidosis diagnosis and monitoring therapy.

Both ACE and angiotensin II were found in the epithelioid cells of sarcoid granuloma, but not in macrophages and monocytes (Pertschuk, Silverstein, and Friedland 1981). In a review article, Studdy and Bird analyzed the value of serum ACE (SACE) in clinical practice. As a diagnostic test for sarcoidosis, SACE demonstrated a 84% positive predictive value and 74% negative predictive value. They described SACE as a useful tool for measuring both pulmonary and extrathoracic sarcoidosis activity. They also suggested SACE as a marker of response to corticosteroid therapy since the SACE level became normal in treated patients within 4-10 weeks. However, an elevated SACE activity is not exclusive to sarcoidosis and a low SACE level does not exclude the disease (Studdy and Bird 1989).

Another large study of SACE level in 1,941 sarcoidosis patients demonstrated a positive predictive value of 90%, negative predictive value of 60%, sensitivity of 57% and specificity of 90% (Baughman, Culver, and Judson 2011).

In addition to sarcoidosis, other diseases associated with elevated SACE levels include disseminated tuberculosis, fungal infections, hyperthyroidism and Gaucher's disease (Baughman, Culver, and Judson 2011). It is believed that the serum ACE level reflects the total granulomatous load. This level may be influenced by the presence of specific or non-specific ACE inhibitors such as albumin and its fragments, fibrinolytic products, insulin including its beta chain (Klauser et al. 1979). Immunoassays of ACE concentration avoid this problem and allow the calculation of the specific activity of ACE. A radio-immune assay was developed and showed a strong correlation with serum ACE activity (Brice et al. 1995). However, another study showed that serum ACE level does not correlate with sarcoidosis severity (Pietinalho et al. 2000).

The controversy is furthered by polymorphisms of the ACE gene which lead to changes in the serum enzyme level. To elucidate the role of the insertion (I)/deletion (D) polymorphism of the ACE gene, a case control study was performed in two different patient populations: Afro-Americans and Caucasians. In Afro–Americans, the increased risk for sarcoidosis was 1.30 (95% confidence interval) for ID heterozygotes and 3.17 (95% confidence interval CI: 1,50-6,71) for DD homozygotes (Maliarik et al. 1998). In the study of a European white population, no association was found between the ACE I/D polymorphism and pulmonary disease activity, fibrosis or progression. The I/D polymorphism is not a regulatory variant in this disease (McGrath et al. 2001).

A non-invasive marker of airway inflammation, especially in patients with asthma, is the fraction of end tidal exhaled nitric oxide (FeNO). In a feasibility pilot study, FeNO was used to detect and monitor therapy response in patients with sarcoidosis (Choi et al. 2009). These exhaled NO measurements were not useful for monitoring disease progression in sarcoidosis.

An ideal biomarker for sarcoidosis does not exist yet. The main limitation is the insufficient sensitivity and specificity of the biomarker. Practically, ACE activity is still the most often used marker for disease activity despite its limitations. It is relatively cheap and easy to perform in a standard laboratory and may support the clinical and radiologic features suggestive of a sarcoidosis diagnosis. Its value as a marker for therapeutic response in those treated with corticosteroids is debatable.

4. Histology

Sarcoidosis is defined as a systemic disorder of non-necrotizing granulomatous inflammation in affected organs. Almost any organ may be involved but the lungs and intrathoracic lymph nodes are by far the most commonly affected (Saldana 1994). In addition to the careful correlation of clinical and radiologic features, the diagnosis requires the histologic confirmation of granulomatous inflammation and the exclusion of known causes of systemic granulomatous disorders. It is not an easy task for the pathologist.

Sarcoidosis is one of modern medicine's "great mimicker's." In addition to important alternative diagnoses such as lymphoma, tuberculosis, fungal and other infections, unusual presentations include the Guillain-Barre syndrome (Shah and Lewis 2003), metastatic Crohn's disease (Emanuel and Phelps 2008), and even pulmonary embolism (Morello, Ali, and Cesani 1998). In the retrospective analysis of 30,000 surgical pathology reports, 3% revealed granulomatous lesions of which only 1/3 were considered relevant to the clinical diagnosis. Of the primary granulomatous disorders, an estimated 1/3 were attributable to infection and sarcoidosis (Woodard et al. 1982).

This section will focus on the histologic features which support the diagnosis of sarcoidosis and available methods in obtaining histologic specimens.

4.1 Granulomatous inflammation

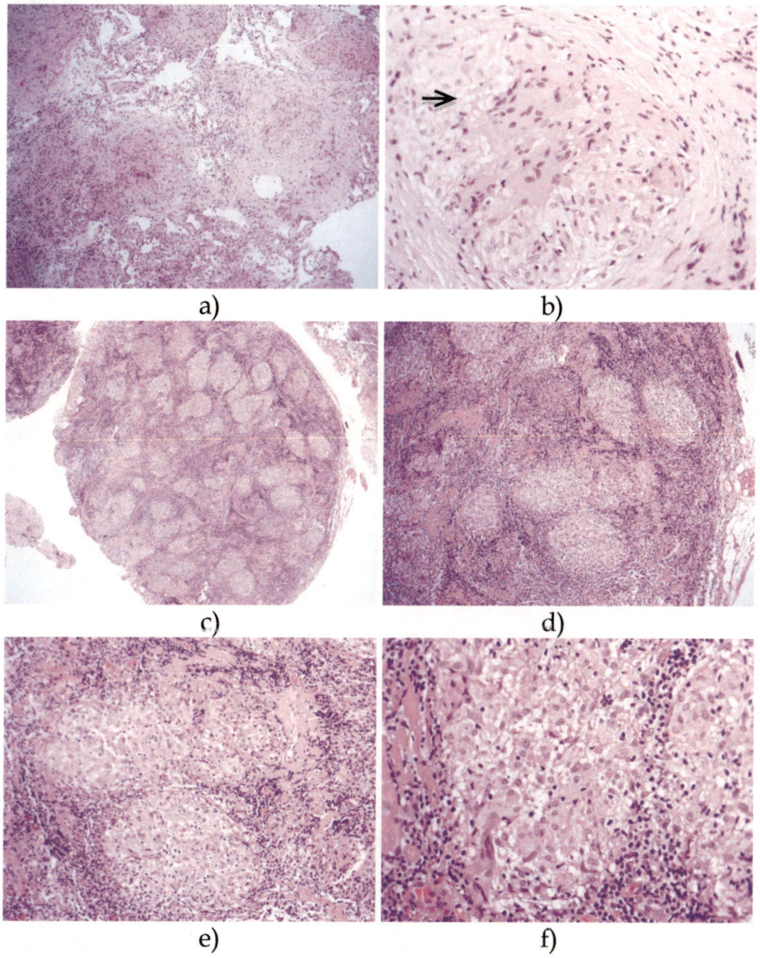

Fig. 5. Lung and lymph node biopsies at different magnification demonstrating the typical non-necrotizing granulomatous lesions of sarcoidosis (contributed by Marina Perlman, M.D., Department of Pathology, The Chaim Sheba Medical Center, Tel Aviv, Israel)

A granuloma is the compact aggregation of histiocytes (activated macrophages). They are also named "epithelioid" histiocytes because of their indistinct cell borders with elongated nuclei in contrast to typical histiocytes with well-defined borders and round or kidney bean-shaped nuclei (Mukhopadhyay and Gal 2010). The hematoxylin and eosin (H&E) preparation demonstrates the pale pink granular cytoplasm and indistinct cell boundaries which appear to merge into one another. They may fuse to form giant cells in the periphery and, less often, in the center of granulomas. These giant cells comprise a large mass of cytoplasm with many small nuclei arranged peripherally (Langerhans-type giant cell, Figure 5b) or hazardly (foreign-type giant cell).

The two types of granulomas, foreign body granulomas and immune granulomas, are distinguished by both appearance and pathogenesis. Foreign body granulomas are incited by relatively inert foreign bodies. The foreign body is large enough to prevent phagocytosis by a single macrophage but its presence does not incite an immune response exemplified by lipioid pneumonia. Typically, foreign body granulomatosis is a reaction to material such as talc, sutures, or other fibers. The foreign object is often visualized in the center of the granuloma, especially if viewed with polarized light in which it appears retractile.

Immune granulomas, in contrast to foreign body granulomas, incite an immune response. Macrophages engulf the foreign material then process and present it to T lymphocytes. The activated T lymphoctyes produce cytokines, such as IL-2 and IFN-ϒ, which perpetuate the immune response and transform macrophages into epithelioid cells and multinucleate giant cells. These cytokines are essential to both the formation and maintenance of granulomas.

4.2 Granuloma classification

Granulomas are classified as either necrotizing or non-necrotizing. Necrosis occurs when the trigger invokes a significant delayed hypersensitivity response or is highly toxic to the macrophage. According to Rosen (Saldana 1994), caseous necrosis refers to the cheeselike gross appearance and not to microscopic features. The terms "caseous," "caseating" and "noncaseating" have no diagnostic relevance and may be misleading because of the association with tuberculosis. For this reason, granulomas are best reported as necrotizing, non-necrotizing, or exhibiting minimal necrosis.

4.3 Histologic features of sarcoidosis

Sarcoidosis is classically characterized by discrete, well-formed non-necrotizing epithelioid granulomas tightly uniform in their size and stage of development (Saldana 1994). Macroscopically, granulomas may coalesce to form small nodules which may be palpable as 1-2 cm non-caseating consolidations. In chronic disease, the granuloma may be surrounded by concentric, lamellated fibrous rims or even replaced by fibrous scars. Classic sarcoidosis is also supported by the absence of certain features. For example, the absence of interstitial inflammation in areas without granulomas, the absence of organizing pneumonia, and the absence of granulomas within alveoli further characterize classic sarcoidosis.

The classic granulomas in sarcoidosis are non-necrotizing but the presence of necrosis is not uncommon. When necrosis is present, however, it is usually "minute, spotty and inconspicuous" affecting the central core of a small proportion of granulomas. The necrosis seen in tuberculosis and other infectious diseases may be indistinguishable from that seen in sarcoidosis (Saldana 1994).

"Sarcoid reactions" deserve special mention. These are non-caseating granulomas which are morphologically identical to those seen in sarcoidosis yet secondary to a primary process. Such reactions have been reported in patients with lymphoma, non-small carcinoma of the lung, draining lymph nodes of germ cell neoplasm and even in remote lymph node stations (Mehrotra and Dhingra 2010). Indeed, sarcoidosis may precede malignancy in hematologic malignancies (the sarcoidosis-lymphoma syndrome), the full spectrum of solid tumors, and as a paraneoplastic syndrome for the associated cancer (Cohen and Kurzrock 2007).

Intracytoplasmic inclusions are frequently found in sarcoidosis. Schaumann bodies are calcified structures often present within the giant cells. Colorless, birefringent crystals may also be seen within the cytoplasm and often together with Schaumann bodies (Saldana 1994). They are reported in up to 88% of cases of sarcoidosis but are nonspecific findings and also seen in 62% of beryliosis, and 6% of tuberculosis cases.(Saldana 1994)

Asteroid bodies are star-like inclusions with 30 or more rays originating from the central core. Less frequent than Schaumann bodies, they are reported in 2-9% of sarcoidosis specimens (Saldana 1994). Hamazaki-Wesenberg bodies are giant intracellular and extracellular lysosomes seen in both granulomatous and nongranulomatous lymph nodes of sarcoidosis as well as other etiologies. They may be mistaken for fungi because the yellow-brown pigment may stain positive with methenamine silver and may demonstrate a yeast-like budding appearance (Ro et al. 1987; Saldana 1994)

These inclusions, while described in sarcoidosis, are found in many other granulomatous diseases such as hypersensitivity pneumonitis, berylliosis, fungal infection, talc, tuberculosis and nontuberculosis mycobacterial infection. (Mukhopadhyay and Gal 2010; Reid and Andersen 1988). The online atlas of granulomatous diseases by Yale Rosen, M.D is an excellent resource to visualize all these features (http://granuloma.homestead.com/).

In summary, sarcoid granulomatous lesions are compact, uniform non-necrotizing epithelioid granulomas which may exhibit a mild degree of focal necrosis and a variety of inclusion bodies. However, no morphologic feature is specific or diagnostic of sarcoidosis.

4.4 Pulmonary sarcoidosis

Although any organ may be affected, lung or intrathoracic lymph node involvement is present in more than 90 percent of patients with sarcoidosis. It is the most common noninfectious cause of lung granulomas observed by surgical pathologists (Mukhopadhyay and Gal 2010). While no finding is pathognomonic for pulmonary sarcoidosis, classic features may support the diagnosis while their absence encourages the search for an alternative diagnosis. The varied presentations of pulmonary disease will be described.

Granulomas are typically found bilaterally in the upper two thirds of the lungs and in areas rich in lymphatics (the peribronchial, perivascular and septal regions). This "lymphatic" distribution explains the radiographic appearance which may "mimic" primary neoplasm or lymphangitic spread. It also explains the effectiveness of trans-bronchial biopsies in demonstrating sarcoid granulomas. In addition, the alveoli, bronchi, pulmonary blood vessels, and the pleura may all be involved.

Alveolitis is the earliest pulmonary lesion and is characterized by a lymphocyte-predominant interstitial pneumonitis. A high proportion of CD-4 positive cells are found in bronchoalveolar lavage (BAL) (Baughman, Lower, and du Bois 2003). In one study, a lymphocyte CD4/CD8 ratio greater than 3.5 showed 53% sensitivity but 94% specificity for the diagnosis of sarcoidosis (Costabel 1997). These CD4+ T cells, activated by a complex network of cytokines and chemokines, infiltrate at sites of disease and may play a role in the sarcoid granuloma formation. In a recent study of sarcoid patients with and without intense alveolitis, the percentage of a CD4+ effector T cell was much higher in patients with active disease as compared with inactive sarcoidosis (Facco et al. 2011).

The bronchi may be affected by four different mechanism: 1) extrinsic compression by enlarged lymph nodes, 2) granulomatous infiltration in the bronchial mucosa, submucosa and peribronchial tissue, 3) endobronchial mass lesion and 4) fibrotic scarring causing narrowing and distortion of bronchi. The entire spectrum of the airway may be involved from supraglottic structures and larynx to central and distal airways.

The supraglottic airway including the nasal passages, oropharynx, supraglottic structures and larynx are affected in approximately 6% of sarcoid patients (Baughman et al. 2001). Nasal ulceration may cause anosmia while infiltrative nodular sarcoidosis of supraglottic structures may cause stridor or cough. Isolated laryngeal involvement may be misdiagnosed as asthma (Bower et al. 1980). In the larynx, compression of the left pharyngeal nerve by enlarged lymph nodes may cause vocal cord paralysis (Jaffe, Bogomolski-Yahalom, and Kramer 1994).

Involvement of the trachea and main bronchi infrequently cause obstructive symptoms. In a retrospective analysis of 2,500 sarcoidosis patients, only 18 patients were identified with significant (defined as >50% of the lumen) endoluminal stenosis of proximal bronchi (ESPB). Despite the small number of patients, it is important to note that the group with early diagnosis and treatment (<3 months from onset of symptoms) were associated with good prognosis in contrast to patients with delayed diagnosis and treatment (>3 months from onset of symptoms)(Chambellan et al. 2005).

In the bronchi, granulomatous lesions most frequently involve the distal bronchial tree and develop along the bronchovascular bundle or near the airway with predominance for the upper and mid-lung regions. Various airway abnormalities develop and will be described.

The most common endobronchial abnormality is mucosal edema, erythema or granularity but normal-appearing mucosa does not exclude disease. Classic endobronchial sarcoidosis is characterized by mucosal islands of nodules which appear a waxy yellow or dull gray. Coalescence of these nodules is responsible for the cobblestone appearance while endoluminal occlusion may mimic an obstructing mass.

Bronchiolitis may occur early in disease without parenchymal involvement. However, airway distortion and bronchiectasis is more prevalent with progression of parenchymal disease. In advanced fibrotic disease, cystic lesions and cavitary disease predispose to Aspergillus infection. The development of an aspergilloma may cause hemoptysis and massive, life-threatening hemoptysis may occur (Stevens et al. 2000)

Airway Hyperactivity in patients with sarcoidosis is well described. In the prospective evaluation of 42 patients with newly diagnosed sarcoidosis and pulmonary symptoms, 20% demonstrated AHR by methacholine challenge. Endobronchial biopsies demonstrated nonecrotizing granulomas in 100% of these AHR-positive patients but only 45.5% of patients without AHR (Shorr, Torrington, and Hnatiuk 2001).

In the pulmonary vascular system, sarcoid lesions involve the veins much more frequently than the arteries and damage may range from destructive change in the media to stenosis or complete obliteration of the lumen (Saldana 1994). Although vascular involvement is common, the overall prevalence of pulmonary hypertension is low (5%). Although most affected patients have stage IV radiographic disease, two distinct phenotypes of sarcoidosis and pulmonary hypetension (PH) may exist depending on the presence or absence of pulmonary fibrosis.

In the study of 22 patients with sarcoidosis and pulmonary hypertension, 1/3 developed pulmonary hypertension in the absence of pulmonary fibrosis and no other known cause of secondary pulmonary hypertension (Nunes et al. 2006). These patients had near normal or mild restrictive spirometry but severely reduced DLCO. These findings suggest that PH in these patients may be explained by a specific vasculopathy independent of fibrotic destruction of the vascular bed. According to the authors, the presence of septal lines and ground glass opacities on HRCT suggest the possibility of pulmonary vascular occlusive disease from granulomatous involvement of the venous walls. These radiographic features are shared by pulmonary histiocytosis X, a granulomatous disease with intrinsic venopathy.
Honeycombing is the end stage of many interstitial diseases including sarcoidosis. In contrast to UIP, honeycombing in sarcoidosis is found predominantly in the upper lung zones. Bronchiectasis and emphysematous change may be seen but few granulomas are evident at this late stage. An important complication of the cystic parenchymal disease is the development of aspergillomas, which may cause life-threatening hemoptsysis (Rumbak et al. 1996; Wollschlager and Khan 1984).

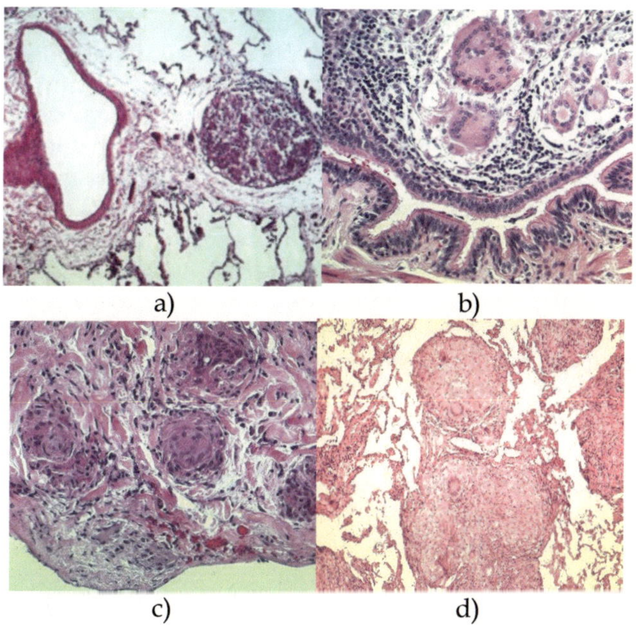

Fig. 6. Pulmonary sarcoidosis affecting a) the lymphatics b) the bronchiole c) the visceral pleura and d) coalescing to form nodular disease. (Contributed by Yale Rosen, M.D.)

4.5 The diagnostic approach

Special clinical situations may preclude the need for tissue biopsy. These include the Lofgren and Heerfodt syndrome as well as isolated bilateral hilar lymphadenopathy in asymptomatic patients. As mentioned, the "panda" sign (Heerfodt syndrome) and the "lambda" sign (Lofgren syndrome) on Gallium-67 scanning further support the diagnosis of sarcoidosis and avoid the need for tissue confirmation. Excluding these unique clinical syndromes, histologic confirmation is required.
In general, the easiest accessible site is used for tissue biopsy which may include the skin, an enlarged superficial lymph node or lacrimal gland. Non-necrotizing granulomas on a liver

or bone marrow biopsy are non-specific and support the diagnosis of sarcoidosis only when competing diagnoses such as infection, malignancy or drug reaction have been excluded.

Pulmonary involvement is seen in 90% of patients with sarcoidosis in which intrathoracic lymphadenopathy is the most common finding (Hughes and Hill 2009). In the absence of an easily accessible biopsy site, fibroscopic bronchoscopy is preferred for its relative safety and high yield. The various techniques include bronchoscopic alveolar lavage (BAL), transbronchial lung biopsy (TBLB), transbronchial needle aspiration (TBNA), and endobronchial ultrasound (EBUS)-guided TBNA and will be discussed below.

In the lung, 75% of granulomas are distributed near or within the connective tissue sheath of bronchioles and subpleural spaces, "following the lymphatics" as authors describe (Mukhopadhyay and Gal 2010). For this reason, the 1999 Statement on Sarcoidosis recommends transbronchial biopsy (TBB) as the procedure of choice in most cases. Diagnostic yield ranges from 40 to 90% depending on operator experience, the presence of pulmonary infiltrates and if at least four biopsies are performed.

Endobronchial biopsy may detect noncaseating granulomas in 40-60% of cases even in the absence of endobronchial nodules or cobblestone appearance (Bjermer et al. 1991). Bronchial washing is recommended for microbiologic evaluation while bronchoalveolar lavage (BAL) may provide the study of lymphocyte subpopulations. In one study, a CD4/CD8 ratio >3.5 supports the diagnosis with 94% specificity and 53% sensitivity (Costabel 1997; Bjermer et al. 1991). However, its utility is unclear since some report a low yield of 47%(Garwood et al. 2007) while authorities report overlap with other etiologies such as infection, malignancy, and other inflammatory disorders (Fishman 2008).

When traditional bronchoscopic procedures such as EBB and TBB are nondiagnostic, further investigation has traditionally included mediastinoscopy for patients with mediastinal adenopathy and video-assisted thoracoscopic surgical lung biopsy (VATS) or open lung biopsy for patients with pulmonary infiltrates. However, advances in conventional and endobronchial ultrasound (EBUS)-assisted transbronchial needle aspiration (TBNA) may now avoid the need for surgical biopsy in most patients. Comparison of these techniques will be discussed.

The potential of EBUS-TBNA was demonstrated in a experienced, tertiary care center (Garwood et al. 2007). Fifty consecutive patients with suspected sarcoidosis underwent EBUS-TBNA with rapid on-site cytologic evaluation (ROSE). Results demonstrate safety (no major complications) and efficacy with 85% diagnostic yield. Lymph node size was not limited to >1cm and included nine nodes <1cm with 89% successful aspiration. Such results are impressive and comparable to studies of combined modalities (conventional TBNA and TBLB) but without the increased risk of pneumothorax and bleeding. However, these results are limited to experienced tertiary-care centers with the availability of ROSE.

A randomized controlled trial compared conventional TBNA with EBUS-assisted TBNA in patients with clinically suspected Stage I and Stage II sarcoidosis (Baughman et al. 2001). ROSE was not provided and lymph node size was limited to >1cm (short axis on CT scan). The EBUS-assisted TBNA procedure increased the diagnostic yield by an absolute 30% ($p<0.05$). It was 10.2 minutes longer and more patients (26.9%) received propofol for sedation. Complications were limited to moderate bleeding in two conventional TBNA attempts. Two observations deserve mention. First, the increased diagnostic yield was limited to patients with Stage 1 disease. Second, only 24% of patients in the follow-up period received specific treatment for sarcoidosis. These findings question the need to seek tissue confirmation in all patients (to be discussed further).

A large prospective, "implementation" study was designed to assess the yield of EBUS-assisted TBNA only after routine bronchoscopic procedures (EBB, TBB and conventional

TBNA) were nondiagnostic (Tournoy et al. 2010). ROSE was not available. Bronchial washing was routinely performed for microbiologic evaluation. A definitive diagnosis was obtained in 59% by routine bronchoscopy (72% TBB, 26% EBB, 14% TBNA) and 77% by EBUS-TBNA following nondiagnostic routine bronchoscopy. In other words, EBUS-TBNA following negative flexible bronchoscopy avoided a surgical procedure in 47 out of 80 patients. Overall, this implementation strategy provided a definitive diagnosis in 92% of patients. Minor complications included minor bleeding, intolerance to the procedure and one pneumothorax.

Despite the advancement in these techniques, the decision to pursue tissue diagnosis must be carefully considered especially when the diagnosis of sarcoidosis will not initiate treatment. For example, in asymptomatic patients with isolated bilateral hilar lymphadenopathy (Stage I disease), the main alternative diagnoses include lymphoma, malignancy, tuberculosis and fungal infections.

The likelihood of these alternative diagnoses may be narrowed. The probability of fungal infections is increased only when travel exposure and geographic location are suggestive. Second, the presentation of tuberculosis as bilateral hilar lymphadenopathy is rare (<1%) and systemic symptoms are invariably present. Likewise, the presentation of lymphoma is rarely asymptomatic nor limited to hilar lymphadenopathy. In fact, the *number needed to diagnosis* Hodgkin's and Non-Hodgkin's lymphoma in such patients with asymptomatic, isolated hilar lymphadenopathy is estimated at 1 in 3,600 and 1 in 33,000, respectively (Reich et al. 1998). For those who underwent mediastinoscopy, 18 patients would experience major morbidity and 36 require hospitalization.

4.6 Summary

Sarcoidosis is a disorder of unknown origin and definitive diagnosis is never certain. Typical cases of Lofgren's and Heerfodt syndrome do not require histologic confirmation. Furthermore, the risk/benefit ratio of histologic confirmation should be carefully considered when the likelihood of an alternative diagnosis is low. When histologic confirmation is desired, routine bronchoscopic procedures followed by EBUS or EUS-assisted TBNA, when needed, is a relatively safe and effective strategy applicable in most institutions.

5. Conclusion

Sarcoidosis is defined as a systemic (multiorgan) granulomatous disease of unknown cause. The diagnosis is traditionally established by (1) compatible clinical and radiographic features, (2) histologic confirmation of granulomatous inflammation with evidence of systemic (multiorgan) disease and (3) the exclusion of systemic granulomatous diseases of known cause. Although histologic evidence is needed from only a single site, clinical involvement of more than one system helps exclude local granulomatous reactions to foreign bodies, tumor or infections.

In a consensus opinion of the members of the Steering Committee of the ACCESS study, a subjective instrument for determining organ involvement in sarcoidosis was proposed (Judson et al. 1999). Criteria for organ involvement in patients with biopsy confirmed sarcoidosis were described for commonly involved sites (lung, skin, eyes, liver) and those less affected (nervous system, kidney, heart, bone marrow, spleen, salivary glands, ear-nose-throat area, non thoracic lymph nodes , muscle). Although not validated in large scale prospective studies, this instrument helps define the systemic nature of disease without the necessity to histologically confirm the presence of non-necrotizing granulomatous inflammation outside the lungs.

The clinician and the pathologist must work together. The pathologist's dilemma is the differentiation of sarcoidosis from an alternative cause of granulomatous inflammation.
While infection (both fungal and mycobacterial) may be easier to diagnose today with molecular-based techniques, other illnesses such as sarcoid-like related granulomatous disease, vasculitis, granulomatous lesions of unknown significance (GLUS) or the Blau syndrome may be difficult to differentiate.
The clinician must diligently search for the clinical syndromes described that may provide a diagnosis without the need for histologic confirmation. In addition, the clinician must consider both the likelihood of an alternative diagnosis and the indications for treatment prior to recommending invasive procedures for histologic confirmation. Finally, our goal is to limit the degree of uncertainty to the best of our ability since the etiology of sarcoidosis is still unknown. This requires a careful, step-wise approach. We propose a practical algorithm based on the data provided and our experience that most patients will be referred to the pulmonologist because of abnormal findings on chest imaging.

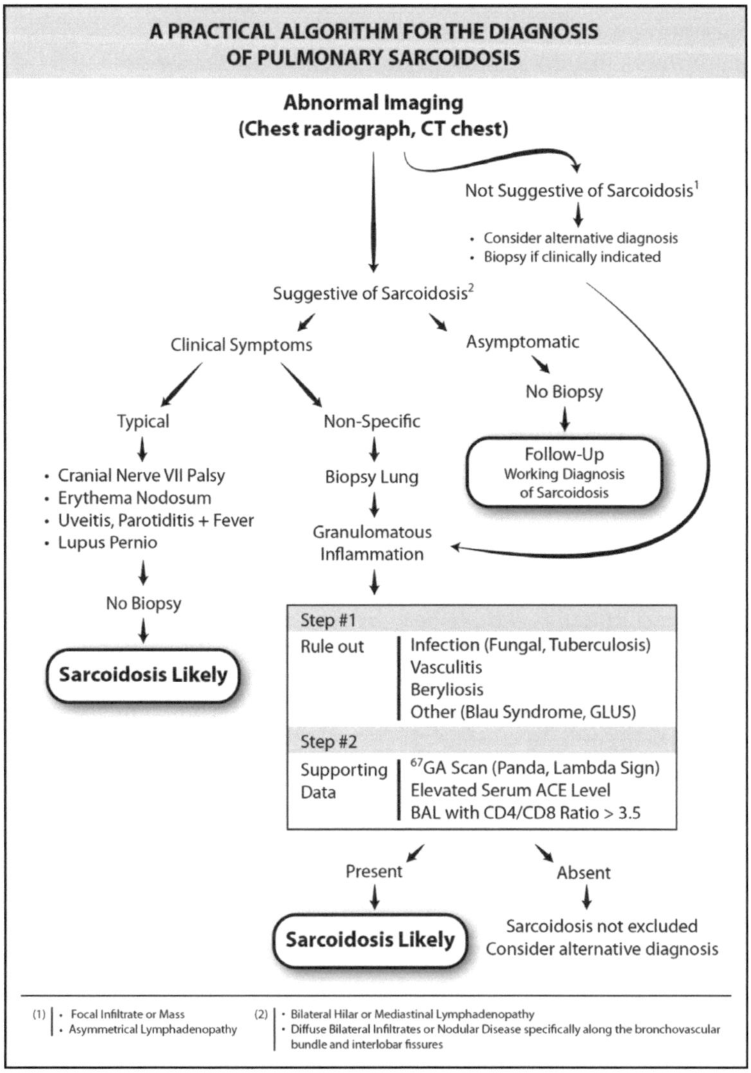

6. Acknowledgments

We wish to thank Dr. Judith Rozenman and Dr. Marina Perlman for their contribution to the pictures provided of radiographic and histologic features of sarcoidosis. Additional pictures are contributed via personal communication with Yale Rosen, MD and we encourage readers to visit the excellent website, http://granuloma.homestead.com.

7. References

Abehsera, M., D. Valeyre, P. Grenier, H. Jaillet, J. P. Battesti, and M. W. Brauner. 2000. Sarcoidosis with pulmonary fibrosis: CT patterns and correlation with pulmonary function. *AJR. American journal of roentgenology* 174 (6):1751-7.

Albert, R. H., and J. J. Russell. 2009. Evaluation of the solitary pulmonary nodule. *American family physician* 80 (8):827-31.

Alhamad, E. H., S. A. Shaik, M. M. Idrees, M. O. Alanezi, and A. C. Isnani. 2010. Outcome measures of the 6 minute walk test: relationships with physiologic and computed tomography findings in patients with sarcoidosis. *BMC pulmonary medicine* 10:42.

Arcasoy, S. M., J. D. Christie, A. Pochettino, B. R. Rosengard, N. P. Blumenthal, J. E. Bavaria, and R. M. Kotloff. 2001. Characteristics and outcomes of patients with sarcoidosis listed for lung transplantation. *Chest* 120 (3):873-80.

Baughman, R. P., D. A. Culver, and M. A. Judson. 2011. A concise review of pulmonary sarcoidosis. *American journal of respiratory and critical care medicine* 183 (5):573-81.

Baughman, R. P., E. E. Lower, and R. M. du Bois. 2003. Sarcoidosis. *Lancet* 361 (9363):1111-8.

Baughman, R. P., R. Shipley, S. Desai, M. Drent, M. A. Judson, U. Costabel, R. M. du Bois, M. Kavuru, R. Schlenker-Herceg, S. Flavin, K. H. Lo, and E. S. Barnathan. 2009. Changes in chest roentgenogram of sarcoidosis patients during a clinical trial of infliximab therapy: comparison of different methods of evaluation. *Chest* 136 (2):526-35.

Baughman, R. P., B. K. Sparkman, and E. E. Lower. 2007. Six-minute walk test and health status assessment in sarcoidosis. *Chest* 132 (1):207-13.

Baughman, R. P., A. S. Teirstein, M. A. Judson, M. D. Rossman, H. Yeager, Jr., E. A. Bresnitz, L. DePalo, G. Hunninghake, M. C. Iannuzzi, C. J. Johns, G. McLennan, D. R. Moller, L. S. Newman, D. L. Rabin, C. Rose, B. Rybicki, S. E. Weinberger, M. L. Terrin, G. L. Knatterud, and R. Cherniak. 2001. Clinical characteristics of patients in a case control study of sarcoidosis. *American journal of respiratory and critical care medicine* 164 (10 Pt 1):1885-9.

Bjermer, L., M. Thunell, L. Rosenhall, and N. Stjernberg. 1991. Endobronchial biopsy positive sarcoidosis: relation to bronchoalveolar lavage and course of disease. *Respiratory medicine* 85 (3):229-34.

Bower, J. S., J. E. Belen, J. G. Weg, and D. R. Dantzker. 1980. Manifestations and treatment of laryngeal sarcoidosis. *The American review of respiratory disease* 122 (2):325-32.

Bradley, B., H. M. Branley, J. J. Egan, M. S. Greaves, D. M. Hansell, N. K. Harrison, N. Hirani, R. Hubbard, F. Lake, A. B. Millar, W. A. Wallace, A. U. Wells, M. K. Whyte, and M. L. Wilsher. 2008. Interstitial lung disease guideline: the British Thoracic Society in collaboration with the Thoracic Society of Australia and New Zealand and the Irish Thoracic Society. *Thorax* 63 Suppl 5:v1-58.

Braun, J. J., R. Kessler, A. Constantinesco, and A. Imperiale. 2008. 18F-FDG PET/CT in sarcoidosis management: review and report of 20 cases. *European journal of nuclear medicine and molecular imaging* 35 (8):1537-43.

Brice, E. A., W. Friedlander, E. D. Bateman, and R. E. Kirsch. 1995. Serum angiotensin-converting enzyme activity, concentration, and specific activity in granulomatous interstitial lung disease, tuberculosis, and COPD. *Chest* 107 (3):706-10.

Chambellan, A., P. Turbie, H. Nunes, M. Brauner, J. P. Battesti, and D. Valeyre. 2005. Endoluminal stenosis of proximal bronchi in sarcoidosis: bronchoscopy, function, and evolution. *Chest* 127 (2):472-81.

Choi, J., L. A. Hoffman, J. M. Sethi, T. G. Zullo, and K. F. Gibson. 2009. Multiple flow rates measurement of exhaled nitric oxide in patients with sarcoidosis: a pilot feasibility study. *Sarcoidosis, vasculitis, and diffuse lung diseases : official journal of WASOG / World Association of Sarcoidosis and Other Granulomatous Disorders* 26 (2):98-109.

Cohen, P. R., and R. Kurzrock. 2007. Sarcoidosis and malignancy. *Clinics in dermatology* 25 (3):326-33.

Costabel, U. 1997. CD4/CD8 ratios in bronchoalveolar lavage fluid: of value for diagnosing sarcoidosis? *The European respiratory journal : official journal of the European Society for Clinical Respiratory Physiology* 10 (12):2699-700.

Devaraj, A., N. Griffin, A. G. Nicholson, and S. P. Padley. 2007. Computed tomography findings in fibrosing mediastinitis. *Clinical radiology* 62 (8):781-6.

Dunn, T. L., L. C. Watters, C. Hendrix, R. M. Cherniack, M. I. Schwarz, and T. E. King, Jr. 1988. Gas exchange at a given degree of volume restriction is different in sarcoidosis and idiopathic pulmonary fibrosis. *The American journal of medicine* 85 (2):221-4.

Emanuel, P. O., and R. G. Phelps. 2008. Metastatic Crohn's disease: a histopathologic study of 12 cases. *Journal of cutaneous pathology* 35 (5):457-61.

Facco, M., A. Cabrelle, A. Teramo, V. Olivieri, M. Gnoato, S. Teolato, E. Ave, C. Gattazzo, G. P. Fadini, F. Calabrese, G. Semenzato, and C. Agostini. 2011. Sarcoidosis is a Th1/Th17 multisystem disorder. *Thorax* 66 (2):144-50.

Fishman. 2008. Fishman's Pulmonary Diseases and Disorders.1282.

Garwood, S., M. A. Judson, G. Silvestri, R. Hoda, M. Fraig, and P. Doelken. 2007. Endobronchial ultrasound for the diagnosis of pulmonary sarcoidosis. *Chest* 132 (4):1298-304.

Hawtin, K. E., M. E. Roddie, F. A. Mauri, and S. J. Copley. 2010. Pulmonary sarcoidosis: the 'Great Pretender'. *Clinical radiology* 65 (8):642-50.

Hollister, D., Jr., M. S. Lee, R. N. Eisen, C. Fey, and C. S. Portlock. 2005. Variable problems in lymphomas: CASE 2. Sarcoidosis mimicking progressive lymphoma. *Journal of clinical oncology : official journal of the American Society of Clinical Oncology* 23 (31):8113-6.

Huang, C. T., A. E. Heurich, Y. Rosen, S. Moon, and H. A. Lyons. 1979. Pulmonary sarcoidosis: roentgenographic, functional, and pathologic correlations. *Respiration; international review of thoracic diseases* 37 (6):337-45.

Huggins, J. T., P. Doelken, S. A. Sahn, L. King, and M. A. Judson. 2006. Pleural effusions in a series of 181 outpatients with sarcoidosis. *Chest* 129 (6):1599-604.

Hughes, M., and J. Hill. 2009. Left vocal cord paralysis in systemic lupus erythematosus. *Modern rheumatology / the Japan Rheumatism Association* 19 (4):441-2.

Hunninghake, G. W., U. Costabel, M. Ando, R. Baughman, J. F. Cordier, R. du Bois, A. Eklund, M. Kitaichi, J. Lynch, G. Rizzato, C. Rose, O. Selroos, G. Semenzato, and O. P. Sharma. 1999. ATS/ERS/WASOG statement on sarcoidosis. American Thoracic Society/European Respiratory Society/World Association of Sarcoidosis and other Granulomatous Disorders. *Sarcoidosis Vasc Diffuse Lung Dis* 16 (2):149-73.

Jaffe, R., V. Bogomolski-Yahalom, and M. R. Kramer. 1994. Vocal cord paralysis as the presenting symptom of sarcoidosis. *Respiratory medicine* 88 (8):633-6.

Judson, M. A. 1998. Lung transplantation for pulmonary sarcoidosis. *The European respiratory journal : official journal of the European Society for Clinical Respiratory Physiology* 11 (3):738-44.

Judson, M. A., R. P. Baughman, A. S. Teirstein, M. L. Terrin, and H. Yeager, Jr. 1999. Defining organ involvement in sarcoidosis: the ACCESS proposed instrument. ACCESS Research Group. A Case Control Etiologic Study of Sarcoidosis. *Sarcoidosis, vasculitis, and diffuse lung diseases : official journal of WASOG / World Association of Sarcoidosis and Other Granulomatous Disorders* 16 (1):75-86.

Judson, M. A., G. E. Gilbert, J. K. Rodgers, C. F. Greer, and S. I. Schabel. 2008. The utility of the chest radiograph in diagnosing exacerbations of pulmonary sarcoidosis. *Respirology* 13 (1):97-102.

Kabitz, H. J., F. Lang, S. Walterspacher, S. Sorichter, J. Muller-Quernheim, and W. Windisch. 2006. Impact of impaired inspiratory muscle strength on dyspnea and walking capacity in sarcoidosis. *Chest* 130 (5):1496-502.

Kaira, K., N. Oriuchi, Y. Otani, N. Yanagitani, N. Sunaga, T. Hisada, T. Ishizuka, K. Endo, and M. Mori. 2007. Diagnostic usefulness of fluorine-18-alpha-methyltyrosine positron emission tomography in combination with 18F-fluorodeoxyglucose in sarcoidosis patients. *Chest* 131 (4):1019-27.

Klauser, R. J., C. J. Robinson, D. V. Marinkovic, and E. G. Erdos. 1979. Inhibition of human peptidyl dipeptidase (angiotensin I converting enzyme: kininase II) by human serum albumin and its fragments. *Hypertension* 1 (3):281-6.

Kobayashi, J., and S. Kitamura. 1996. Serum KL-6 for the evaluation of active pneumonitis in pulmonary sarcoidosis. *Chest* 109 (5):1276-82.

Lenique, F., M. W. Brauner, P. Grenier, J. P. Battesti, A. Loiseau, and D. Valeyre. 1995. CT assessment of bronchi in sarcoidosis: endoscopic and pathologic correlations. *Radiology* 194 (2):419-23.

Lewis, P. J., and A. Salama. 1994. Uptake of fluorine-18-fluorodeoxyglucose in sarcoidosis. *Journal of nuclear medicine : official publication, Society of Nuclear Medicine* 35 (10):1647-9.

Lieberman, J. 1975. Elevation of serum angiotensin-converting-enzyme (ACE) level in sarcoidosis. *The American journal of medicine* 59 (3):365-72.

Maliarik, M. J., B. A. Rybicki, E. Malvitz, R. G. Sheffer, M. Major, J. Popovich, Jr., and M. C. Iannuzzi. 1998. Angiotensin-converting enzyme gene polymorphism and risk of sarcoidosis. *American journal of respiratory and critical care medicine* 158 (5 Pt 1):1566-70.

Mana, J. 2002. Magnetic resonance imaging and nuclear imaging in sarcoidosis. *Current opinion in pulmonary medicine* 8 (5):457-63.

Manolio, T. 2003. Novel risk markers and clinical practice. *The New England journal of medicine* 349 (17):1587-9.

McGrath, D. S., P. J. Foley, M. Petrek, L. Izakovicova-Holla, V. Kolek, S. Veeraraghavan, P. A. Lympany, P. Pantelidis, A. Vasku, A. U. Wells, K. I. Welsh, and R. M. Du Bois. 2001. Ace gene I/D polymorphism and sarcoidosis pulmonary disease severity. *American journal of respiratory and critical care medicine* 164 (2):197-201.

Medinger, A. E., S. Khouri, and P. K. Rohatgi. 2001. Sarcoidosis: the value of exercise testing. *Chest* 120 (1):93-101.

Mehrotra, R., and V. Dhingra. 2010. Cytological diagnosis of sarcoidosis revisited: A state of the art review. *Diagnostic cytopathology*.

Mehta, D., S. A. Lubitz, Z. Frankel, J. P. Wisnivesky, A. J. Einstein, M. Goldman, J. Machac, and A. Teirstein. 2008. Cardiac involvement in patients with sarcoidosis: diagnostic and prognostic value of outpatient testing. *Chest* 133 (6):1426-35.

Miyoshi, S., H. Hamada, T. Kadowaki, N. Hamaguchi, R. Ito, K. Irifune, and J. Higaki. 2010. Comparative evaluation of serum markers in pulmonary sarcoidosis. *Chest* 137 (6):1391-7.

Morello, F. A., S. A. Ali, and F. Cesani. 1998. Sarcoid: an unusual mimicker of classic pulmonary embolus. *Clinical nuclear medicine* 23 (10):654-6.

Mukhopadhyay, S., and A. A. Gal. 2010. Granulomatous lung disease: an approach to the differential diagnosis. *Arch Pathol Lab Med* 134 (5):667-90.

Muller-Quernheim, J. 1998. Sarcoidosis: immunopathogenetic concepts and their clinical application. *The European respiratory journal : official journal of the European Society for Clinical Respiratory Physiology* 12 (3):716-38.

Nakatsu, M., H. Hatabu, K. Morikawa, H. Uematsu, Y. Ohno, K. Nishimura, S. Nagai, T. Izumi, J. Konishi, and H. Itoh. 2002. Large coalescent parenchymal nodules in pulmonary sarcoidosis: "sarcoid galaxy" sign. *AJR. American journal of roentgenology* 178 (6):1389-93. New England of Medicine June 2011 Reduced Lung Cancer Mortality with Low Dose Computed Tomography Screening (on-line)

Ng, K. K., and J. R. Vane. 1967. Conversion of angiotensin I to angiotensin II. *Nature* 216 (5117):762-6.

Nishino, M., K. S. Lee, H. Itoh, and H. Hatabu. 2010. The spectrum of pulmonary sarcoidosis: variations of high-resolution CT findings and clues for specific diagnosis. *European journal of radiology* 73 (1):66-73.

Nunes, H., P. Y. Brillet, D. Valeyre, M. W. Brauner, and A. U. Wells. 2007. Imaging in sarcoidosis. *Seminars in respiratory and critical care medicine* 28 (1):102-20.

Nunes, H., M. Humbert, F. Capron, M. Brauner, O. Sitbon, J. P. Battesti, G. Simonneau, and D. Valeyre. 2006. Pulmonary hypertension associated with sarcoidosis: mechanisms, haemodynamics and prognosis. *Thorax* 61 (1):68-74.

Pertschuk, L. P., E. Silverstein, and J. Friedland. 1981. Immunohistologic diagnosis of sarcoidosis. Detection of angiotensin-converting enzyme in sarcoid granulomas. *American journal of clinical pathology* 75 (3):350-4.

Pietinalho, A., M. Ohmichi, A. B. Lofroos, Y. Hiraga, and O. Selroos. 2000. The prognosis of pulmonary sarcoidosis in Finland and Hokkaido, Japan. A comparative five-year study of biopsy-proven cases. *Sarcoidosis, vasculitis, and diffuse lung diseases : official journal of WASOG / World Association of Sarcoidosis and Other Granulomatous Disorders* 17 (2):158-66.

Reich, J. M., M. C. Brouns, E. A. O'Connor, and M. J. Edwards. 1998. Mediastinoscopy in patients with presumptive stage I sarcoidosis: a risk/benefit, cost/benefit analysis. *Chest* 113 (1):147-53.

Reid, J. D., and M. E. Andersen. 1988. Calcium oxalate in sarcoid granulomas. With particular reference to the small ovoid body and a note on the finding of dolomite. *American journal of clinical pathology* 90 (5):545-58.

Ro, J. Y., M. A. Luna, B. Mackay, and O. Ramos. 1987. Yellow-brown (Hamazaki-Wesenberg) bodies mimicking fungal yeasts. *Archives of pathology & laboratory medicine* 111 (6):555-9.

Rohatgi, P. K., and L. E. Schwab. 1980. Primary acute pulmonary cavitation in sarcoidosis. *AJR. American journal of roentgenology* 134 (6):1199-203.

Rothkrantz-Kos, S., M. P. van Dieijen-Visser, P. G. Mulder, and M. Drent. 2003. Potential usefulness of inflammatory markers to monitor respiratory functional impairment in sarcoidosis. *Clinical chemistry* 49 (9):1510-7.

Rumbak, M., G. Kohler, C. Eastrige, H. Winer-Muram, and M. Gavant. 1996. Topical treatment of life threatening haemoptysis from aspergillomas. *Thorax* 51 (3):253-5.

Saldana. 1994. *Pathology of Pulmonary Disease.*

Saldana, Mario. 1994. *Pathology of Pulmonary Disease.*

Scadding, J. G. 1961. Prognosis of intrathoracic sarcoidosis in England. A review of 136 cases after five years' observation. *British medical journal* 2 (5261):1165-72.

Shadid, S., and J. C. ter Maaten. 2002. Sarcoidosis--a great mimicker. *Journal of internal medicine* 251 (2):174-6.

Shah, J. R., and R. A. Lewis. 2003. Sarcoidosis of the cauda equina mimicking Guillain-Barre syndrome. *Journal of the neurological sciences* 208 (1-2):113-7.

Sharma, O. P., and S. Alam. 1995. Diagnosis, pathogenesis, and treatment of sarcoidosis. *Current opinion in pulmonary medicine* 1 (5):392-400.

Sharma, O. P., and R. Johnson. 1988. Airway obstruction in sarcoidosis. A study of 123 nonsmoking black American patients with sarcoidosis. *Chest* 94 (2):343-6.

Shorr, A. F., K. G. Torrington, and O. W. Hnatiuk. 2001. Endobronchial involvement and airway hyperreactivity in patients with sarcoidosis. *Chest* 120 (3):881-6.

Stevens, D. A., V. L. Kan, M. A. Judson, V. A. Morrison, S. Dummer, D. W. Denning, J. E. Bennett, T. J. Walsh, T. F. Patterson, and G. A. Pankey. 2000. Practice guidelines for diseases caused by Aspergillus. Infectious Diseases Society of America. *Clinical infectious diseases : an official publication of the Infectious Diseases Society of America* 30 (4):696-709.

Studdy, P. R., and R. Bird. 1989. Serum angiotensin converting enzyme in sarcoidosis--its value in present clinical practice. *Annals of clinical biochemistry* 26 (Pt 1):13-8.

Sulavik, S. B., R. P. Spencer, D. A. Weed, H. R. Shapiro, S. T. Shiue, and R. J. Castriotta. 1990. Recognition of distinctive patterns of gallium-67 distribution in sarcoidosis. *Journal of nuclear medicine : official publication, Society of Nuclear Medicine* 31 (12):1909-14.

Terasaki, H., K. Fujimoto, N. L. Muller, J. Sadohara, M. Uchida, T. Koga, H. Aizawa, and N. Hayabuchi. 2005. Pulmonary sarcoidosis: comparison of findings of inspiratory and expiratory high-resolution CT and pulmonary function tests between smokers and nonsmokers. *AJR. American journal of roentgenology* 185 (2):333-8.

Tournoy, K. G., A. Bolly, J. G. Aerts, P. Pierard, R. De Pauw, D. Leduc, A. Leloup, T. Pieters, H. Slabbynck, A. Janssens, K. Carron, L. Schrevens, K. Pat, T. De Keukeleire, and C.

Dooms. 2010. The value of endoscopic ultrasound after bronchoscopy to diagnose thoracic sarcoidosis. *The European respiratory journal : official journal of the European Society for Clinical Respiratory Physiology* 35 (6):1329-35.

Tzouvelekis, A., G. Kouliatsis, S. Anevlavis, and D. Bouros. 2005. Serum biomarkers in interstitial lung diseases. *Respiratory research* 6:78.

Winterbauer, R. H., and J. F. Hutchinson. 1980. Use of pulmonary function tests in the management of sarcoidosis. *Chest* 78 (4):640-7.

Wollschlager, C., and F. Khan. 1984. Aspergillomas complicating sarcoidosis. A prospective study in 100 patients. *Chest* 86 (4):585-8.

Woodard, B. H., S. I. Rosenberg, R. Farnham, and D. O. Adams. 1982. Incidence and nature of primary granulomatous inflammation in surgically removed material. *The American journal of surgical pathology* 6 (2):119-29.

Yeager, H., M. D. Rossman, R. P. Baughman, A. S. Teirstein, M. A. Judson, D. L. Rabin, M. C. Iannuzzi, C. Rose, E. A. Bresnitz, L. DePalo, G. Hunninghakes, C. J. Johns, G. McLennan, D. R. Moller, L. S. Newman, B. Rybicki, S. E. Weinberger, P. C. Wilkins, and R. Cherniack. 2005. Pulmonary and psychosocial findings at enrollment in the ACCESS study. *Sarcoidosis, vasculitis, and diffuse lung diseases : official journal of WASOG / World Association of Sarcoidosis and Other Granulomatous Disorders* 22 (2):147-53.

Ziegenhagen, M. W., M. E. Rothe, M. Schlaak, and J. Muller-Quernheim. 2003. Bronchoalveolar and serological parameters reflecting the severity of sarcoidosis. *The European respiratory journal : official journal of the European Society for Clinical Respiratory Physiology* 21 (3):407-13.

5

Imaging in Sarcoidosis

M. Reza Rajebi[1], Nicole A. Zimmerman[1], Roozbeh Sharif[2], Ernest M. Scalzetti[1], Stuart A. Groskin[3] and Rolf A. Grage[1]
[1]SUNY Upstate Medical University,
[2]University of Texas Health Science Center at Houston,
[3]Crouse Hospital,
USA

1. Introduction

Sarcoidosis is an enigmatic systemic granulomatous disease of unknown etiology. It was first described in 1877 by Jonathon Hutchinson, an English physician (Hutchinson, 1877). Caesar Boeck used the term sarkoid originally in 1899 because he felt that the lesions resembled sarcoma (Boeck, 1899). Kuznitsky and Bittorf reported the cardinal patient with enlarged hilar nodes and pulmonary infiltrates on chest radiograph, describing the principle case of sarcoidosis (Kuznitsky & Bittorf, 1915).

Sarcoidosis primarily affects the lung and lymphatic system. The patients are usually young to middle-aged adults, appearing more commonly in individuals of African descent. Bilateral hilar lymphadenopathy, pulmonary involvement, and ocular and cutaneous lesions are classic findings, however sarcoidosis can affect many other organs. Clinical and imaging findings are helpful in establishing the diagnosis. Histologic demonstration of noncaseating epithelioid cell granulomas is confirmatory for diagnosis. In 1958, Wurm and colleagues proposed a radiographic staging system, which still remains in widespread clinical use (Table 1) (Wurm et al., 1958).

Stage	Radiographic findings
0	Normal
1	Bilateral hilar adenopathy
2	Bilateral hilar adenopathy with parenchymal opacities
3	Parenchymal opacities
4	Advanced lung disease with fibrosis

Table 1. Radiographic stages of pulmonary sarcoidosis as defined by chest radiograph.

This chapter reviews the imaging findings of sarcoidosis based on the involved organ systems and recommends the principle imaging study contingent upon the diagnostic capabilities of different modalities. Options for radiologic evaluation of sarcoidosis include plain radiography, ultrasonography, scintigraphy, computed tomography (CT), and magnetic resonance imaging (MRI). Until the 1970s, evaluation of sarcoidosis was limited to plain chest radiographs. Radionuclide imaging is occasionally used to assess lymphatic, cardiac, and musculoskeletal involvement. With the development of CT in the early 1970s, cross-sectional imaging became available. The multiplanar and multisequential capabilities of MRI have enhanced the characterization of sarcoid lesions involving different organs.

2. Thoracic sarcoidosis

Classically, thoracic involvement of sarcoidosis presents as bilateral hilar adenopathy which may occur in combination with parenchymal opacities. The chest roentgenogram is still the most commonly used method for detecting lung involvement, however various other modalities are being used with increased frequency. Pulmonary involvement is present in 90% of patients with sarcoidosis.

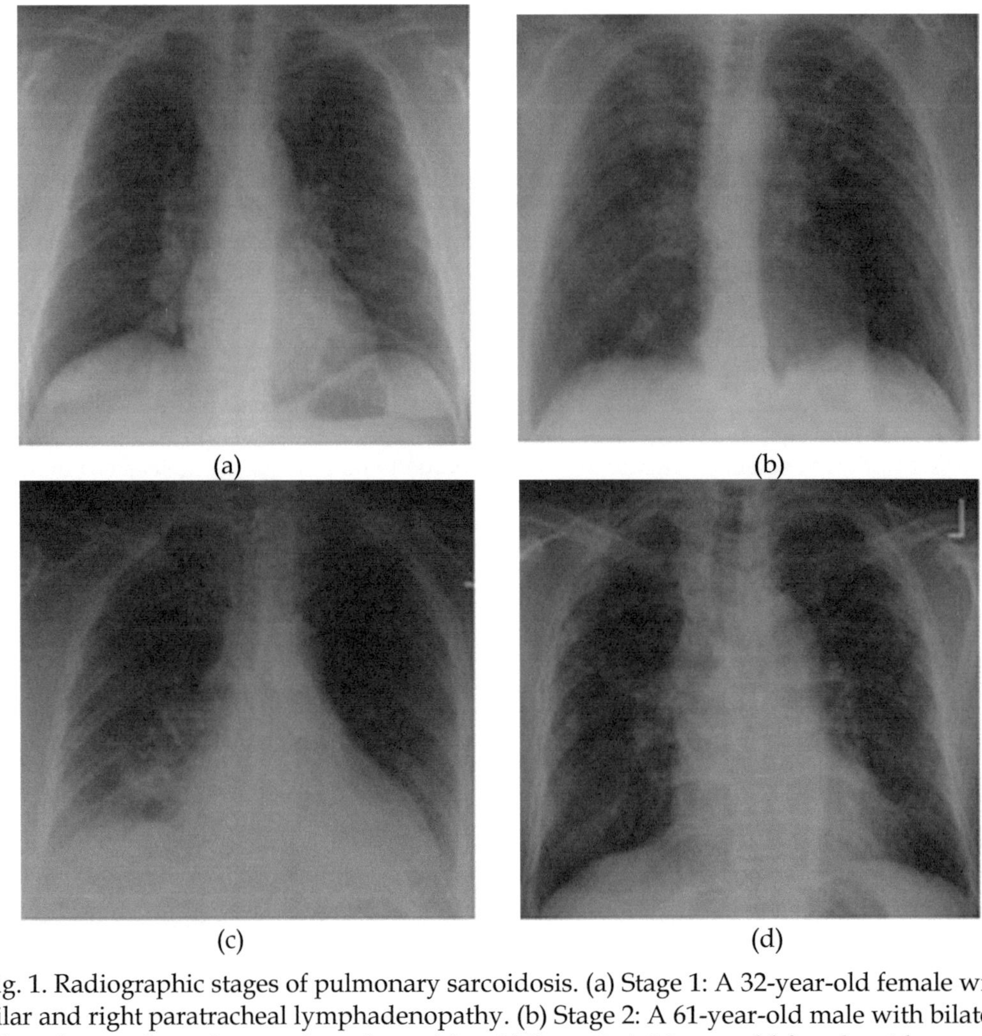

Fig. 1. Radiographic stages of pulmonary sarcoidosis. (a) Stage 1: A 32-year-old female with hilar and right paratracheal lymphadenopathy. (b) Stage 2: A 61-year-old male with bilateral hilar adenopathy and parenchymal opacities. (c) Stage 3: A 54-year-old female with parenchymal opacities in the right lower lung. (d) Stage 4: A 51-year-old female with extensive increased interstitial markings.

2.1 Radiography

Simple radiographs are sufficient for diagnosing and follow-up of sarcoidosis, although high-resolution CT without intravenous contrast is helpful in characterizing interstitial lung disease and the extent of adenopathy. It is also suitable in determining the lung involvement stage, amount and type of reversible versus irreversible lung damage, and the overall prognosis.

Pulmonary involvement can be categorized into five radiographic stages (Figure 1) (Silzbach, 1967). Pulmonary function test findings such as restrictive pattern and decreased carbon monoxide diffusing capacity worsen as the disease progresses from stages zero to four (Criado et al., 2010).

Lymphadenopathy is the most common finding in patients with pulmonary sarcoidosis; it is seen in 80% of patients. Bilateral hilar lymphadenopathy is the typical pattern of involvement. Additionally, right paratracheal lymphadenopathy is also common. Lymph nodes can be of different sizes ranging from subtle enlargement to conglomerate masses.

In 20% of patients, parenchymal infiltration can be identified on radiographs. Reticulonodular opacities are the most common findings and are primarily seen in the upper lung zones. Large nodules are seen in patients with alveolar sarcoidosis. In cases with advanced disease and fibrosis, honeycombing and traction bronchiectasis may be seen. The upper lobes and superior segments of the lower lobes are usually involved in this presentation. Occasionally, cavitary lesions and pleural effusion can be demonstrated.

2.2 Computed tomography

High-resolution CT is more sensitive in detecting adenopathy and parenchymal involvement as well as differentiating reversible inflammatory features from irreversible fibrotic changes. The most common CT findings of pulmonary sarcoidosis are symmetric lymphadenopathy, micronodules with lymphagitic spread, fibrotic changes, and bilateral perihilar opacities. Reversible inflammatory changes consist of nodules and uncommonly, alveolar densities and patchy ground-glass opacities. Irreversible changes due to pulmonary fibrosis include honeycombing, architectural distortion, bullae formation and tractional bronchiectasis.

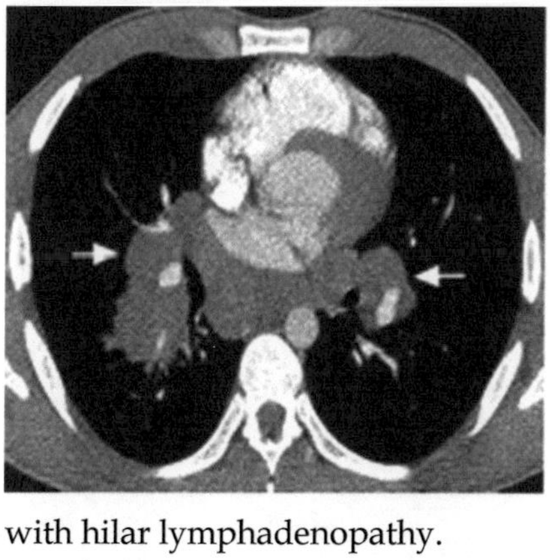

Fig. 2. A 56-year-old female with hilar lymphadenopathy.

Typically, hilar and right paratracheal lymph nodes are enlarged (Figure 2). Furthermore, as the disease progresses to a chronic state, nodes can become calcified (Figure 3). A symmetric bilateral perilymphatic micronodular distribution, commonly referred to as lymphangitic spread, is the most common pattern in patients with parenchymal involvement in pulmonary sarcoidosis (Lynch et al., 1997). Lymphangitic spread can include peribronchovascular, subpleural, and interlobular septal distribution of the nodules (Figure

4). Micronodules are defined as round nodules measuring 2-4 mm and usually seen in the upper and middle zones. Bilateral perihilar opacities are one of the common findings in thoracic sarcoidosis; these opacities are confluent nodular consolidations with irregular borders and central predilection (Figure 5).

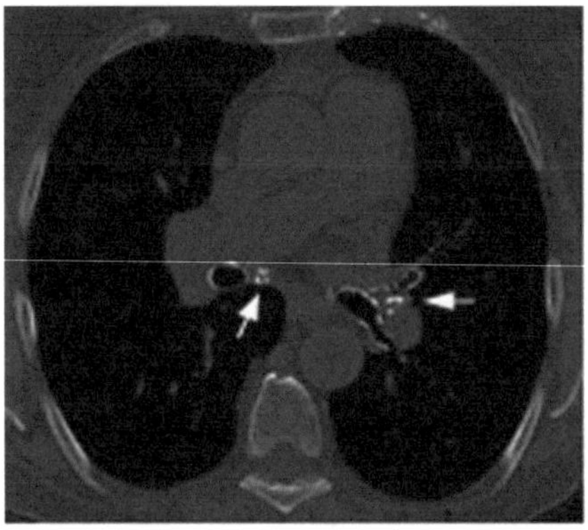

Fig. 3. A 69-year-old female with calcified hilar lymph nodes.

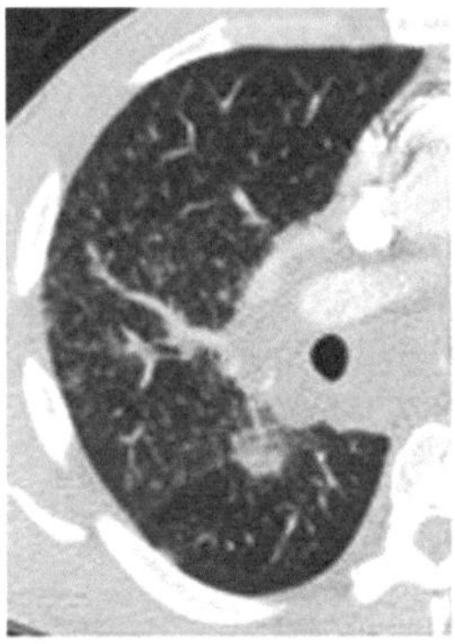

Fig. 4. A 56-year-old female with pulmonary sarcoidosis. CT of the chest demonstrates micronodules with peribronchovascular distribution.

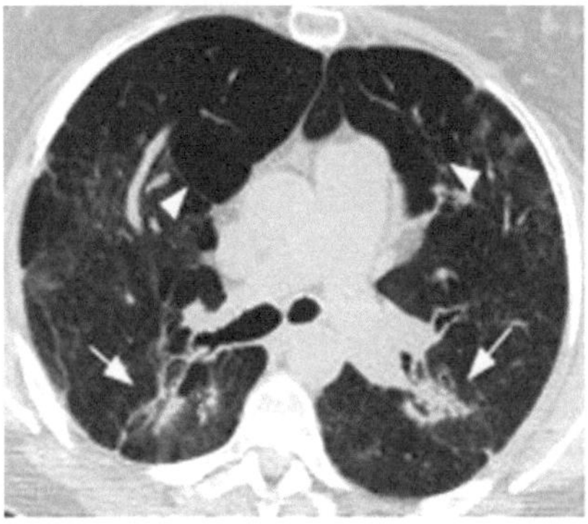

Fig. 5. A 51-year-old female with sarcoidosis. CT of the chest shows bilateral perihilar densities (arrows). Areas of air trapping and mosaic attenuation pattern are also identified (arrowheads)

In 20% of patients, the initial inflammatory phase leads to fibrotic changes such as honeycombing, linear densities, architectural distortion and secondary traction bronchieactasis (Figure 6). Honeycombing refers to "destroyed and fibrotic lung tissue containing numerous cystic airspaces with thick fibrous walls, representing the late stage of various lung diseases, with complete loss of acinar architecture" (Hansell et al., 2008). Upper and middle zones are usually involved in a patchy distribution. Abehsera et al described three major patterns of pulmonary involvement in patients with fibrosis: bronchial distortion in 47% of patients; honeycombing in 29% of patients; and diffuse linear opacities in 24% of patients (Abehsera et al., 2000).

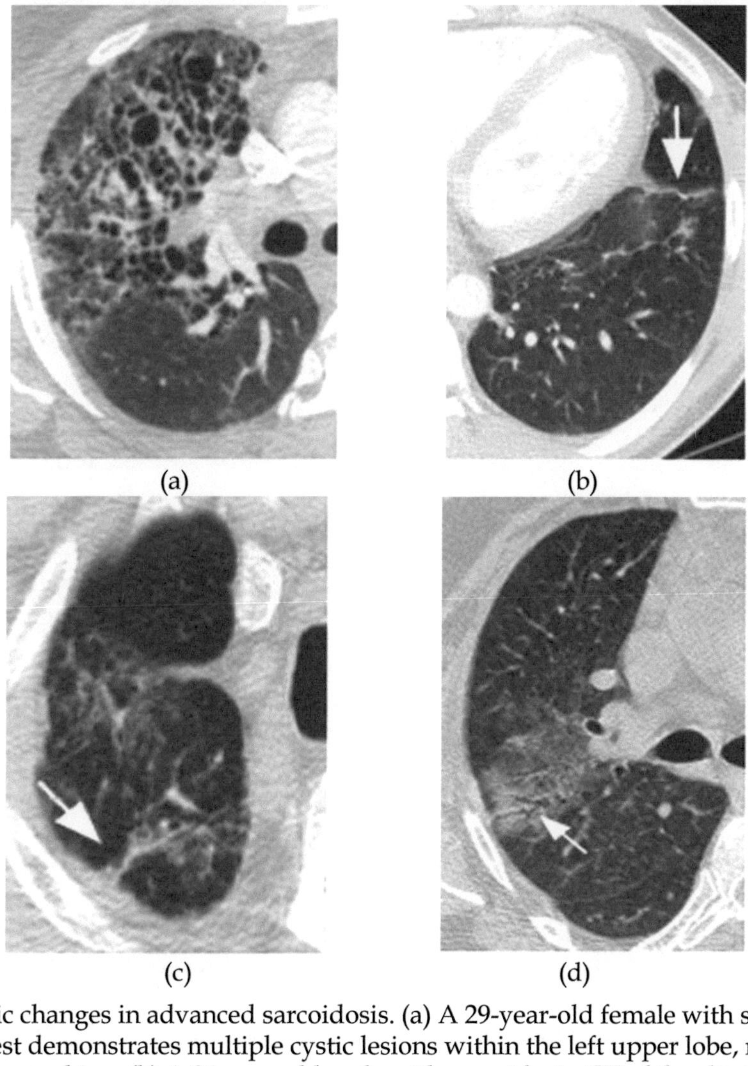

(a) (b) (c) (d)

Fig. 6. Fibrotic changes in advanced sarcoidosis. (a) A 29-year-old female with sarcodidosis. CT of the chest demonstrates multiple cystic lesions within the left upper lobe, representing areas of honeycombing. (b) A 34-year-old male with sarcoidosis. CT of the chest shows areas of linear densities (arrow) in the left lower lobe compatible with linear scarring. (c) A 49-year-old male with sarcoidosis. CT of the chest demonstrates architectural distortion in the right lung apex (arrow). (d) A 54 year-old female with sarcoidosis. CT of the chest shows bronchiectasis in the right upper lobe.

Atypical features of pulmonary involvement include unilateral lymphadenopathy, unusual location of lymphadenopathy, nodules and masses, patchy airspace, ground-glass, and linear opacities, airway involvement, fibrocystic changes, miliary opacities, and pleural disease. Unusual manifestations of mediastinal lymphadenopathy in a minority of patients may contribute to challenging diagnostic dilemmas.

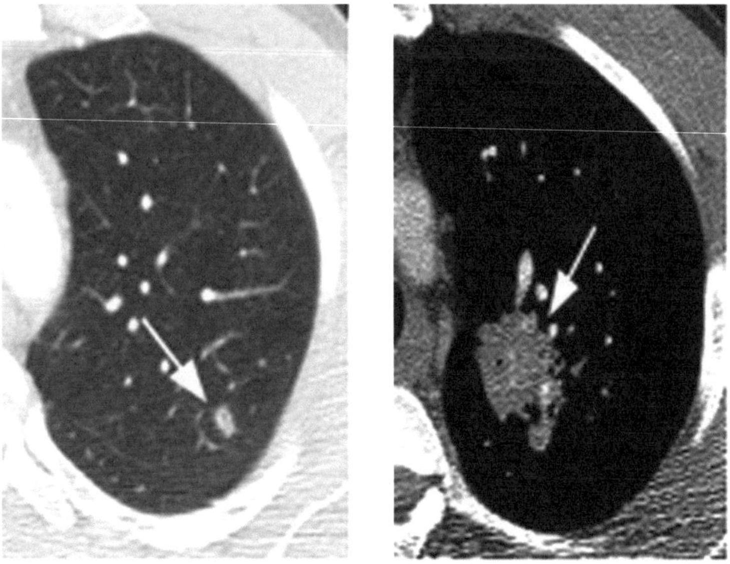

(a) (b)

Fig. 7. Pulmonary macronodules and masses in sarcoidosis. (a) A 34-year-old male. CT of the chest shows a 12 mm nodule in the left upper lobe. (b) A 39-year-old male. CT of the chest demonstrates a large soft tissue mass in the left upper lobe. Biopsy confirmed non-caseating granulomatous disease in both patients.

Nodules and masses are predominantly bilateral and multiple (Figure 7). Nevertheless, these lesions can occasionally present in varying manners. "Galaxy sign" refers to multiple small nodules around a larger mass (Figure 8). A conglomerate of multiple micronodules is called a "sarcoid cluster". Acinar or alveolar sarcoidosis refers to alveolar opacities, which are composed of multiple nodules causing adjacent alveoli compression and can easily be mistaken as pneumonia, tuberculosis, or cryptogenic organizing pneumonitis (Figure 9). Patchy ground-glass opacities are more commonly seen as compared to diffuse ground-glass opacities (Figure 10). Interlobular and intralobular septal thickening may lead to a linear reticular pattern (Figure 11). Honeycomb-like cysts, cavitations and mycetoma formations are considered fibrocystic changes.

Airway involvement is indicative of a poor prognosis (Handa et al., 2006). It can present as mosaic attenuation pattern, air trapping (Figure 5), tracheobronchial abnormalities, and atelectasis. Miliary pattern is a rare presentation of pulmonary sarcoidosis, found in less than one percent of cases (Figure 12). Pleural effusion, hemorrhagic or chylous pleural effusion, pneumothorax (Figure 12), pleural thickening, plaque-like opacities and pleural calcification occur in 1-4% of patients (Soskel & Sharma, 1992).

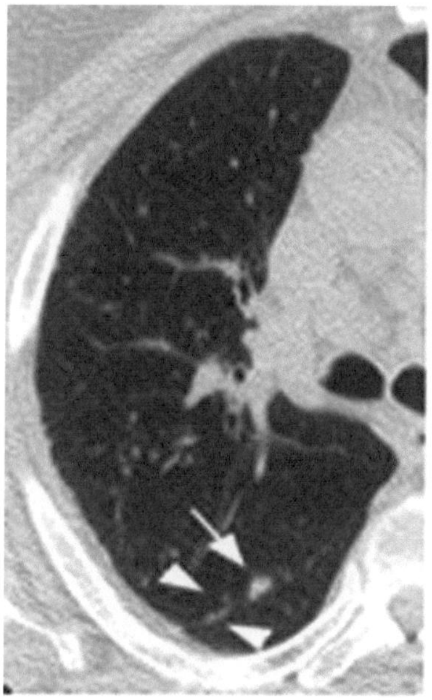

Fig. 8. "Galaxy sign". A 49-year-old female. CT of the chest shows a 7 mm nodule in the left lower lobe (arrow) as well as multiple adjacent 2 mm nodules (arrowhead).

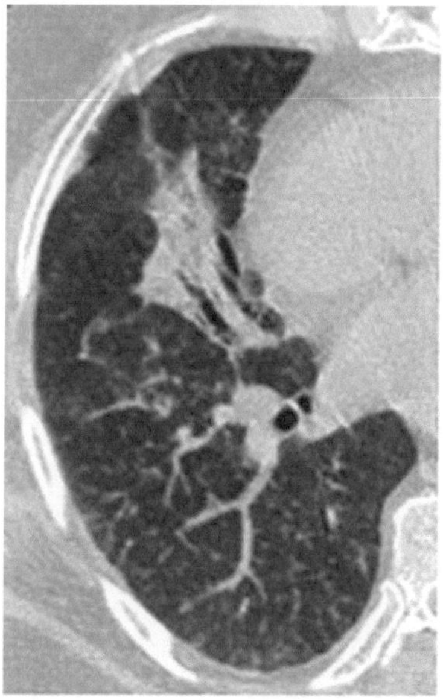

Fig. 9. A 54-year-old female with sarcoidosis. CT of the chest shows a large alveolar density in the right middle lobe

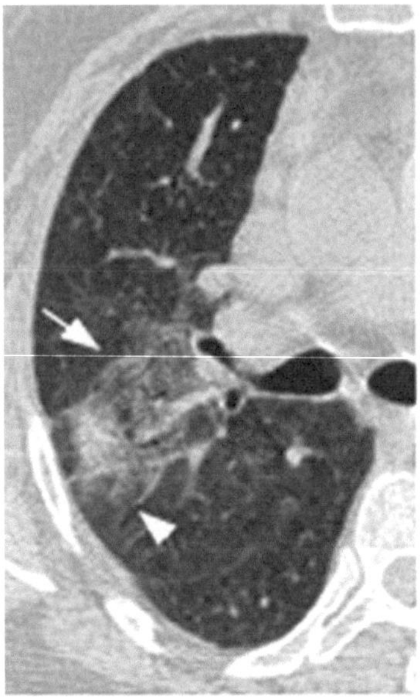

Fig. 10. A 54-year-old female with sarcoidosis. CT of the chest shows an area of patchy groundglass opacity (arrow) in the right upper lobe. A confluent opacity (arrowhead) lateral to this area is also identified.

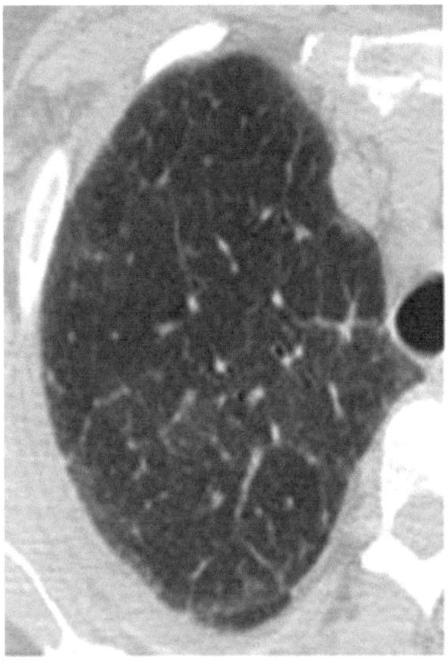

Fig. 11. A 56-year-old female with sarcoidosis. CT of the chest demonstrates intralobular septal thickening in the right upper lobe.

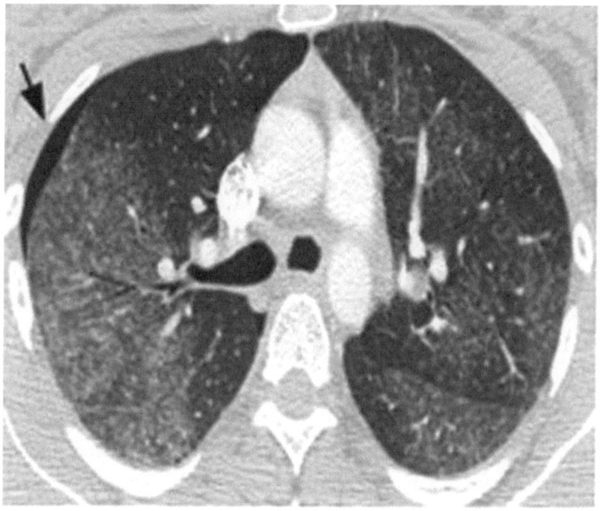

Fig. 12. A 66-year-old male. CT of chest reveals innumerable micronodules with a miliary pattern. A small right-sided pneumothorax (arrow) is also noted.

One study compared the high-resolution CT and pulmonary function test findings of smokers and nonsmokers with pulmonary sarcoidosis. 46 patients (23 smokers and 23 lifelong nonsmokers) with histologically proven sarcoidosis were included. Air trapping and small nodules were the most common findings. The extent of emphysema was greater in smokers although no significant difference was seen in the extent of airway involvement between smokers and nonsmokers (Terasaki et al., 2005).

2.3 Nuclear medicine

Gallium-67 (^{67}Ga) scintigraphy shows a relatively specific pattern of abnormal radiopharmaceutical uptake in thoracic lymph nodes of patients with pulmonary sarcoidosis referred to as "lambda sign". This is a distinctive pattern of increased ^{67}Ga uptake in the hilar and right paratracheal lymph nodes resembling the Greek letter lambda (λ). Sulivak et al evaluated 65 patients with sarcoidosis and compared ^{67}Ga scintigraphy findings in these patients with 540 patients with other disorders. Lambda sign was seen in 72% of patients with sarcoidosis and none of the patients in the comparison group (Sulavik et al., 1990).

2.4 Ultrasonography

Endobronchial ultrasound (EBUS) with transbronchial needle aspiration (TBNA) is a promising minimally invasive technique, which recently has been used for diagnosis of a wide variety of pulmonary disorders ranging from sarcoidosis to lung cancer. In one study, EBUS-TBNA is performed for diagnosis of sarcoidosis in 50 patients with suspected pulmonary sarcoidosis. Non-caseating granuloma was demonstrated in 41 of 48 patients (85%) with a final diagnosis of sarcoidosis (Garwood et al., 2007).

In summary, plain radiographs are sufficient for diagnosis of pulmonary sarcoidosis and subsequent follow-up. High resolution CT without intravenous contrast may be helpful to characterize interstitial lung disease and the extent of adenopathy.

3. Cardiac sarcoidosis

Although clinical cardiac involvement in sarcoidosis is uncommon, it is still a major contributing factor in disease prognosis (Perry & Vuitch, 1995). Acute cardiac failure, ventricular arrhythmias, heart blockage, and sudden cardiac death are several complications of sarcoidosis in the cardiovascular system. Myocardial involvement is more common than pericardial disease. The basal and lateral walls of the left ventricle as well as the septum are typically involved, while the endocardium is usually spared. As with any other organ, cardiac sarcoidosis can be divided into three stages including initial edema, granulomatous infiltration and scarring.

3.1 Nuclear medicine

Resting Thallium-201 and Tc-99m-methoxyisobutylisonitrile (Tc-99m-MIBI) scintigraphy demonstrate segmental regions of decreased radiopharmaceutical uptake in the myocardium although these foci do not correspond to histologic findings for an unknown reason. Reverse distribution has been described in patients with cardiac sarcoidosis as indicated by increased uptake in Thallium-201 on stress images.

^{67}Ga scintigraphy is useful for diagnosis of the active inflammatory phases of cardiac sarcoidosis including the initial edema and granulomatous infiltration phases. Presence of areas of increased uptake in ^{67}Ga scintigraphy correlates with a favorable response to corticosteroid treatment.

18F-fluorodeoxyglucose (FDG) accumulates in inflammatory cells and although it is nonspecific, FDG-Positron Emission Tomography (PET) may be a useful modality for detecting inflammatory processes such as sarcoidosis. Okumura et al (Okumura et al., 2004) described that fasting FDG-PET can detect cardiac sarcoidosis in earlier stages in comparison to other radiopharmaceuticals.

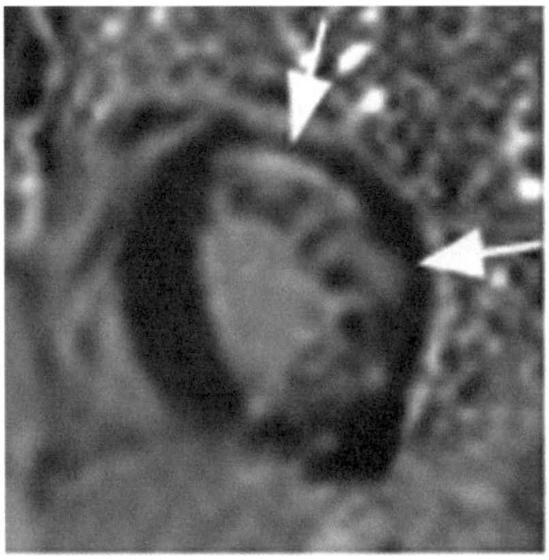

Fig. 13. Short-axis gadolinium-enhanced T1-weighted image shows an area of diffuse enhancement (arrows) in the lateral wall of the left ventricle representing edema in the early stage of cardiac sarcoidosis. (Courtesy of Prof. Olivier Vignaux, University René Descartes, Paris, France)

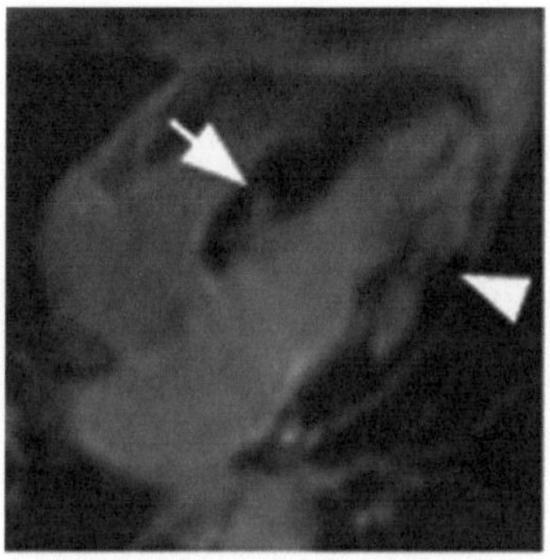

Fig. 14. Four-chamber delayed gadolinium-enhanced T1-weighted image demonstrates an area of nodular enhancement (arrow) in the septum compatible with granulomatous infiltration. Diffuse lateral wall enhancement (arrowhead) is also noted. (Courtesy of Prof. Olivier Vignaux, University René Descartes, Paris, France)

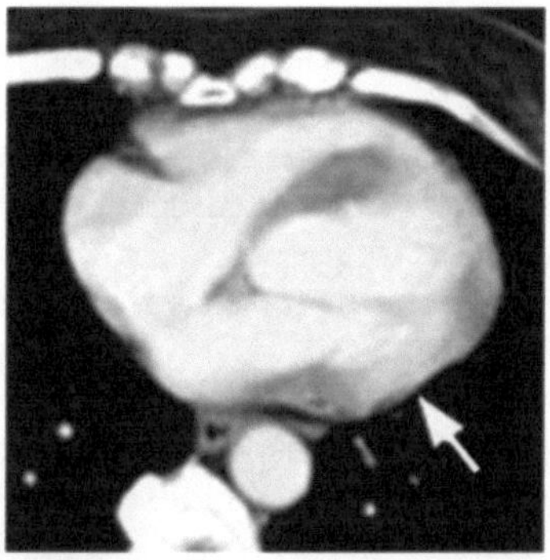

Fig. 15. Axial CT image of the chest in a patient with sarcoidosis shows an area of diffuse enhancement in the lateral wall of the left ventricle, representing presumed cardiac involvement. (Courtesy of Dr. Takashi Koyama, Kyoto University of Medicine, Kyoto, Japan)

3.2 Magnetic resonance imaging

Magnetic resonance imaging is a sensitive method for diagnosis of cardiac sarcoidosis. Initial edema will present as regions of increased signal intensity on T2-weighted sequences and early contrast enhancement within the myocardium (Figure 13). Granulomatous infiltration can be visualized as nodular areas of signal intensity on T2-weighted images with delayed contrast enhancement (Figure 14). Eventually focal areas of wall thinning and hypokinesis may appear representing a progression into the third phase, scarring. These lesions correspond to foci of delayed enhancement in the subepicardial layer. Segmental contraction abnormalities can be seen, however severe disease can lead to diffuse contraction abnormalities and wall thickening.

Ichinose et al performed delayed contrast-enhanced cardiac MRI in 40 patients with sarcoidosis, 11 having cardiac involvement (Ichinose et al., 2008). Myocardial enhancement was present in 91% of patients with cardiac sarcoidosis (10 of the 11), whereas none of the 29 patients without cardiac sarcoidosis showed enhancement. They concluded that myocardial lesions can be predominantly localized in the basal and subepicardial myocardium.

Clinically, cardiac sarcoidosis is found in five percent of patients, however it is present in approximately 20-30% of autopsy studies indicating that often it can be asymptomatic. In those patients that display clinical symptoms, cardiac sarcoidosis can be life-threatening and detection by MRI becomes increasingly important. MRI with gadolinium is the forefront modality in following cardiac sarcoidosis (Vignaux, 2005). CT is not a commonly used modality for evaluation of cardiac sarcoidosis. Nevertheless, in a few case reports, CT reveals a similar pattern of myocardial enhancement as in MRI (Figure 15).

4. Abdominal sarcoidosis

Abdominal visceral involvement is frequently reported in autopsy series of patients with sarcoidosis (Iwai et al., 1988). Nonetheless, most of these patients are asymptomatic and organ dysfunction is uncommon. Abdominal lymphadenopathy as well as genitourinary, pancreatic, and gastrointestinal sarcoidosis have been documented with the liver and spleen being the most frequently affected abdominal organs.

4.1 Liver and spleen

Hepatomegaly is the most common imaging finding of hepatic sarcoidosis. Liver dysfunction is occasionally seen; however end stage liver disease manifesting as cirrhosis or portal hypertension is rarely reported. On ultrasonography, hepatic sarcoidosis could represent as diffuse or patchy areas of increased echogenicity although the enlarged liver might remain homogenous. Another frequently seen pattern of involvement presents as multiple low-density lesions throughout the liver. These lesions can range from 1-2 millimeters to several centimeters. Sarcoidosis nodules could present as hypoechoic or hyperechoic lesions on sonographic examination. These nodules remain unenhanced on contrast-enhanced CT (Figure 16) and present as low signal intensity nodules with no evidence of enhancement on MRI. Rarely, cirrhosis can be seen with involvement of intrahepatic biliary ducts. When involvement includes the extrahepatic ducts, granulomatous infiltration can lead to obstructive jaundice.

Splenomegaly is a common finding of sarcoidosis, reported in up to 33% of patients (Warshauer & Lee, 2004). Hypodense nodular disease is frequently seen while calcified lesions have also been reported (Figure 17). Nodular splenic disease has similar imaging characteristic as hepatic nodular disease (Figure 18).

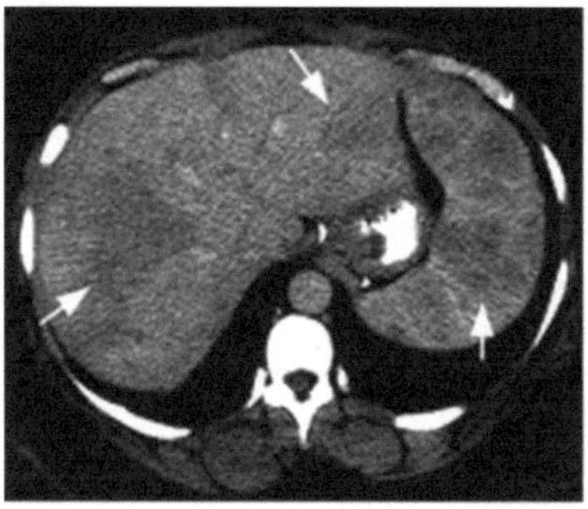

Fig. 16. A 41-year-old female with upper abdominal pain. Axial contrast-enhanced CT image of the abdomen at the level of the T11 vertebra reveals low attenuating geographic lesions (arrows) in the liver and spleen. Splenomegaly is also present. Biopsy confirmed non-caseating granulomas.

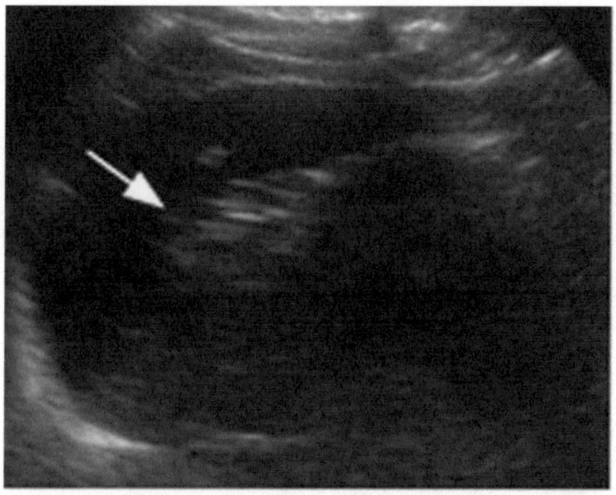

Fig. 17. A 47-year-old female with systemic sarcoidosis. Ultrasonography image of the spleen shows a hyperechoic lesion withon the parenchyma compatible with a calcified splenic granuloma.

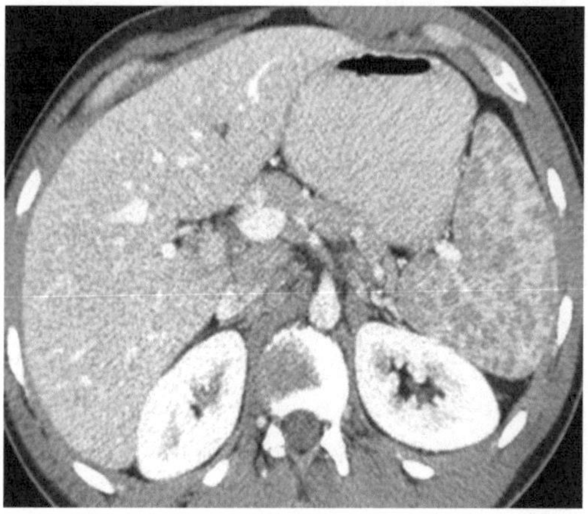

Fig. 18. A 30-year-old male with systemic sarcoidosis. Axial contrast-enhanced CT image shows multiple small low attenuating nodules throughout the spleen.

4.2 Lymph nodes

Lymphadenopathy is another common finding of abdominal sarcoidosis. Constitutional symptoms such as fever, fatigue and weight loss have been reported. In comparison with lymphoma, one study showed smaller nodes and less conglomerate mass formation in abdominal lymphadenopathy of sarcoidosis (Britt et al., 1991). Enlarged lymph nodes can compress on adjacent organs causing obstruction of hollow organs such as the biliary ducts or ureters leading to obstructive jaundice or hydronephrosis. These nodes appear hypoechoic on ultrasonography (Figure 19a), of soft tissue density on CT (Figure 19b), and mildly enhancing with increased T2 signal intensity on MRI.

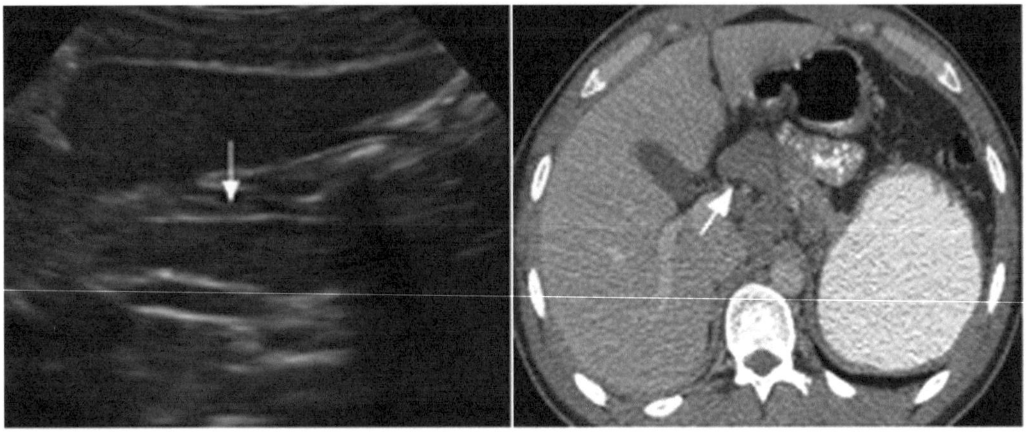

(a) (b)

Fig. 19. Abdominal lymphadenopathy. (a) A 34-year-old male with jaundice and systemic sarcoidosis. An ultrasonography image of the midline upper abdomen shows an enlarged lymph node (arrow) near the porta hepatis. (b) Axial contrast-enhanced CT image of the upper abdomen confirms intrabdominal lymphadenopathy (arrow).

4.3 Pancreas

Pancreatitis due to granulomatous infiltration of the pancreatic duct secondary to sarcoidosis is an uncommon manifestation of sarcoidosis. Additionally, focal pancreatic masses have been reported. These masses appear hypoechoic on ultrasonography and hypodense on CT. These lesions typically do not enhance or enhance minimally on CT.

4.4 Gastrointestinal tract

Sarcoidosis can involve any part of the gastrointestinal tract. In the stomach focal nodular involvement with wall thickening is a classic finding. Gastric wall ulceration is another manifestation of sarcoidosis. Duodenal, colonic and appendiceal involvement have also been reported. Focal wall thickening is the most common imaging presentation.

4.5 Genitourinary tract

Hypercalcemia and hypercalciuria in the setting of sarcoidosis can lead to nephrocalcinosis, nephrolithiasis, and interstitial calcium deposition, which can be visualized on CT and ultrasonography. On CT, multiple isodense lesions with relative hypo-enhancement compared to normal renal parenchyma has been reported. Testicular involvement is rare, appearing as hypodense lesions on CT and hypoechoic areas on ultrasonography (Figure 20).

Organomegaly and nodular disease are the common manifestations of abdominal sarcoidosis. However, these findings are generally nonspecific and could be present in other settings such as neoplasms and infectious diseases. A combination of imaging findings and clinical signs and symptoms will help with further delineation of the disease process and possible need for tissue biopsy.

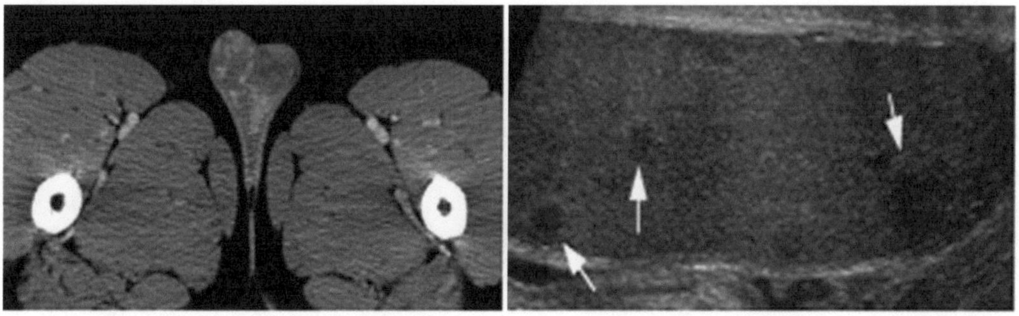

(a) (b)

Fig. 20. A 30-year-old male with sarcoidosis. (a) Axial contrast-enhanced CT image incidentally shows hypodense lesions within the testes. (b) Subsequent sagittal ultrasonography image of the testes show multiple small round hypoechoic lesions (arrow).

5. Neurosarcoidosis

Symptomatic involvement of the nervous system is reported in 5% of patients with sarcoidosis. However, asymptomatic neurosarcoidosis has been reported in up to 25% of cases in postmortem studies (Johns & Michele, 1999). Isolated neurosarcoidosis is rarely seen. Although sarcoidosis can involve the entire nervous system and its supportive tissues, Central Nervous System (CNS) involvement is far more common. Clinical symptoms of neurosarcoidosis are nonspecific; the involved region of the CNS determines the presenting symptoms. Vision loss, facial nerve involvement, headache, neck stiffness and seizure have all been described as correlated symptoms. Imaging characteristics of neurosarcoidosis are nonspecific so a lesion biopsy is occasionally performed to reach a definite diagnosis.

5.1 Leptomeningeal involvement

Enhancing thickened leptomeninges on contrast-enhanced T1-weighted sequences are the most common imaging finding of CNS involvement with sarcoidosis; it has been reported in 40% of patients with neural involvement (Nowak & Widenka, 2001). Nodular and diffuse patterns have been described with the basilar meninges being most commonly involved (Figure 21). Some authors have hypothesized that parenchymal involvement is an extension of leptomeningeal disease via the perivascular spaces (Junger et al., 1993). In the spinal cord linear and nodular enhancing extramedullary lesions are also common. Hydrocephalus secondary to adhesions or abnormal CSF resorption can be seen in patients with leptomeningeal sarcoidosis.

5.2 Parenchymal disease

Multiple high signal intensity lesions on T2-weighted sequences are the most common finding in patients with parenchymal involvement. In the brain, these lesions are mainly located in the periventricular white matter. Although non-enhancing lesions are typical, contrast enhancement can also be seen (Figure 22). Occasionally, low signal intensity masses on T2-weighted sequences have been reported.

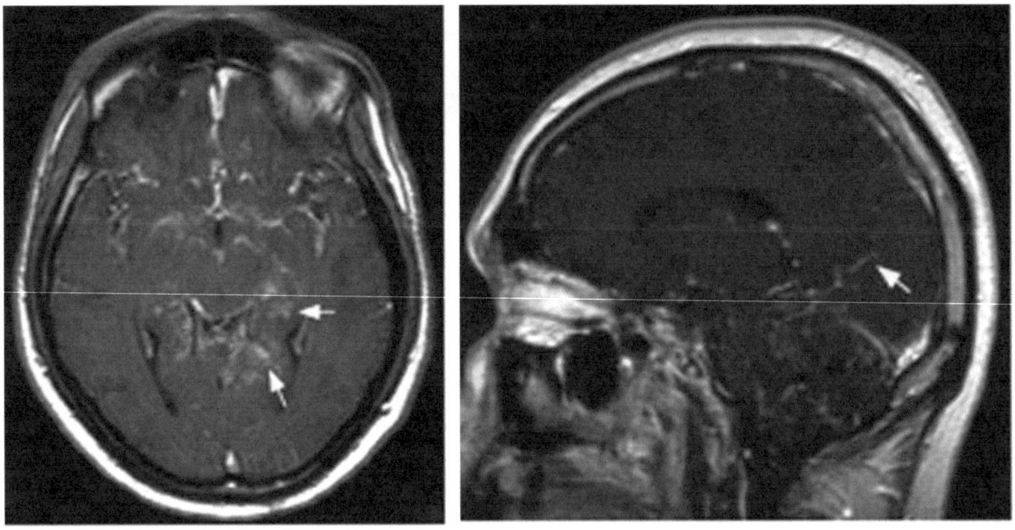

(a) (b)

Fig. 21. Leptomeningeal sarcoidosis. (a) A gadolinium-enhanced axial T1-weighted image in a 27-year-old male and (b) a gadolinium-enhanced sagittal T1-weighted image in a 38-year-old male with systemic sarcoidosis show curvilinear areas of abnormal enhancement along the sulci and basal cisterns, representing leptomeningeal sarcoidosis.

In the spinal cord, intramedullary sarcoidosis presents as fusiform high T2-signal intensity segmental lesions with decreased signal intensity on T1-weighted sequences. Patchy enhancement on contrast-enhanced T1-weighted sequences is common (Figure 23). One study evaluated clinical, laboratory, and MRI profiles in 31 patients with spinal cord sarcoidosis (Cohen-Aubart et al., 2010). Spinal cord MRIs performed in 26 patients with spinal cord involvement revealed intramedullary T2-hyperintensities that were extensive and heterogeneous with a central distribution in axial slides. They concluded that a spinal cord MRI study may be a useful tool in the diagnosis of spinal cord sarcoidosis.

Cranial nerve involvement is another feature of parenchymal sarcoidosis with contrast enhancing nerve enlargement being typical. Optic nerve involvement is frequently seen and can be bilateral or unilateral (Figure 24). In MRI scans of 15 patients with orbital or optic pathway involvement, eight patients had MR evidence of optic nerve involvement by sarcoid granuloma (Carmody et al., 1994). Optic chiasmal involvement, periventricular white matter abnormalities, perineural enhancement, and optic nerve enlargement were commonly identified. Less frequently, optic nerve atrophy, increased T2 signal intensity in the optic radiations, and orbital masses with MR signal characteristics similar to a pseudotumor were reported.

Additionally, other orbital structures such as orbital fat, muscles, globe and lacrimal glands can be involved (Figure 25). Mass-like lacrimal and muscle infiltration, pseudotumor-like intraorbital masses and rarely uveal and scleral nodularity have been reported. Facial nerve paralysis can be seen with facial nerve (VII) involvement. Nevertheless, there is no correlation between imaging findings and clinical presentation.

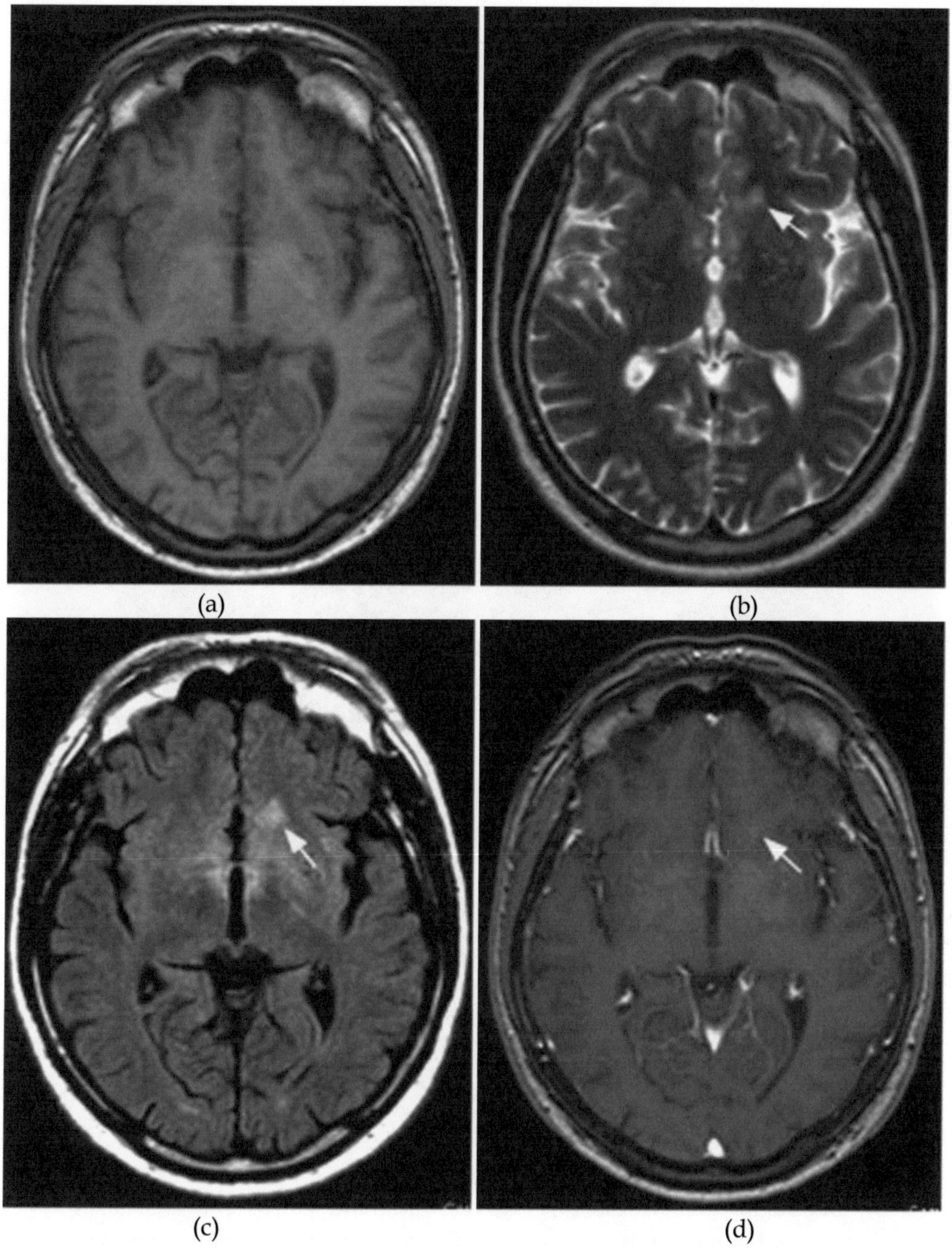

Fig. 22. A 40-year-old male with memory loss, confusion, disorientation and multisystemic sarcoidosis. (a) Axial T1-weighted MR image at the level of the basal ganglia is unremarkable. (b) Axial T2 and (c) axial FLAIR images show areas of increased signal intensity within the white matter of the medial frontal lobes, left being greater than right. (d) Axial gadolinium-enhanced image shows minimal enhancement in the medial frontal lobes.

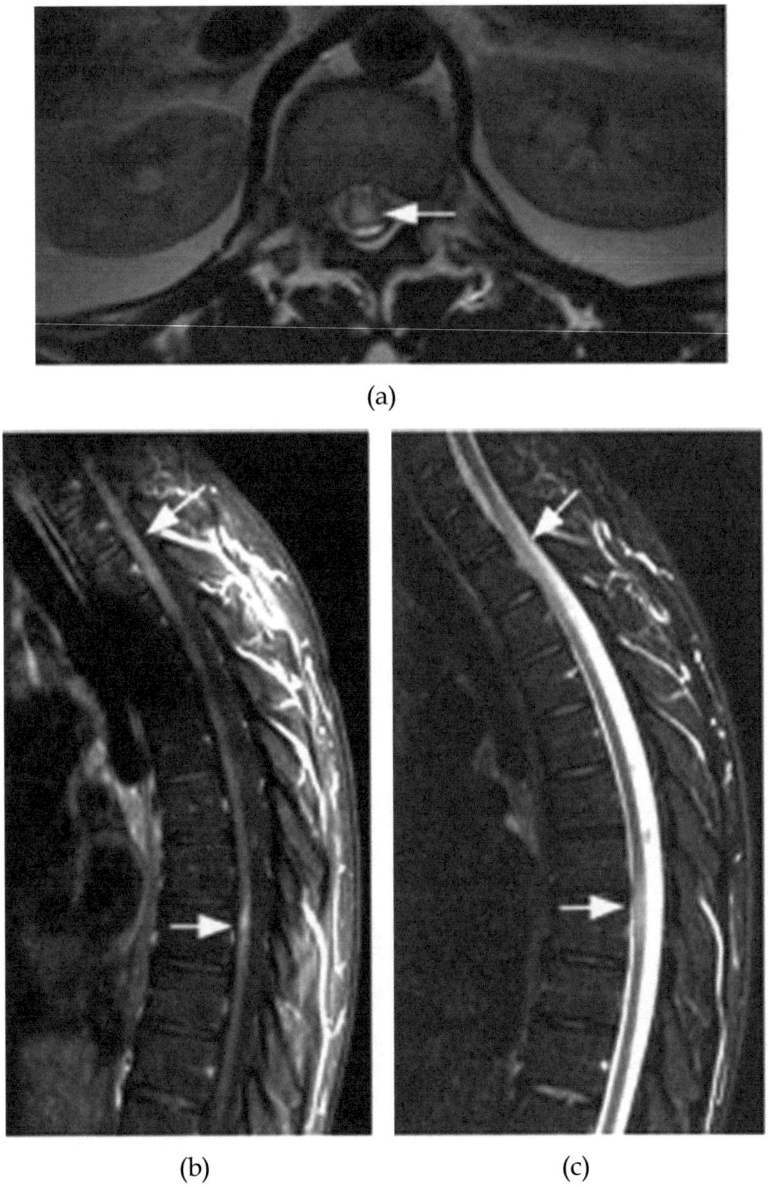

Fig. 23. Intramedullary sarcoidosis. (a) A 27-year-old male with sarcoidosis. Axial T2-weighted image at the level of the conus medullaris shows an area of increased signal intensity within the conus (arrow) representing intramedullary involvement. (b) A 27-year-old male with systemic sarcoidosis presented with paraplegia. A T2-weighted sagittal image shows patchy increased signal intensity within the spinal cord at the C7-T2 level as well as T6-T7 level (arrows) and (c) a sagittal gadolinium-enhanced T1-weighted image shows abnormal enhancement of these lesions (arrows), representing intramedullary involvement.

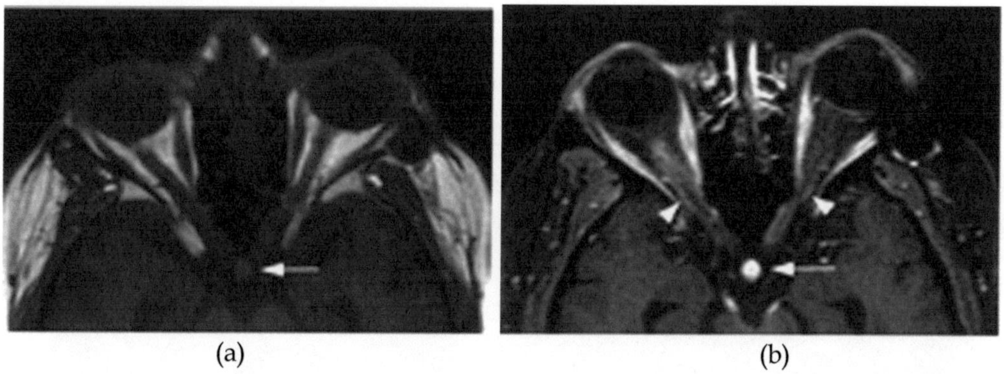

Fig. 24. A 39-year-old male with vision loss and systemic sarcoidosis. (a) T1-weighted image shows thickened pituitary infundibulum (arrow). (b) Gadolinium-enhanced T1-weighted image shows enhancement of the optic nerves (arrowheads) and pituitary infundibulum (arrow).

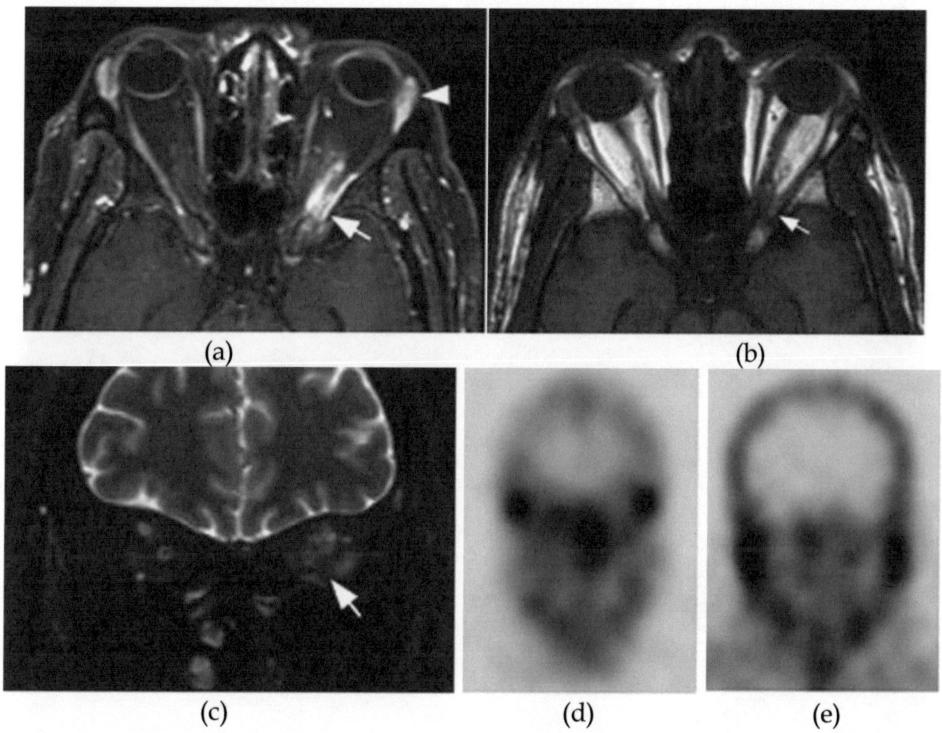

Fig. 25. A 44-year-old male with pulmonary sarcoidosis, left eye pain and sixth nerve palsy. (a) Axial T1-weighted image shows a low signal intensity lesion in the left orbital apex (arrow). (b) Gadolinium-enhanced fat suppressed T1-weighted image shows enhancement of the previously seen lesion (arrow). Slight enlargement of the left lacrimal gland is noted (arrowhead). (c) Coronal fat suppressed T2-weighted image shows diffuse increased signal intensity with in the left intraconal fat, representing an inflammatory process (arrow). (d) and (e) ^{67}Gallium SPECT images show increased radiopharmaceutical activity in the lacrimal and parotid glands respectively.

5.3 Dural Involvement

Diffuse thickening of the dura and focal nodular dural masses are common manifestations of dural sarcoidosis. Dural involvement with sarcoidosis is much more commonly found in the brain rather than in the spine. In the brain, these lesions appear dark on T2-weighted sequences and enhance diffusely on contrast-enhanced T1-weighted sequences (Figure 26). Unlike in leptomeningeal disease, involvement of the basal cisterns and perivascular spaces are not seen. When seen in the spine, dural-based high signal intensity masses on T2-weighted sequences are characteristic (Figure 27).

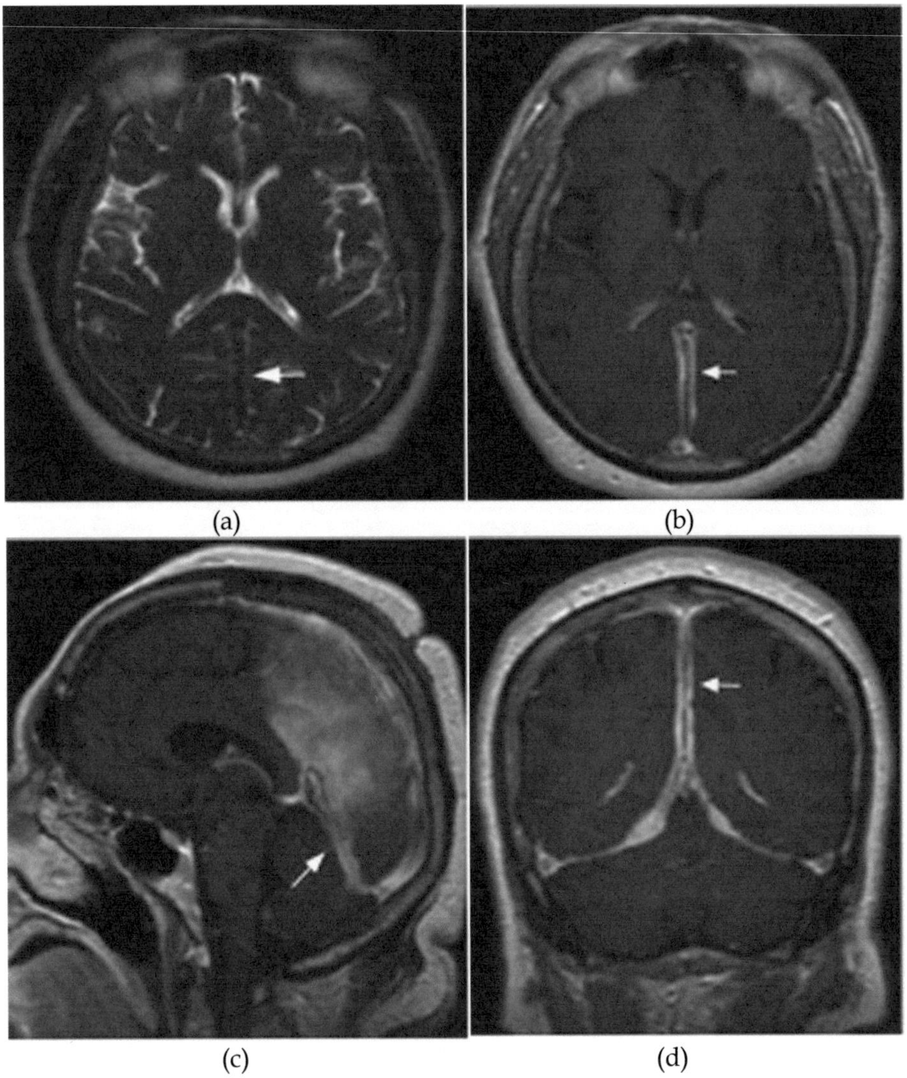

Fig. 26. A 66-year-old male with worsening headaches and sarcoidosis. (a) A T2-weighted image shows diffuse low signal intensity in the dura. (b), (c), and (d) Axial, sagittal and coronal gadolinium-enhanced images demonstrate diffuse and nodular enhancement of the dura respectively (arrows).

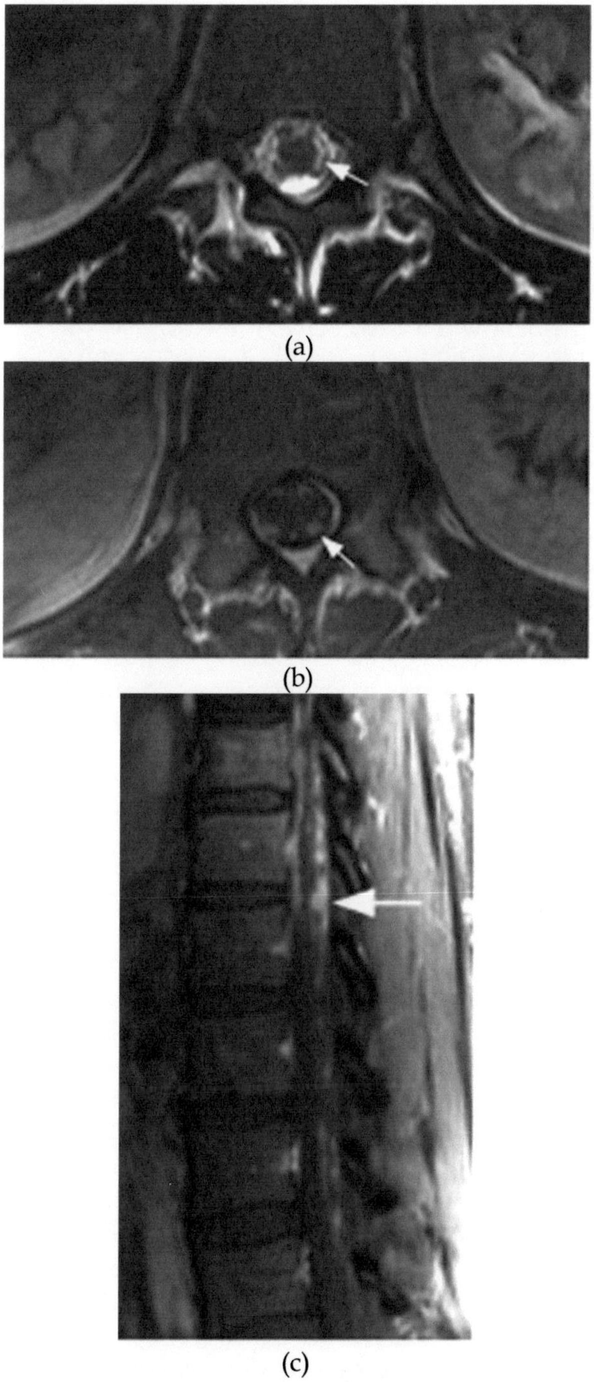

Fig. 27. A 27-year-old male with confusion and thoracic sarcoidosis. (a) T2-weighted image shows irregular areas of increased signal intensity (arrow) at the surface of the cauda equina. (b) Axial and (c) sagittal gadolinium enhanced T1-weighted images show nodular enhancement (arrows) compatible with dural involvement.

Refractory and recurrent CNS sarcoidosis is common (Christoforidis et al., 1999). Imaging characteristics of neurosarcoidosis are nonspecific and correlation between a response to treatment and resolution of imaging findings is not well established. Nonetheless, imaging can be useful for follow-up in patients with known CNS sarcoidosis. Lexa et al evaluated the role of MRI in the diagnosis and treatment of 24 patients with neurosarcoidosis. White matter and periventricular high signal intensity on T2-weighted sequences, leptomeningeal enhancement, parenchymal mass, lacrimal gland mass, hydrocephalus, ventriculomegaly, periventricular enhancement, extraaxial mass, optic chiasmal enhancement, nerve root enhancement, enlarged pituitary infundibulum, and pontine infarct were identified. They concluded that enhancement was a useful clue to the diagnosis in 15 of 17 cases in which gadolinium was used (88%). Additionally, it was shown that MRI is useful in the evaluation of treatment response in patients with neurosarcoidosis particularly in the leptomeningeal and parenchymal lesions (Lexa & Grossman, 1994).

Symptomatic neurosarcoidosis may be present in 3%-5% of patients with sarcoidosis. Although imaging findings are nonspecific, recognition of common patterns may be helpful in the planning for further diagnostic tests and disease surveillance. MRI with gadolinium is the study of choice for initial diagnosis as well as follow-up evaluation of neurosarcoidosis.

6. Musculoskeletal sarcoidosis

Although sarcoidosis can involve any organ, symptomatic musculoskeletal involvement is uncommon. More specifically, muscular, articular and osseous sarcoidosis can be seen. Imaging findings are nonspecific in most cases.

6.1 Muscular involvement

Symptomatic myopathy is an extremely rare manifestation of sarcoidosis, which is seen in less than 0.5% of patients (Douglas et al., 1973). However, asymptomatic granulomatous disease is seen commonly in up to 80% of patients (Baydur et al., 1993). Chronic myopathy, palpable lesions and acute myositis are different presentations of symptomatic muscular involvement with sarcoidosis. Typically, sarcoid myopathy has a symmetrical pattern with bilateral involvement of the proximal muscles of the extremities. Nevertheless, any muscular structure including the respiratory muscles can be involved.

Oval nodules with a central area of low signal intensity surrounded by an area of increased signal intensity in T2-weighted images are characteristic for nodular sarcoidosis. Evaluation of sonographic and MRI findings in three cases of the nodular type of muscular sarcoidosis revealed intramuscular hypoechoic well-defined nodules in all three patients (Tohme-Noun et al., 2004). On MRI, the nodules were iso- or hyperintense on T1-weighted sequences. On T2-weighted images and STIR sequences, intramuscular nodules of homogeneous high signal intensity were observed. Homogeneous enhancement in all nodules on gadolinium-enhanced T1-weighted sequences was characteristic.

In chronic myopathy, MRI and CT occasionally show muscle atrophy. With acute myositis, on MR imaging diffuse increased T2 signal intensity of involved muscles may be noted. CT may show thickening of the involved musculature (Figure 28). ^{67}Ga scintigraphy reveals nonspecific diffuse increased radiopharmaceutical uptake in the involved musculature in both acute myositis and chronic myopathy.

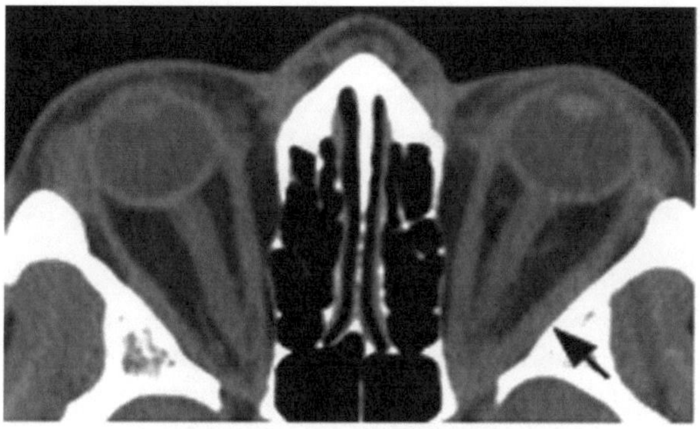

Fig. 28. A 44-year-old male with left eye pain and sarcoidosis. Axial CT image shows mild thickening of the left lateral rectus muscle (arrow) compatible with granulomatous infiltration.

6.2 Joint involvement

Arthralgia with polyarticular involvement of the distal joints of the extremities is a common early finding of sarcoidosis. Additionally, MRI findings such as synovitis, bursitis, tenosynovitis, and tendonitis have been reported in patients with sarcoidosis (Figure 29). Tissue biopsy might be necessary for definite diagnosis as these findings are nonspecific.

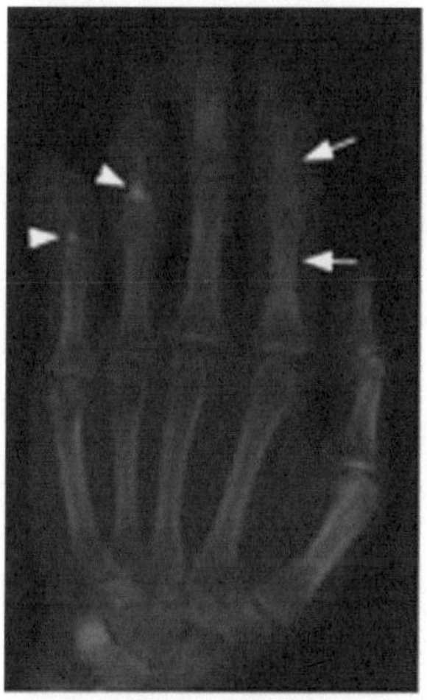

Fig. 29. Posteroanterior radiograph of the right hand shows sausage-like dactylitis of the second to fifth digits in a patient with sarcoidosis, representing synovitis. Multiple classic osteolytic bony lesions (arrows) as well as sclerotic foci at the base of the middle phalanges of the forth and fifth digits (arrowheads) are also noted. (Courtesy of Drs. Shipley, Weinstein and Wissman. University of Cincinnati, Ohio, USA)

6.3 Osseous involvement

Osseous sarcoidosis has been reported in about 5% of patients (Johns & Michele, 1999). Plain radiographs are the first imaging modality for diagnosis of osseous sarcoidosis. Osteolysis with a lacy trabecular pattern is the characteristic findings on radiographs (Figure 30).

Typically, small bones of the hand and foot are involved although the vertebral body (Figure 31), skull, and long bones may also be affected rarely. Cyst formation with a "punched out" pattern appearing as well-circumscribed lytic lesions with nonsclerotic margins is also common. Pathologic fractures secondary to extensive bony erosion have been reported (Figure 32). Periosteal reaction is usually not present. Furthermore, osseous sarcoidosis can also present as osteosclerosis, as evidenced by nodular opacities in the medullary cavity on plain radiographs (Figure 29).

^{99m}Tc-pyrophosphate scintigraphy is more sensitive in detecting osseous sarcoidosis in comparison to plain radiographs. Areas of increased radiopharmaceutical activity correspond to active granulomatous infiltration. Nuclear imaging findings are nonspecific for sarcoidosis; however ^{99m}Tc bone scintigraphy can be used effectively for monitoring disease activity.

MRI is the most sensitive imaging modality for detecting osseous sarcoidosis. Typically, sarcoid bony lesions appear hypointense on T1-weighted sequences and hyperintense on T2-weighted, inversion-recovery, and fat-saturated proton-density-weighted MR sequences. Occasionally, the lesions can have low signal intensity.

Occult lesions, soft tissue involvement and cortical disruption may also be identified with MR imaging in osseous sarcoidosis. In the long bones, sarcoidosis can be seen as well-defined discrete masses, infiltrative marrow lesions and ill-defined mass-like lesions, which may enhance after administration of contrast. These lesions can be replaced with fat or fibrotic tissues, indicating the chronicity of the disease.

In vertebral bodies lytic lesions with sclerotic margins are typical which may extend into the pedicles. Sclerotic or mixed lytic and sclerotic involvement as well as disc involvement is all relatively rare. In the skull, sarcoid lesions are usually well-defined expansile lytic areas with a "punched out" pattern, which can be visualized on CT. Skull lesions are seldom seen alone and are customarily associated with other bony lesions when osseous involvement of sarcoidosis is present (Yaghmai, 1983).

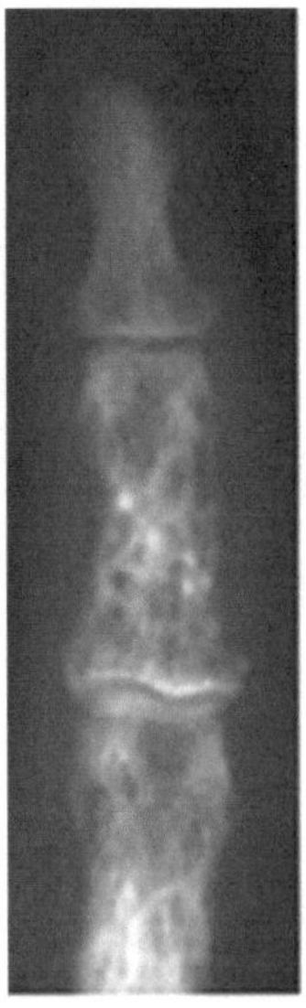

Fig. 30. Coned-down posteroanterior radiograph of the right hand in a patient with sarcoidosis shows osteolytic lesions with a lacy pattern within the middle phalanx of the second digit. (Courtesy of Drs. Shipley, Weinstein and Wissman, University of Cincinnati, Cincinnati, Ohio, USA)

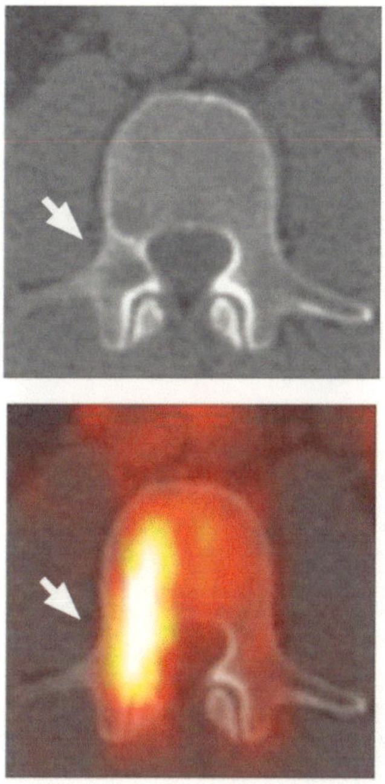

Fig. 31. A 50-year-old male with sarcoiodosis. PET/CT images show a lytic lesion with increased FDG activity within the posterior aspect of the L3 vertebral body. (Rajebi et al. Uncommon osseous involvement in multisystemic sarcoidosis. *Ann Saudi Med.* 2009;29:485-6)

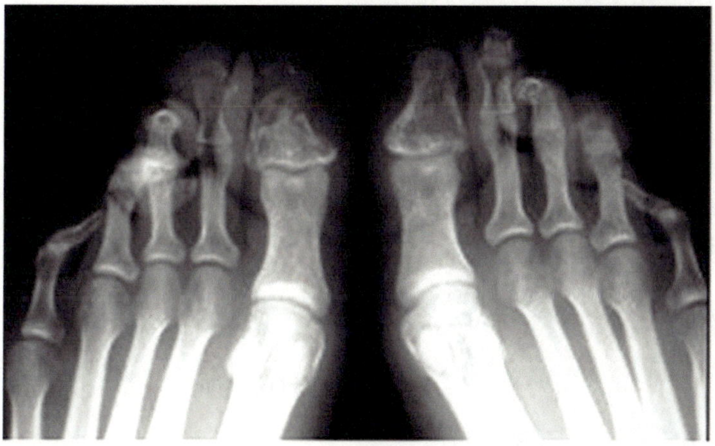

Fig. 32. Coned-down posteroanterior radiograph of the feet in a patient with sarcoidosis shows a large osteolytic lesion in the distal phalanx of the right first digit causing a pathological fracture. (Courtesy of Dr. Hojnowski, SUNY Upstate Medical University, Syracuse, New York, USA)

Compared to conventional radiography and nuclear scintigraphy, MRI with gadolinium is more sensitive in detection of lesions in patients with musculoskeletal sarcoidosis. Nonetheless, in most cases these findings are nonspecific and correlation with clinical and laboratory findings is essential.

7. FDG-PET and PET/CT

FDG-PET and PET/CT identify areas of abnormally increased glucose transport and metabolism. This capability makes FDG-PET imaging a suitable modality in conditions with increased glucose metabolism such as cancer and inflammatory disease. However, pattern and intensity of FDG uptake are nonspecific in multisystemic disorders such as sarcoidosis and can be mistaken with lymphoma and diffuse metastatic diseases (Figure 31 and 33) (Rajebi et al., 2009). Despite this, FDG uptake value can decrease after treatment of sarcoidosis and FDG-PET and PET/CT can be useful for monitoring the disease and efficacy of the treatment (Brundin et al., 1994).

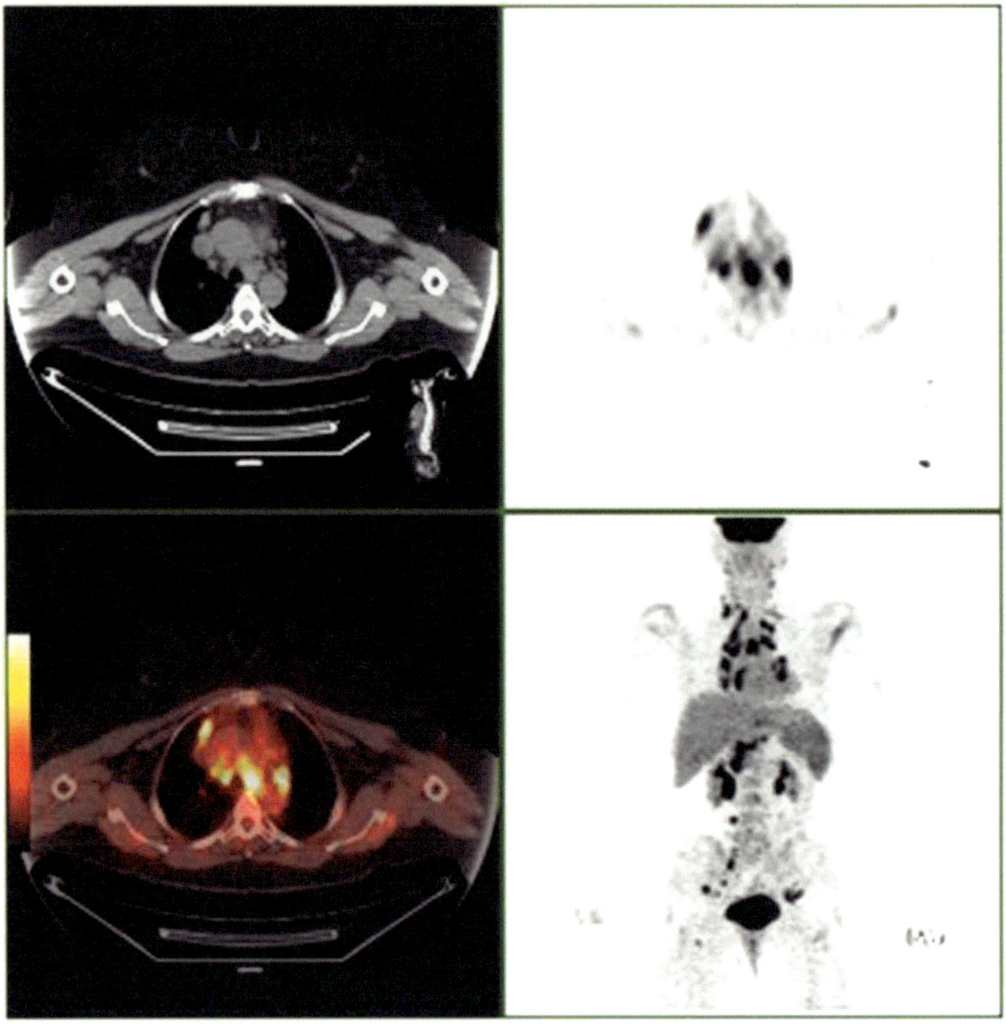

Fig. 33. A 37-year-old female with mediastinal lymphadenopathy on chest radiograph (not shown). An FDG-PET/CT shows extensive FDG-avid hilar, mediastinal, intrabdominal and inguinal lymphadenopathy. Biopsy confirmed the diagnosis of sarcoidosis. (Courtesy of Dr. McGrath, SUNY Upstate Medical University, Syracuse, New York, USA)

It has been shown that persistent retention of FDG correlates with refractory disease. Umeda et al evaluated the prognostic value of dual time point FDG-PET in patients with pulmonary sarcoidosis. In this study, twenty-one patients with pulmonary sarcoidosis underwent an early FDG-PET at 60 minutes and a delayed FDG-PET scan at 180 minutes after the injection of FDG. Standardized uptake values (SUVs) at the two time points and the retention index (RI-SUV) calculated from these were assessed. To evaluate disease progression, all patients underwent chest CT one year after the initial FDG-PET. RI-SUV was significantly higher in patients with increased or unchanged pulmonary lesions at follow-up CT than in patients with improved pulmonary lesions indicating that RI-SUV can be a good indicator of disease progression (Umeda et al 2011).

With FDG-PET/CT, it is postulated that the addition of typical CT findings in patients with multisystemic disease such as hilar and paratracheal lymphadenopathy and parenchymal involvement in pulmonary sarcoidosis, can increase usefulness of this modality in evaluation of treatment response in sarcoidosis.

8. Conclusion

Sarcoidosis is a multisystemic disease, which can involve any organ in the body. Similar to presenting signs and symptoms, imaging findings of sarcoidosis are diverse. Conventional radiography is useful in initial evaluation of pulmonary and musculoskeletal sarcoidosis. Ultrasonography is playing an emerging role in the diagnosis of pulmonary involvement. The modality of choice for evaluation of the parenchymal lung disease is CT. MRI findings in cardiac sarcoidosis are relatively specific and advantageous in diagnosis. Furthermore, MRI is an extremely invaluable tool for initial diagnosis and treatment response in neurosarcoidosis. Extent of musculoskeletal sarcoidosis is also best evaluated with MRI. Although the imaging findings in abdominal sarcoidosis are nonspecific, CT and ultrasonography are helpful in evaluation of organ involvement and lymphadenopathy. FDG-PET/CT may be useful in evaluating disease progress and treatment efficacy.

Clinicians and radiologists should be familiar with typical as well as atypical imaging findings of sarcoidosis. This may decrease the unnecessary workup and prevent needless patient discomfort.

9. References

Abehsera M, Valeyre D, Grenier P, Jaillet H, Battesti JP, & Brauner MW. (2000). Sarcoidosis with pulmonary fibrosis: CT patterns and correlation with pulmonary function. *AJR Am J Roentgenol*, Vol. 174, No. 6, (June 2000), pp. 1751-7, ISSN 0361-803X

Baydur A, Pandya K, Sharma OP, Kanel GC, & Carlson M. (1993). Control of ventilation, respiratory muscle strength, and granulomatous involvement of skeletal muscle in patients with sarcoidosis. *Chest*, Vol. 103, No. 2, (February 1993), pp. 396-402, ISSN 0012-3692

Boeck, C. (1899). Multiple benign sarkoid of the skin. *J. Cutan. Genitourinary Dis*, Vol. 17, pp. 543–550

Britt AR, Francis IR, Glazer GM, & Ellis JH.(1991). Sarcoidosis: abdominal manifestations at CT. *Radiology,* Vol.178, No. 1, (January 1991), pp. 91–94, ISSN 0033-8419

Brudin LH, Valind SO, Rhodes CG, Pantin CF, Sweatman M, Jones T, & Hughes JM. (1994). Fluorine-18 deoxyglucose uptake in sarcoidosis measured with positron emission tomography. *Eur J Nucl Med,* Vol. 21, No. 4, (April 1994), pp. 297-305, ISSN 0340-6997

Carmody RF, Mafee MF, Goodwin JA, Small K, & Haery C. (1994). Orbital and optic pathway sarcoidosis: MR findings. *AJNR Am J Neuroradiol,* Vol. 15, No. 4, (April 1994), pp. 775-83, ISSN 0195-6108

Christoforidis GA, Spickler EM, Reccio MV, & Mehta BM. (1999). MR of CNS sarcoidosis: correlation of imaging features to clinical symptoms and response to treatment. *AJNR Am J Neuroradiol,* Vol. 20, No. 4, (April 1999), pp. 655–669, ISSN 0195-6108

Cohen-Aubart F, Galanaud D, Grabli D, Haroche J, Amoura Z, Chapelon-Abric C, Lyon-Caen O, Valeyre D, & Piette JC.(2010). Spinal cord sarcoidosis: clinical and laboratory profile and outcome of 31 patients in a case-control study. *Medicine (Baltimore),* Vol. 89, No. 2, (March 2010), pp. 133-40, ISSN 0025-7974

Criado E, Sánchez M, Ramírez J, Arguis P, de Caralt TM, Perea RJ, & Xaubet A.(2010). Pulmonary sarcoidosis: typical and atypical manifestations at high-resolution CT with pathologic correlation. *Radiographics,* Vol. 30, No. 6, (October 2010), pp.1567-86, ISSN 1527-1323

Douglas AC, Macleod JG, & Matthews JD. (1973). Symptomatic sarcoidosis of skeletal muscle. *J Neurol Neurosurg Psychiatry,* Vol. 36, No. 6, (December 1973), pp. 1034-40, ISSN 0022-3050

Garwood S, Judson MA, Silvestri G, Hoda R, Fraig M, & Doelken P. (2007). Endobronchial ultrasound for the diagnosis of pulmonary sarcoidosis. *Chest,* Vol. 132, No. 4, (October 2007), pp. 1298-304, ISSN 0012-3692

Handa T, Nagai S, Fushimi Y, et al. (2006). Clinical and radiographic indices associated with airflow limitation in patients with sarcoidosis. *Chest,* Vol. 130, No. 6, (December 2006), pp. 1851–1856, ISSN 0012-3692

Hansell DM, Bankier AA, MacMahon H, McLoud TC, Muller NL, & Remy J. (2008). Fleischner Society: glossary of terms for thoracic imaging. *Radiology,* Vol. 246, No. 3, (March 2008), pp. 697-722, ISSN 1527-1315

Hutchinson, J. (1877). Case of livid papillary psoriasis. *In Illustrations of Clinical Surgery,* Vol. 1, pp. 42–43, J&A Churchill, London, UK

Ichinose A, Otani H, Oikawa M, Takase K, Saito H, Shimokawa H, & Takahashi S. (2008). MRI of cardiac sarcoidosis: basal and subepicardial localization of myocardial lesions and their effect on left ventricular function. *AJR Am J Roentgenol,* Vol. 191, No. 3, (September 2008), pp.862-9, ISSN 1546-3141

Iwai K, Tachibana T, Hosoda Y, & Matsui Y. (1988). Sarcoidosis autopsies in Japan: frequency and trend in the last 28 years. *Sarcoidosis,* Vol. 5, No. 1, (March 1988), pp. 60–65, ISSN 0393-1447

Johns CJ & Michele TM. (1999). The clinical management of sarcoidosis. A 50-year experience at the Johns Hopkins Hospital. *Medicine (Baltimore),* Vol. 78, No. 2, (March 1999), pp. 65-111, ISSN 0025-7974

Junger SS, Stern BJ, Levine SR, Sipos E, & Marti-Masso JF. (1993). Intramedullary spinal sarcoidosis: clinical and magnetic resonance imaging characteristics. *Neurology*, Vol. 43, No. 2, (February 1993), pp. 333–337, ISSN 0028-3878

Kuznitsky, E. & A. Bittorf. (1915). Sarkoid mit Beteiligung innerer Organe. *Munch. Med. Wochenschr*, pp.1349–1353

Lexa FJ & Grossman RI. (1994). MR of sarcoidosis in the head and spine: spectrum of manifestations and radiographic response to steroid therapy. *AJNR Am J Neuroradiol*, Vol. 15, No. 5, (May 1994), pp. 973-82, ISSN 0195-6108

Lynch JP 3rd, Kazerooni EA, & Gay SE. (1997). Pulmonary sarcoidosis. *Clin Chest Med*, Vol. 18, No. 4, (December 1997), pp. 755–785, ISSN 0272-5231

Nowak DA & Widenka DC. (2001). Neurosarcoidosis: a review of its intracranial manifestation. *J Neurol*, Vol. 248, No. 5, (May 2001), pp. 363–372, ISSN 0340-5354

Okumura W, Iwasaki T, Toyama T, Iso T, Arai M, Oriuchi N, Endo K, Yokoyama T, Suzuki T, & Kurabayashi M. (2004). Usefulness of fasting 18F-FDG PET in identification of cardiac sarcoidosis. *J Nucl Med*, Vol. 45, No. 12, (December 2004), pp. 1989-98, ISSN 0161-5505

Perry A & Vuitch F. (1995). Causes of death in patients with sarcoidosis: a morphologic study of 38 autopsies with clinicopathologic correlations. *Arch Pathol Lab Med*, Vol. 119, No. 2, (February 1995), pp. 167–172, ISSN 0003-9985

Rajebi MR, Shahrokni A, & Chaisson M. (2009). Uncommon osseous involvement in multisystemic sarcoidosis. *Ann Saudi Med*, Vol 29, No. 6, (Nov-Dec 2009), pp. 485-6, ISSN 0975-4466

Siltzbach LE. (1967). Sarcoidosis: clinical features and management. *Med Clin North Am*, Vol. 51, No. 2, (March 1967), pp. 483–502, ISSN 0025-7125

Soskel NT & Sharma OP. (2000). Pleural involvement in sarcoidosis. *Curr Opin Pulm Med*, Vol. 6, No. 5, (September 2000), pp. 455-468, ISSN 1070-5287

Sulavik SB, Spencer RP, Weed DA, Shapiro HR, Shiue ST, & Castriotta RJ.(1990). Recognition of distinctive patterns of gallium-67 distribution in sarcoidosis. *J Nucl Med*, Vol. 31, No. 12 (December 1990), pp. 1909-14, ISSN 0161-5505

Tohme-Noun C, Le Breton C, Sobotka A, Boumenir ZE, Milleron B, Carette MF, & Khalil A. (2004). Imaging findings in three cases of the nodular type of muscular sarcoidosis. *AJR Am J Roentgenol*, Vol. 183, No. 4, (October 2004) pp. 995-9, ISSN 0361 803X

Terasaki H, Fujimoto K, Müller NL, Sadohara J, Uchida M, Koga T, Aizawa H, & Hayabuchi N. (2005). Pulmonary sarcoidosis: comparison of findings of inspiratory and expiratory high-resolution CT and pulmonary function tests between smokers and nonsmokers. *AJR Am J Roentgenol*, Vol. 185, No. 2, (August 2005), pp. 333-8, ISSN 0361-803X

Umeda Y, Demura Y, Morikawa M, Ameshima S, Tsuchida T, Fujibayashi Y, Okazawa H, Ishizaki T. (2011) Prognostic value of dual time point (18) F-fluorodeoxyglucose positron emission tomography in patients with pulmonary sarcoidosis. *Respirology*, "Accepted Article"; doi: 10.1111/j.1440-1843.2011.01966.x

Warshauer DM & Lee JK. (2004). Imaging manifestation of abdominal sarcoidosis. *AJR Am J Roentgenol*, Vol. 182, No. 1, (January 2004), pp. 15-28, ISSN 0361-803X

Wurm, K., H. Reindell, & L. Heilmeyer. (1958). *Der Lungenboeck im Röntgenbild*. Thieme, Stuttgart, Germany.

Vignaux O. (2005). Cardiac sarcoidosis: spectrum of MRI features. *AJR Am J Roentgenol*, Vol. 184, No. 1, (January 2005), pp. 249-54, ISSN 0361-803X

Yaghmai I.(1983). Radiographic, angiographic and radionuclide manifestations of osseous sarcoidosis. *Radiographic,* Vol. 3, No. 3, (September 1983), pp. 375-396, ISSN 1527-1323

6

Bronchoalveolar Lavage and Sampling in Pulmonary Sarcoidosis

Edvardas Danila
Clinic of Chest Diseases, Allergology and Radiology of Vilnius University, Centre of Pulmonology and Allergology of Vilnius University Hospital Santariškių klinikos, Lithuania

1. Introduction

Sarcoidosis is a multisystem disorder of unknown cause. It commonly affects young and middle-aged adults and frequently it presents with bilateral hilar lymphadenopathy, pulmonary infiltration, ocular and skin lesions. Other organs may also be involved. The diagnosis is established when clinicoradiological findings are supported by histological evidence of noncaseating epitheloid cell granulomas. Granulomas of known causes and local sarcoid reactions must be excluded. Frequently observed immunological features are depression of cutaneous delayed-type hypersensitivity and increased CD4/CD8 ratio at the site of involvement. Circulating immune complexes along with signs of B-cell hyperactivity may also be detectable. The course and prognosis may correlate with the mode of the onset and the extent of the disease. An acute onset with erythema nodosum or asymptomatic bilateral hilar lymphadenopathy usually heralds a self-limiting course, whereas an insidious onset, especially with multiple extrapulmonary lesions, may be followed by relentless, progressive fibrosis of the lungs or other organs. Corticosteroids relieve symptoms, suppress inflammation and granuloma formation (Grutters et al., 2009). Sarcoidosis is the most frequently observed interstitial lung disease of unknown origin in Europe (Müller-Quernheim, 1998). In young adults, pulmonary sarcoidosis is the second most common respiratory disease after asthma (Rothkrantz-Kos, 2003).

The reported prevalence and presenting symptoms of sarcoidosis vary significantly by sex, racial group, and country. The true prevalence of the disease is difficult to assess because a lot of patients are asymptomatic. Estimation of radiographic population screening programmes indicates a global prevalence of 10-40 per 100 000 and an incidence of 10 per 100 000. The incidence appears to be higher in Northern European countries, Japan and African - Americans (Dements, 2001).

Sarcoidosis is a granulomatous disorder resulting from an uncontrolled cell-mediated immune reaction. Following recognition of unknown antigens, the accumulation of immunocompetent cells in the lungs, i.e. alveolitis, occurs. Although lung parenchyma normally contains only a few lymphoid elements, lymphocyte populations are strikingly compartmentalized in air spaces and interstitium in sarcoidosis. The infiltration of activated CD4 positive T-cells represents the immunological hallmark of sarcoidosis. However, many types of other immune cells, such as macrophages, are involved in the inflammatory

response of the disorder. In the lung, this accumulation in both air spaces and interstitium (alveolitis) precedes and accompanies the development of granulomas (Semenzato, 2005).
Sarcoid granulomas are immune granulomas resulting from a specific cell-mediated immune response to an antigenic antigen. The granulomas of sarcoidosis are well-formed, compact aggregates. They usually are of varying age, ranging from highly cellular lesions to collections with diminishing cellularity, some fibrosis and progressive hyalinization. Two characteristic zones can be seen in a typical, well-developed sarcoid granuloma: 1) a central zone or follicle, which is tightly packed with cells composed primarily of macrophages, multinucleated giant cells and epitheloid cells; 2) a peripheral zone consisting of a collar of loosely arranged lymphocytes, monocytes and fibroblasts. Although many microscopic features may suggest sarcoidosis, the epitheloid granulomas, especially in their earlier stages, are indistinguishable from those of other idiopathic granulomatous disorders or even granulomatous disorders of known origin, such as berylliosis, tuberculosis or hypersensitivity pneumonitis (Müller-Quernheim, 1998).
Sarcoidosis is a worldwide disease with a lifetime incidence rate of 0.85-2.4 %. It generally affects 25-40-year-old people. The clinical phenotype of sarcoidosis can be extremely diverse in terms of presentation, involved organs, duration and severity. Lung involvement is present in 86-92 % of cases according to the chest X-ray, alone or in association with extrapulmonary localizations in about 50 % of cases (Nunes, 2005). International pulmonary registries have illustrated differences in the presentation of sarcoidosis in different countries: in Asia the majority of cases presented with a radiological stage I, and a positive tuberculin skin test was found more frequently than in other countries. However, erythema nodosum has not been reported among the Japanese, is rare among African-Americans, it is the presenting symptom in 18% of cases in Finland and occurs in about 30% of British sarcoidosis patients (Dements, 2001).
Clinical features of sarcoidosis are varied. It may manifest as an acute form (Löfgren's syndrome), chronic sarcoidosis or asymptomatic disease that may be found accidentally. However, even an acute form (e.g. erythema nodosum and joint pain) of disorder, which is the most typical clinical feature of sarcoidosis, is a nonspecific one (Bourke, 2006).
There are five radiologic stages (forms) of intrathoracic changes of sarcoidosis: stage 0, normal chest radiograph; stage 1, only lymphadenopathy; stage 2, lymphadenopathy with parenchyma infiltration; stage 3, only parenchymal disease; stage 4, pulmonary fibrosis (Koyama, 2004). Sarcoidosis may present at any stage. However, a great variation of radiologic appearance in each stage has been noticed. Radiographic features of sarcoidosis may be atypical, especially in older patients (Conant, 1988). Pulmonary sarcoidosis radiologically may be indistinguishable from tuberculosis, lymphangitic carcinomatosis, pulmonary metastases or metastatic lymphadenopathy (Heo, 2005; Kaira, 2007; Thomas 2008). Furthermore, subtle radiologic changes in sarcoidosis (e.g. presence of subpleural micronodules or mild intrathoracic lymphadenopathy) may be similar to those present in healthy adults, especially smokers and/or residents of urban areas (Remy-Jardin, 1990).
Histological features of the disease are varied (Rosen, 1978). Non-necrotising granuloma, a hallmark of morphologic appearance of the disease, is not unique for sarcoidosis. The granulomas in tuberculosis, extrinsic allergic alveolitis (hypersensitivity pneumonitis) and chronic beryllium disease are often identical to those of sarcoidosis (Williams, 1967; Popper, 1999). Even if the pathologic diagnosis of sarcoidosis is confirmed by biopsy, this may not confirm that all the lesions appear because of sarcoidosis (Kaira, 2007). Usage of needle

aspirate, either transbronchial or percutaneous, provides support but never an absolute proof of diagnosis (Baughman, 2000). Sarcoid-like reactions have been reported to be associated with carcinoma and lymphoma (Brincker, 1986; Laurberg, 1975; Tomimaru, 2007). Bronchoalveolar lavage (BAL) is a method of sampling fluid and cells from a large area of the lung tissue by instilling and aspirating saline via a bronchoscope wedged in bronchi. BAL as a method of sampling cells is very useful in the diagnosis and differential diagnosis of sarcoidosis (Drent, 1993; Welker, 2004). High lymphocytosis and CD4/CD8 ratio in bronchoalveolar lavage fluid (BALF) are the main features of sarcoidosis (Poulter, 1992). In patients with a clinical picture typical for sarcoidosis, an elevated CD4/CD8 ratio in BAL fluid may confirm the diagnosis and obviate the need for biopsy (Costabel, 2001; Kvale, 2003). However, CD4/CD8 ratio in BALF is highly variable (Kantrow, 1997). BALF cell patterns, including CD4/CD8 ratio are related to radiographic stage, clinical symptoms of sarcoidosis and previous empiric treatment with corticosteroids. Optimal cutoff point for CD4/CD8 ratio is different in various manifestations of sarcoidosis (Danila et al., 2008, 2009).

Diagnosis of sarcoidosis requires a compatible clinical and radiologic picture. However, there are no specific diagnostic tests and sarcoidosis is therefore a diagnosis of exclusion (Boer, 2010). The diagnosis of sarcoidosis must always be based on summation of clinical and radiological symptoms, results of BALF examination and other findings, which include data of histological examination of the lung or lymph node biopsy material if necessary.

In this chapter the diagnostic role of bronchoalveolar lavage and other sampling methods (including endobronchial biopsy, bronchoscopic lung biopsy, transbronchial lymph node biopsy and mediastinoscopy) in various clinical situations are discussed.

2. Bronchoalveolar lavage

2.1 History of bronchoalveolar lavage

Bronchoalveolar lavage was first used at Yale in 1922 in the management of phosgene poising. This approach has been extended to cystic fibrosis and alveolar proteinosis. In 1961, Myrvik showed how this simple lavage procedure could be used in rabbits to obtain lung macrophages. This seminal observation spawned new discipline, pulmonary cell biology (Gee & Fick, 1980). With the introduction in the mid-1960's of the design of the fiberoptic bronchoscope into clinical medicine by S. Ikeda, bronchoalveolar lavage was widely used for clinical investigations and diagnostic purposes (Zizel & Müller-Quernheim, 1998). Bronchoalveolar lavage was adapted to fiberoptic bronchoscopy by Reynolds and Newball in 1974 (Winterbauer et al., 1993). Bronchoscopy and lavage procedure have been a great stimulus for lung research to have access to normal and disease-affected airways and alveolar surfaces for direct samples (Reynolds, 1992). The observation of characteristic changes in the cytology of the BAL fluid in interstitial lung diseases were first reported by Hunninghake and Crystal in 1981 (Müller-Quernheim, 1998). With the widespread use of fibreoptic bronchoscopy for diagnostic evaluation of patients with interstitial lung diseases, bronchoalveolar lavage has also become part of the procedure (Reynolds, 1992).

2.2 Technique of bronchoalveolar lavage

After the fiberoptic bronchoscope has been inserted and the search for abnormalities in the respiratory tract is complete, the tip of the bronchoscope should be advanced into the desired bronchus as far as possible until well wedged. Biopsy and brushing should be avoided before BAL. The right middle lobe or the lingula of the left lung are the preferred sites for BAL (Emad, 1997). From these lobes, almost 20 % of more fluid and cells are recovered than from the lower lobes. However, in cases of predominant infiltrates in other lobes (e.g. upper lobe), bronchaolaveolar lavage should be done in these lobes or multiple lung segments (Cantin et al., 1983; Ziora et al. 2001).

The fluid used to perform bronchoalveolar lavage is isotonic 0,9 % NaCl solution suitable for intravenous use. Saline fluid is instilled through the working channel of the fiberoptic bronchoscope as a bolus with syringe with aliquots of 20 ml to 100 ml. The volume infused ranges from 100 ml to 300 ml. Overall, the amount of BAL fluid collected is about 40-60 % of the volume instilled (Klech & Pohl, 1989). The first neutrophil-rich aliquot, which contains the airways sample, is usually excluded from analysis of BALF differential cell count.

The information about cell types obtained in volumes of 100-250 ml is comparable, supposedly that cell populations obtained from volumes excess of 120 ml will not add to diagnostic accuracy. In most patients with sarcoidosis lavage at one site gives sufficient clinical information (Klech & Pohl, 1989; Winterbauer et al., 1993).

After measuring the recovered volume and performing total cell counts, the normal method of processing the cells from the BALF for differential counting is to prepare cytospins. The differential counts are assessed by viewing with a light microscope and counting at least 300-500 cells (Klech & Pohl, 1989). Lymphocyte subsets (CD4 and CD8) are evaluated usually using flow cytometry.

2.3 Cellular components of bronchoalveolar lavage fluid in healthy persons

The alveolar macrophages constitute the largest cell population in BALF, about 80-95 % of total recovered cells. Lymphocytes are the second major cell population in BALF .Other cells found in lavage fluid include neutrophils, occasional eosinophils, basophils and mast cells. For practical reasons the following percentages can be expected as normal within nonsmokers: lymphocytes < 20 %, neutrophils < 5 %, eosinophils < 0.5 %. T lymphocytes are the main lymphocytes, and the ratio of T-helper to T-suppressors (CD4/CD8) is approximately 1.0-3.5. Smokers usually have a decreased percentage of lymphocytes and decreased CD4/CD8 ratio (Klech & Pohl, 1989; Zizel & Müller-Quernheim, 1998).

2.4 Cellular components of bronchoalveolar lavage fluid in sarcoidosis

Bronchoalveolar lavage is thought to mirror parenchymal inflammation in the interstitial lung diseases. In sarcoidosis BAL recovers activated lymphocytes and alveolar macrophages, which are the precursors of granuloma formation (Hendricks et al., 1999). A distinct compartmentalization to the lungs of CD4 T cells has been already found in the early 1980s. The characteristic finding of lung-accumulated CD4 T cells in sarcoidosis and resulting increase in the BAL fluid CD4/CD8 ratio has come to be a clinically important marker of the disease and is used for diagnostic purposes (Grunewald & Eklund, 2007). However, cellular components and T lymphocyte profiles are related to clinical presentation, radiological stage, smoking status, and previous treatment with corticosteroids (Danila et al., 2008, 2009). Therefore, the CD4/CD8 ratio in BAL fluid may be highly variable (Kantrow et al., 1997). It should be remembered that advanced sarcoidosis may present with no increase in numbers of BAL fluid lymphocytes, and CD4/CD8 ratio can be normal.

Patients with erythema nodosum and/or arthralgia show the most marked characteristics of alveolitis, including increased percentages of T lymphocytes, the highest CD4/CD8 ratios (up to 30) in BALF samples (Ward et al., 1989; Drent et al., 1993). However, asymptomatic sarcoid patients have significantly lower BAL fluid lymphocytosis and CD4/CD8 ratio comparing with non-treated patients with sarcoidosis-related symptoms. Moreover, previously corticosteroid-treated symptomatic patients have lower BALF lymphocytosis and CD4/CD8 ratio compared to non-treated symptomatic patients (Danila et al., 2009). The increase of the macrophage and neutrophil count, decrease of lymphocyte count and CD4/CD8 ratio with increased radiographic stage of sarcoidosis in BAL fluid in patients with newly diagnosed sarcoidosis have been documented (Danila et al., 2008).

Spontaneous macrophage-lymphocytes rosettes (adherence of lymphocytes to alveolar macrophages) in BALF from active sarcoid patients have been found, probably due to active antigen presentation at the focus of inflammation (Reynolds, 1992). Macrophage-lymphocyte rosettes and giant cells (elements of immune granuloma) are found more often in BAL fluid of symptomatic patient groups compared to asymptomatic patients (Danila et al., 2008). A case of severe pulmonary sarcoidosis with intact granulomas in BAL fluid was described in medical literature (Hendricks et al., 1999). These findings may reflect still on-going inflammation in lung parenchyma.

Acute onset of the disease and high CD4/CD8 ratio is associated with good prognosis. On the other hand, increased neutrophil counts are associated with a more advanced, chronic disease course, impaired lung function, poor response to corticosteroid treatment and persisting abnormal chest radiographs. It is supposed that an increased percentage of BAL fluid neutrophils and eosinophils reflect an ongoing inflammatory process, which may result in progressive loss of lung parenchyma (Lin et al., 1985; Dren et al., 1999; Ziegenhagen et al., 2003). However, BALF lymphocyte count at diagnosis is not a valuable prognostic factor in patients with newly diagnosed sarcoidosis (Greening et al., 1984; Laviolette et al., 1991). Moreover, high lymphocyte count and high CD4 lymphocyte count (as percentage of lymphocytes) reflect an intense alveolitis at the time of the procedure, but they are not indicators of poor prognosis on which therapeutic decisions can be based (Verstraeten et al., 1990) and may be a favorable prognostic factor for lung function in pulmonary sarcoidosis (Foley et al., 1989).

Sarcoidosis patients may present with extrapulmonary lesions due to the multisystem character of the disease. In patients presenting with extrapulmonary sarcoid lesions interstitial pulmonary changes with or without hilar adenopathy may be present. There may be a normal chest X-ray film, but conclusions from roentgenographic examination may underestimate the alveolitis already present. Moreover, typical sarcoid changes in BAL fluid samples can be found even without lung field involvement shown by high-resolution computed tomography, for example in patients with only ocular findings (ocular sarcoidosis) (Hoogsteden et al., 1988; Takahashi et al., 2001).

Cigarette smoking modifies the immunologic BAL fluid sample profile and alveolitis is found to be less pronounced in smokers. Smoking results in increased total cell counts, increased CD8 lymphocytes, and less increased CD4/CD8 ratios in the BAL fluid samples in sarcoid patients. CD4/CD8 ratios are lower in smoking than in non-smoking patients (Valeyre et al., 1988; Drent et al., 1993).

2.5 Clinical role of bronchoalveolar lavage in pulmonary sarcoidosis

Several groups of investigators examined diagnostic value of the CD4/CD8 ratio of BAL lymphocytes for differentiating sarcoidosis from other causes of lung diseases. Costabel *et al.* reported that a ratio of 3.5 or greater had a sensitivity of 52 % and specificity of 94 % in 117 consecutive patients with biopsy-proven sarcoidosis (Costabel et al., 1992). Winterbauer *et al.* described that a ratio of 4.0 or greater distinguished patients with sarcoidosis from patients with other interstitial lung diseases with a sensitivity of 59 % and a specificity of 96 % (Winterbauer et al., 1993). Thomeer & Demedts found that a CD4/CD8 ratio of greater than 4.0 had a sensitivity of 55 % and a specificity of 94 % (Thomeer & Demedts, 1997). Welker *et al.* found that when the CD4/CD8 ratio is combined with lymphocyte and granulocyte numbers, the probability of sarcoidosis could exceed 85 % (Welker et al., 2004).

Group	Selected cutoff	Sensitivity (95% CI), %	Specificity (95% CI), %	PPV %	NPV %
All patients	3.5	80	90	96	64
	4.0	76	93	97	59
	5.0	66	95	97	50
	8.0	58	99	99	37
	10.0	26	100	100	33
Asymptomatic	3.5	62	90	86	68
	4.0	57	93	89	67
	5.0	49	97	94	62
	8.0	21	99	99	54
	10.0	10	100	100	51
Symptomatic non-treated	3.5	86	90	92	90
	4.0	84	93	94	85
	5.0	81	95	95	79
	8.0	52	99	98	61
	10.0	37	100	100	55
Symptomatic treated	3.5	83	91	73	94
	4.0	77	93	77	93
	5.0	70	96	86	91
	8.0	50	99	98	85
	10.0	33	100	100	83

CI – confidence interval. PPV – positive predicted value. NPV – negative predicted value.

Table 1. Diagnostic value of sarcoid patients' bronchoalveolar lavage fluid CD4/CD8 ratio in relation to clinical symptoms (Danila et al., 2009)

Comparable results were reported by other authors (Fireman et al., 1999). CD4/CD8 ratio of less than 1.0 virtually excludes the diagnosis of sarcoidosis (Winterbauer et al., 1993).
We have found that optimal cutoff points for CD4/CD8 ratio are 3.5 and 4.0 for asymptomatic and symptomatic patients, respectively (Danila et al., 2009). Sensitivity of the optimal cutoff points (3.5 and 4.0) of CD4/CD8 ratio were lower in the asymptomatic patient groups compared to the symptomatic (non-treated and treated) patients. Sensitivity of the optimal cutoff points decreased with increased stage of sarcoidosis. The values of sensitivity, specificity and predicted values are presented in Tables 1 and 2. Normal BALF

cell counts were found in 7 % of 318 consecutive sarcoid patients with newly diagnosed disease. However, typical sarcoid BAL fluid cellular pattern (lymphocytosis and CD4/CD4 >3.5) was found in 6.2 % of all control subjects. Additionally, in 3.8 % of all control subjects BALF CD4/CD8 ratios of more than 3.5 without lymphocytosis were found.
Maximum value of BALF CD4/CD8 ratio for non-sarcoid subjects was 5.6, except for one patient with non-Hodgkin's lymphoma of low-grade malignancy (CD4/CD4 ratio = 8.8). According to the world-leading expert in interstitial lung disorders Professor U. Costabel examination of bronchoalveolar lavage fluid may be of diagnostic value in sarcoidosis, obviating need of biopsy in 40-60 % of patients (Costabel, 1997). The author's experience is in agreement with this statement. Having in mind that significant part of sarcoid patients, at least in European countries, manifested with an acute form of the disease (Löfgren's syndrome of fever, erythema nodosum, arthralgias, and bilateral hilar lymphadenopathy), even more of the patients due to very typical clinical-radiological symptoms and signs may obviate need of biopsy.

Group	Selected cutoff	Sensitivity (95% CI), %	Specificity (95% CI), %	PPV %	NPV %
Stage 1	3.5	88	90	94	81
	4.0	85	92	95	77
	5.0	78	96	97	69
	8.0	47	99	99	52
	10.0	33	100	100	46
Stage 2	3.5	74	91	84	83
	4.0	69	92	87	80
	5.0	57	95	89	78
	8.0	25	99	95	67
	10.0	18	100	100	65
Stage 3	3.5	46	90	59	85
	4.0	42	92	64	84
	5.0	34	96	66	83
	8.0	15	99	95	80
	10.0	5	100	100	77

CI – confidence interval. PPV – positive predicted value. NPV – negative predicted value.

Table 2. Diagnostic value of sarcoid patients' bronchoalveolar lavage fluid CD4/CD8 ratio in relation to a Stage (Danila et al., 2009)

So CD4/CD8 ratio has an important role in personal diagnostic algorithms of many clinicians, although the best use of this test requires considerable experience in its application (Wells, 2010). In summary, an increased lymphocyte count with CD4/CD8 ratio > 3.5 is regarded as typical for pulmonary sarcoidosis, and is considered generally sufficient to secure the diagnosis of sarcoidosis in the appropriate clinical setting (Spagnolo et al., 2009).

2.6 Side-effects of bronchoalveolar lavage

One of the reasons why bronchoalveolar lavage is enjoying its general acceptance among scientists and clinicians is its noninvasiveness. This makes bronchoalveolar lavage possible to perform in virtually all patients with few exceptions. Bronchoalaveolar lavage is a very safe procedure. Serious complications like significant bleeding, pneumothorax and other are extremely rare (Klech et al., 1992). Fever occurred some hours after BAL in about one fifth of all patients that underwent the procedure. Side-effects can be minimized by not exceeding lavage volume of 250 ml (Klech & Pohl, 1989). At the Department headed by the author only one serious complication of bronchoalveolar lavage (performed in a patient with tuberculosis) - pneumothorax, occurred during the last fifteen years. So, the rate of serious complications is extremely small, less than 0.1 %. Usually we do not perform BAL in patients with blood platelet count below 20000 / µl. Through its safety bronchoalveolar lavage does not raise any special ethical considerations (Rennard et al., 1992).

3. Endobronchial biopsy

3.1 Airway involvement in sarcoidosis

Bronchoscopic abnormalities have been observed in up to 60 % of patients with sarcoidosis (Shorr et al., 2001). These include "retinalization" of mucosa from increased mucosal vascularity, mucosal coarseness, pallor, flat yellow mucosal plaques, wartlike excrescences, "bleb-like" formations, irregular mucosal thickening, ulceration, and atrophic mucosa. The three common findings were bronchial mucosal hyperemia or edema, distortion of the bronchial anatomy, and bronchial narrowing (due to extrinsic compression of airways by the enlarged lymphnodes, various types of mucosal involvement or airway distortion caused by parenchymal changes). The classic endobronchial sarcoidosis is characterized by mucosal islands of waxy yellow mucosal nodules, 2 to 4 mm in diameter. Bronchoscopy may reveal endobronchial occlusion by sarcoid granulomas in the submucosa or an endobronchial polyp caused by sarcoid granulomas. Lobar, segmental, subsegmental, and more distal bronchi as well as bronchioles are affected more frequently than the trachea and main bronchi (Polychronopoulos & Prakash, 2009). Rarely, sarcoidosis manifested with endoluminal stenosis of proximal bronchi (Chambellan et al., 2005). The presence of endobronchial sarcoid lesions significantly increases the risk for airway obstruction and airway hyperreactivity in patients with sarcoidosis (Lavergne et al., 1999; Shorr et al., 2001).

3.2 Technique of endobronchial biopsy

After satisfactory anesthesia is established, the lesion is visualized, biopsy forceps are passed through the working channel of the fiberoptic bronchoscopy until the forceps are just beyond the tip of the bronchoscope. The forceps are opened, advanced into the area to be biopsed, and closed firmly. The forceps should be withdrawn slowly to avoid its slipping from the tissue. The forceps may then be withdrawn through the bronchoscope (Cortese & McDougall, 1994). Biopsy is taken from most prominent lesions. If bronchial mucosa seems normal, biopsy is usually taken from the carina of segmental, subsegmental or subsubsegmental bronchus. Usually from 4 to 6 biopsy samples are taken.

3.3 Diagnostic yield of endobronchial biopsy in sarcoidosis

Although airway appearance affects the results of endobronchial biopsy (EBB), this biopsy technique may demonstrate non-necrotizing granulomas even if the airways are normal on visual inspection. EBB resulted in diagnostic tissue in 50-70 % of cases (Puar et al., 1985; Shorr et al., 2001). The results of EBB correlated with airway appearance. EBB result is more likely to be positive if the endobronchial mucosa is abnormal. However, a normal-appearing airway mucosa does not exclude the presence of granulomas. EBB is positive in approximately 35 % of subjects with normal airway mucosa. Endobronchial biopsy increased in about 20 % in diagnostic value of fiberoptic bronchoscopy (Shorr et al., 2001).

3.4 Side-effects of endobronchial biopsy

Endobronchial biopsy is an extremely safe procedure. To the best of the author's knowledge there are no publications addressed specifically to the side-effects to endobronchial biopsy in sarcoidosis. The risk of the major complications during endobronchial biopsy, such as significant bleeding, is extremely small when a patient's blood platelets count is 50000 / μl or more. However, it should be remembered that massive or even fatal bleeding may occur after endobronchial biopsy in case of an abnormal bronchial artery of Dieulafoy's disease of the bronchus (Sweerts et al., 1995; Werf et al., 1999; Maxeiner, 2001; Stoopen et al., 2001), which may appear as submucosal smooth elevated non-pulsating lesion. At the Department for which the author works only one massive bleeding after endobronchial biopsy (presumably due to abnormal located bronchial artery) occurred during the last twenty years. There happened no other with endobronchial biopsy associated to serious complications during this period. Thus, the rate of serious complications after this procedure is less than 0.05 %.

4. Bronchoscopic lung biopsy

4.1 History of bronchoscopic lung biopsy

The ability to obtain lung tissue without subjecting a patient to an open lung biopsy is a major advance in diagnostic bronchoscopy. Bronchoscopic lung biopsy (also named as transbronchial lung biopsy) was first performed by H. Andersen in 1963, using the rigid bronchoscope. In 1974 first results of the BLB via the flexible bronchoscope were published (McDougall & Cortese, 1994). After introduction of the fiberoptic bronchoscope into clinical practice, bronchoscopic lung biopsy (BLB) during fibrobronchoscopy became a standard procedure. BLB is utilised to sample alveolar parenchyma beginning at the bronchiolar, noncartilaginous segment of the airway (Leslie et al., 2000).

4.2 Technique of bronchoscopic lung biopsy

After the inspection of the tracheobronchial tree, a bronchoscope is inserted to subsegmental or smaller bronchus until the wedging position. Under fluoroscopic control, biopsy forceps (a crocodile type biopsy forceps are usually used) are pushed forward until a peripheral position. The position of biopsy forceps is controled by two directions of chest fluoroscopy. Afterwards, the forceps are withdrawn about 2-3 cm, then opened and pushed forward. Usually this maneuver is repeated once or twice, and then the forceps are closed and withdrawn. If the patient indicates ipsilateral chest or shoulder pain then forceps are closed, and should be opened and withdrawn a few centimeters before closing or introducing to other segment or subsegment of the lung. The bronchoscope should not be removed from a wedge position until there is no evidence of significant bleeding. The BLB is usually performed after a patient's inhale (Zavala, 1978; McDougall & Cortese, 1994; Dierkesmann & Dobbertin, 1998). In the Department for which the author works for about 6 biopsies are performed in cases of suspected sarcoidosis. Most of the samples are of 1-3 mm in diameter.

4.3 Diagnostic yield of bronchoscopic lung biopsy in sarcoidosis

The specimens obtained during bronchoscopic lung biopsy are small, but in most cases permit accurate histological diagnosis. Although some authors (Roethe et al., 1980) indicated that 10 are optimal for obtaining the diagnosis in stage I and 5 biopsies in stages II and III. Most investigators (*Gilman & Wang, 1980;* Harber, 1981, Cavazza et al., 2009*)* found that 3-5 biopsies are enough when biopsy is performed by an experienced bronchoscopist.

Bronchoscopic lung biopsy has diagnostic yield of 50 % to 97 % (Mitchell et al., 1980; Roethe et al., 1980; Puar et al., 1985; Leonard et al., 1997; Boer et al., 2009). Density of the granulomas in the lung is not uniform (Rosen et al., 1977). Rosen et al. have found that nongranulomatous, nonspecific interstitial pneumonitis were predominant or prominent histopathologic findings in 62% of 128 granuloma-containing specimens from open lung biopsies obtained from patients with sarcoidosis (Rosen et al., 1978). Diagnostic accuracy is increased when biopsy is taken from the lobes with predominant involvement by chest X-ray or computed tomography scanning (Roethe et al., 1980; Boer et al., 2009).

Although the rate of positive findings on BLB is high among patients with sarcoidosis who have radiological evidence of pulmonary infiltration, it is also high (about 60 %) among patients with or even without hilar lymphadenopathy whose chest radiographs show normal lung fields (Mitchell et al., 1980; Ohara et al., 1993).

A generous transbronchial biopsy may show numerous compact, coalescent, non-necrotizing granulomas embedded within hyaline collagen, i.e. features almost diagnostic of sarcoidosis. Frequently, however, not only bronchial but also transbronchial biopsies show just a tiny granuloma, or even a single giant cell or a Schaumann body, that may be enough for the diagnosis but require a more robust clinical support. Sarcoid granulomas, although classically non-necrotizing, may show necrosis. It generally consists of tiny foci of central fibrinoid ("rheumatoid-like") necrosis, but rarely larger areas of fibrinoid, infarct, or suppurative ("Wegener-like") necrosis may be seen (Cavazza et al., 2009*)*.

Two characteristic zones can be seen in a typical, well-developed sarcoid granuloma: 1) a central zone or follicle which is tightly packed with cells composed primarily of macrophages, multinucleated giant cells and epitheloid cells; 2) a peripheral zone consisting of a collar of loosely arranged lymphocytes, monocytes and fibroblasts. Taken alone granulomas do not confirm the diagnosis of sarcoidosis, since it may also occur in tuberculosis, lymphoma or other malignant disease, berylliosis, brucellosis, extrinsic allergic alveolitis, histoplasmosis, collagen disorders, and other (Müller-Quernheim, 1998).

Specificity of noncaseating epithelioid cell granuloma in transbronchial biopsy for the distinction between sarcoidosis and other forms of diffuse lung disease may be high – about 90 % (Winterbauer et al., 1993). However, specificity of noncaseating granuloma may be less in countries with moderate or high prevalence of pulmonary tuberculosis. Our findings show that the sensitivity of non-necrotizing epithelioid cell granuloma in bronchoscopic biopsy for the diagnosis of sarcoidosis is high (94 %), as well as the negative predictive value (92 %) of this type of epithelioid cell granuloma for the exclusion of sarcoidosis. However, the specificity of epithelioid cell granuloma without necrosis in our investigated group was relatively low-only 60 %. We have found a significant overlap in types of granulomatous inflammation between tuberculosis and sarcoidosis. Moreover, non-necrotizing granulomas were found in several cases of adenocarcinoma and hematological disorder (Danila & Žurauskas, 2008).

4.4 Side-effects of bronchoscopic lung biopsy

Bronchoscopic lung biopsy is a relatively safe diagnostic method. The pneumothorax rate after BLB is 1-5% (Zavala, 1978; Cortese & McDougall, 1997; Becker et al., 1998; Ensminger & Prakash, 2006). Bleeding after the BLB for carefully selected patients is rare and not intensive. Life-threatening haemoptysis occurred in 2-5% of the BLB (Cortese & McDougall, 1997; Dierkesmann & Dobbertin, 1998). Lethal outcome mostly due to the massive bleeding, or pneumothorax, is rare, and it occurred in 0-0.2% of the cases (Schulte & Costabel, 1998).Uremia increased the risk of bleeding.

In author's institution of all the bronchoscopic lung biopsies, serious complications occurred in 2.6 % patients. Clinically significant pneumothorax requiring chest tube treatment occurred in 1.6 % patients. Non-significant pneumothorax not requiring the chest tube treatment occurred in 0.7% patients. Severe bleeding occurred in 1 % out of all BLBs. In all the cases the bleeding was stopped during the same procedure, after the bronchoscope tip in bronchus was occluded for several minutes (Danila et al., 2008). There was no lethal outcome related to BLB performed to more than 500 patients during the last fifteen years.

5. Transbronchial needle aspiration biopsy and endosonography guided needle aspiration biopsy

5.1 Standard transbronchial needle aspiration biopsy

The history of transbronchial needle aspiration (TBNA) goes back to 1949 when Eduardo Schieppat presented his new technique of endoscopical puncturing mediastinal lymph nodes across the tracheal spur (Leonard et al., 1997). In 1978, Wang with colleagues first described needle aspiration of paratracheal masses. In 1979, Oho and colleagues reported use of the first needle adapted for the flexible bronchoscope (Midthun & Cortese, 1994). To obtain cytology specimens, 20–22-gauge needles are usually used, while 19-gauge needles are needed to obtain a "core" of tissue for histology. TBNA can be performed safely and successfully during routine flexible bronchoscopy under local anaesthesia.

Selection of the proper site for needle insertion to increase diagnostic yield may be facilitated by reviewing the CT scan of the chest. The bevelled end of the needle must be secured within the metal hub during its passage through the working channel. The needle is advanced and locked in place only after the metal hub is visible beyond the tip of the working channel. The catheter can then be retracted, keeping the tip of the needle distal to the end of the fibrebronchoscope. The scope is then advanced to the target area and the tip of the needle is anchored in the intercartilaginous space in an attempt to penetrate the airway wall as perpendicularly as possible. With the needle inserted, suction is applied at the proximal port using a syringe. Aspiration of blood indicates inadvertent penetration of a blood vessel. In this case, suction is released, the needle is retracted and a new site is selected for aspiration. When there is no blood in the aspirate, the catheter is moved up and down with continuous suction, in an attempt to shear off cells from the mass or lymph node. The needle is withdrawn from the target site after the suction is released (Herth et al., 2006). Three to five passes in each location are recommended (Tremblay et al., 2009). Whenever possible, sampling of more than one nodal station is advised to increase diagnostic yield (Trisolini et al., 2008).

The diagnostic yield of conventional TBNA ranges from 54 % to 90 % (Wang et al., 1989; Trisolini et al., 2003; Oki et al., 2007; Trisolini et al., 2008; Tremblay et al., 2009).

5.2 Endobronchial ultrasonography guided transbronchial needle aspiration biopsy

The integration of ultrasound technology and flexible fibrebronchoscopy - endobronchial ultrasound (EBUS) enables imaging of lymph nodes, lesions and vessels located beyond the tracheobronchial mucosa. Recently real-time EBUS-TBNA became possible (Herth et al., 2006). EBUS-TBNA is able to sample stations that may be difficult to reach by mediastinoscopy, such as hilar nodes and posterior carinal nodes (Wong et al., 2007). EBUS-TBNA is usually performed under local anaesthesia and conscious sedation using midazolam. TBNA is performed by direct transducer contact with the wall of the trachea or bronchus. When a lesion is outlined, a 22-gauge full-length steel needle is introduced through the biopsy channel of the endoscope. Power Doppler examination may be performed before the biopsy to avoid unintended puncture of vessels. Under real-time ultrasonic guidance, the needle is placed in the lesion. Suction is applied with a syringe, and the needle is moved back and forth inside the lesion (Herth et al., 2006). Three to five passes in each location are recommended (Tremblay et al., 2009).

The diagnostic yield of EBUS-TBNA ranges from 83 % to 96 % (Wong et al., 2007; Garwood et al., 2007; Tremblay et al., 2009). The diagnostic yield significantly increased following the interpretation of the specimens by cytopathologist with expertise in lung disease for both standard and EBUS-guided TBNA (Tremblay et al., 2009).

Both conventional and EBUS-guided TBNA are safe procedures with rare complications, reported as pneumothorax, pneumomediastinum, haemomediastinum, bacteraemia and pericarditis (Herth et al., 2006; Wong et al., 2007; Garwood et al., 2007; Tremblay et al., 2009; Varela-Lema et al., 2009; Tournoy et al., 2010).

5.3 Endosonography guided needle aspiration biopsy

Initially designed for the staging of gastrointestinal malignancies, transoesophageal ultrasound-guided fine needle aspiration (EUS-FNA) has proven to be an accurate diagnostic method for the diagnosis and staging of lung cancer and the assessment of sarcoidosis. Lymph nodes in the following areas can be detected by EUS: paratracheally to the left (station 4L); the aortopulmonary window (station 5); lateral to the aorta (station 6); in the subcarinal space (station 7); adjacent to the lower oesophagus (station 8); and near the pulmonary ligament (station 9) (Herth et al., 2006). Usually, EUS-FNA is incapable of reaching lymph nodes located in the anterior mediastinum and the rest of the thorax beyond the mediastinum (Wong et al., 2007).

EUS-FNA is usually performed under local anaesthesia and conscious sedation using midazolam. The echo-endoscope is initially introduced up to the level of the coeliac axis and gradually withdrawn upwards for a detailed mediastinal imaging. Since the ultrasound waves are emitted parallel to the long axis of the endoscope, the entire needle can be visualised approaching a target in the sector-shaped sound field. Pulse and color Doppler ultrasonography imaging can be performed in cases of suspected vascular structures. For the aspirations, 22-gauge needles are standard, although smaller (25-gauge) and larger needles (19-gauge) can be used as well (Herth et al., 2006).

The diagnostic yield of EUS-FNA is of about 80 % (Annema et al., 2005), sensitivity of 89-100 % and specificity of 94-96 % (Fritscher-Ravens et al., 2000; Wildi et al., 2004).

EUS-FNA is a safe procedure with rare complications (Wildi et al., 2004; Annema et al., 2005).

It should be noted that the presence of non-necrotizing epitelioid granulomas in the specimens of the lymph nodes is not diagnostic *per se* for sarcoidosis. Specificity of the non-necrotizing epitelioid granulomas depends on prevalence of sarcoidosis and other granulomatous disorders (such as tuberculosis) in a specific geographic region.

6. Mediastinoscopy

Mediastinoscopy is a common procedure used for the diagnosis of thoracic disease and the staging of lung cancer. Since its introduction by Carlens in 1959, mediastinoscopy has become the standard to which all other methods of evaluating the mediastinum are compared (Hammound et al., 1999). Mediastinoscopy is effective in assessment of the mediastinum. Porte et al. have found that sensitivity of the mediastinoscopy was 97 % in 400 mediastinoscopes performed in 398 patients with undiagnosed mediastinal lesions (Porte et al., 1998). It is important to remember that non-necrotizing epithelioid cell granulomas may be related to carcinoma of the lung and other malignant disease. Sarcoid reactions in malignant disease appear in close association with tumors, in regional lymph nodes, or in more distant locations. They have been reported to occur in a variety of malignant diseases, with particularly high incidences in lymphoproliferative disorders (Laurberg, 1975; Brincker, 1986; Segawa et al., 1996; Tomimaru et al., 2007).

Mediastinoscopy is more invasive diagnostic method for sampling of the mediastinal lymp nodes comparing with transbronchial or transoesophageal ultrasound-guided fine needle aspiration. Carried out under general anaesthesia, it is costly, requires in-patient care (Hammound et al., 1999). Although, mediastinoscopy is a safe procedure (Venissac et al., 2003; Karfis et al., 2008), death related to mediastinoscopy is described in medical literature (Lemaire et al., 2006).

7. Diagnostic approach in suspected sarcoidosis

Presentation of sarcoidosis varied in clinical and radiological patterns. Moreover, comparative epidemiological studies have demonstrated that geographic, ethnic, and genetic factors are linked to the specific clinical characteristics of sarcoid patients (Baughman et al., 2001; Hosoda et al., 2002; Thomas & Hunninghake, 2003). Specificity of the diagnostic findings depends on other dominant diseases (e.g. tuberculosis, extrinsic allergic alveolitis, histoplasmosis) in specific population or a geographic region (Greco et al., 2005; Sibille et al., 2011). Availability of specific diagnostic techniques and patients' insurance policy differ in different countries. Thus, diagnostic pathway, which leads to confirmation of sarcoidosis, may be different.

Pathognomonic criteria or diagnostic "gold standard" are absent (Muller-Quernheim, 1998; Baughman & Iannuzzi, 2000). Most authorities thus include several clinical, radiological, immunological and histological features into their diagnostic criteria since other disease processes can simulate sarcoidosis in many ways (Muller-Quernheim, 1998; Hunninghake et al., 1999).

In principle, diagnosis of sarcoidosis may be based on typical clinical picture (symptoms of acute sarcoidosis) and typical radiological picture (Costabel, 2001; Iannuzzi et al., 2007). For the patients with no symptoms, bilateral hilar lymphadenopathy, and no other worrisome findings, close clinical observation may be sufficient (Reich et al., 1998; Kvale, 2003; Thomas & Hunninghake, 2003; Reich, 2010).

Diagnosis of sarcoidosis may be based on BAL findings (Costabel, 2001; Nunes et al., 2005). In patients with uncertain diagnosis after clinical assessment and high resolution computed tomography scanning, typical BAL cellular profiles may allow a diagnosis of sarcoidosis to be established with greater confidence (Wells et al., 2008).

In author's institution fibreoptic bronchoscopy and bronchoalveolar lavage are the first diagnostic procedures following clinical and radiological examination of the patient. Additional to BAL we perform endobronchial biopsy if bronchial mucosa seems abnormal. Examination of BAL fluid always includes microscopy and cultures for tuberculosis. Routinely, biopsy material is stained for acid-fast bacteria as well. Typical BAL fluid cellular or findings of non-necrotizing epitelioid granulomas in endobronchial biopsy material confirmed diagnosis of sarcoidosis in asymptomatic patients and patients with acute symptoms (Löfgren's syndrome). At least 60 % of all sarcoidosis cases are diagnosed this way. If BAL fluid cellular profile is non-typical and non-necrotizing epitelioid granulomas are not found, bronchoscopic forceps lung biopsy is performed. Finding of non-necrotizing granulomas confirms sarcoidosis. Practically, mediastinoscopy is performed only in exceptional cases when in patients with mediastinal lymphadenopathy the diagnosis was not confirmed by less invasive method. Routinely the 3-6 moths follow-up of our patients lasts at least up to 3 years or longer if necessary.

8. References

Annema, J.T.; Veslic, M. & Rabe, K.F. (2005). Endoscopic ultrasound-guided fine-needle aspiration for the diagnosis of sarcoidosis. *Eur Respir J*, Vol.25, pp. 405-409, ISSN 0903-1936

Baughman, R.P. & Iannuzzi M.C. (2000). Diagnosis of sarcoidosis: when is a peek good enough? Chest, Vol.117, pp. 931-932, ISSN 0012-3692

Baughman, R.P.; Teirstein, A.S.; Judson, M.A.; Rossman, M.D.; Yeager, Jr. H.; Bresnitz, E.A.; Depalo, L.; Hunninghake, G.; Iannuzzi, M.C.; Johns, C.J.; Mclennan, G.; Moller, D.R.; Newman, L.S.; Rabin, D.L.; Rose, C.; Rybicki, B.; Weinberger, S.E.; Terrin, M.L.; Knatterud, G.L. & Cherniak, R. (2001). Clinical characteristics of patients in a case control study of sarcoidosis. *Am J Respir Crit Care Med*, Vol.164, pp. 1885-1889, ISSN 1073-449X

Becker, H.D.; Shirakawa, T.; Tanaka, F.; Muller, K-M.; & Herth F. (1998). Transbronchial (transbronchoscopic) lung biopsy in the immunocompromised patient. *Eur Respir Mon*, Vol.9, pp. 193-2008, ISSN 1025-448x

Boer, S. & Wilsher M. (2010). Sarcoidosis. *Chron Respir Dis, Vol.*7, pp. 247-258, ISSN 1479-9723

Bourke, S.J. (2006). Interstitial lung disease: progress and problems. *Postgrad Med*, Vol.82, pp. 494-499, ISSN 0032-5481

Brincker, H. (1986). Sarcoid reactions in malignant tumours. Cancer Treat Rev, Vol.13, pp. 147-156, ISSN 0305-7372

Cantin, A.; Begin R.; Rola-Pleszczynski, M. & Boileau, R. (1983). Heterogeneity of bronchoalveolar lavage cellularity in stage III pulmonary sarcoidosis. *Chest, Vol.*83, pp. 3 485-486, ISSN 0012-3692

Cavazza, A.; Harari, S.; Caminati, A.; Barbareschi, M.; Carbonelli, C.; Spaggiari, L.; Paci, M.; & Rossi, G. (2009). The histology of pulmonary sarcoidosis: a review with particular emphasis on unusual and underrecognized features. *Int J Surg Pathol, Vol.*17, pp. 219-230, ISSN 1066-8969

Chambellan, A.; Turbie, P.; Nunes, H.; Brauner, M.; Battesti, J-P. & Valeyre, D. (2005). Endoluminal stenosis of proximal bronchi in sarcoidosis: bronchoscopy, function, and evolution. *Chest, Vol.* 127, pp. 2 472-481, ISSN 0012-3692

Conant, E.F.; Glickstein, M.F.; Mahar, P. & Miller, W.T. (1988). Pulmonary sarcoidosis in the older patient: conventional radiographic features. *Radiology,* Vol.169, pp. 315-319, ISSN 0033-8419

Cortese, D.A. & McDougall, J.C. (1997). Bronchoscopy in peripheral and central lesions, In: *Bronchoscopy,* U.B.S. Prakash, (Ed.), 135-140, Lippincott-Raven Publ., ISBN 0-7817-0095-7, Philadelphia, USA

Costabel, U.; Zaiss, A.W. & Guzman, J. (1992). Sensitivity and specificity of BAL findings in sarcoidosis. *Sarcoidosis,* Vol.9 (Suppl. 1), pp. 211-214, ISSN 0393-1447

Costabel, U. (1997). CD4/CD8 ratios in bronchoalveolar lavage fluid: of value for diagnosing sarcoidosis? *Eur Respir J,* Vol.10, pp. 2699-2700, ISSN 0903-1936

Costabel, U. (2001). Sarcoidosis: clinical update. *Eur Respir J,* Vol.18 (Suppl. 32), pp. 56s–68s, ISSN 0903-1936

Danila, E.; Žurauskas, E.; Loskutovienė, G.; Zablockis, R.; Nargėla, R.; Biržietytė, V. & Valentinavičienė, G. (2008). Significance of bronchoscopic lung biopsy in clinical practice. *Adv Med Sci* Vol.53, pp. 11-16, ISSN 1896-1126

Danila, E.; Jurgauskienė, L. & Malickaitė, R. (2008). BAL fluid cells and pulmonary function in different radiographic stages of newly diagnosed sarcoidosis. *Adv Med Sci* Vol. 53, pp. 228-233, ISSN 1896-1126

Danila, E. & Žurauskas, E. (2008). Diagnostic value of epithelioid cell granulomas in bronchoscopic biopsies. *Inter Med* Vol.47, pp. 2121-2126, ISSN 0918-2918

Danila, E.; Jurgauskienė, L.; Norkūnienė, J. & Malickaitė, R. (2009). BAL fluid cells in newly diagnosed pulmonary sarcoidosis with different clinical activity. *Ups J Med Sci,* Vol.114, pp. 26-31, ISSN 0300-9734

Danila, E.; Norkūnienė, J.; Jurgauskienė, L. & Malickaitė, R. (2009). Diagnostic role of BAL fluid CD4/CD8 ratio in different radiographic and clinical forms of pulmonary sarcoidosis. *Clin Respir J,* Vol.3, pp. 214-221, ISSN 17526981

Demedts, M.; Wells, A.U.; Anto, J.M.; Costabel, U.; Hubbard, R.; Cullinan, P.; Slabbynck, H.; Rizzato, G.; Poletti, V.; Verbeken, E.K.; Thomeer, M.J.; Kokkarinen, J.; Dalphin, J.C. & Newman Taylor A. (2001). Interstitial lung diseases: an epidemiological overview. *Eur Respir J.,* Vol.18 (Suppl. 32), pp. 2s-16s, ISSN 0903-1936

Dierkesmann, R. & Dobbertin, I. (1998). Different techniques of bronchoscopy. *Eur Respir Mon,* Vol.9, pp. 1-21, ISSN 1025-448x

Drent, M.; Mulder, P.G.; Wagenaar, S.S.; Hoogsteden, H.C.; Velzen-Blad, H. & van den Bosch, J.M. (1993). Differences in BAL fluid variables in interstitial lung diseases evaluated by discriminant analysis. *Eur Respir J,* Vol.6, pp. 803–810, ISSN 0903-1936

Drent, M.; Velzen-Blad, H.; Diamant, M.; Hoogsteden, H.C. & Bosch, J.M. (1993). Relationship between presentation of sarcoidosis and T lymphocyte profile. A study in bronchoalveolar lavage fluid. *Chest*, Vol.104, pp. 795-800, ISSN 0012-3692

Drent, M.; Jacobs, J.A.; de Vries, J.; Lamens, R.J.S.; Liem, I.H. & Wouters, E.F.M. (1999). Does the cellular bronchoalveolar lavage fluid profile reflect the severity of sarcoidosis? *Eur Respir J*, Vol.13, pp.1338-1344, ISSN 0903-1936

Emad, A. (1997). Bronchoalveolar lavage: a useful method for diagnosis of some pulmonary disorders. *Respir Care*, Vol.42, pp. 765-790, ISSN 0020-1324

Ensminger, S.A. & Prakash, U.B (2006). Is bronchoscopic lung biopsy helpful in the management of patients with diffuse lung disease? *Eur Respir J*, Vol.28, pp. 1081-1084, ISSN 0903-1936

Fireman, E.; Topilsky, I.; Greif, J.; Lerman, Y.; Schwarz, Y.; Man, A. & Topilsky, M. (1999). Induced sputum compared to bronchoalveolar lavage for evaluating patients with sarcoidosis and non-granulomatous interstitial lung disease. *Respir Med*, Vol. 93, pp. 827-834, ISSN 0954-6111

Foley, N.M.; Coral, A.P.; Tung, K.; Hudspith, B.N.; James, D.G. & Johnson, N.M. (1989). Bronchoalveolar lavage cell counts as a predictor of short term outcome in pulmonary sarcoidosis. *Thorax, Vol.44, pp.* 732-738, ISSN 0040-6376

Fritscher-Ravens, A.; Sriram, P.V.J.; Topalidis, T.; Hauber, H.P.; Meyer, A.; Soehendra, N. & Pforte, A. (2000). Diagnosing sarcoidosis using endosonography-guided fine-needle aspiration. *Chest, Vol.*118, pp. 4 928-935, ISSN 0012-3692

Garwood, S.; Judson, M.A.; Silvestri, G.; Hoda, R.; Fraig, M. & Doelken, P. (2007). Endobronchial ultrasound for the diagnosis of pulmonary sarcoidosis. *Chest, Vol.*132, pp. 4 1298-1304, ISSN 0012-3692

Gee, J.B. & Fick Jr, R.B. (1980). Bronchoalveolar lavage. *Thorax, Vol.*35, pp. 1-8, ISSN 0040-6376

Gilman, M.J. & Wang K.P. (1980). Transbronchial lung biopsy in sarcoidosis: an approach to determine the optimal number of biopsies. *Am Rev Respir Dis*, Vol.122, pp. 721-724, ISSN 0003-0805

Greco, S.; Marruchella, A.; Massari, M. & Saltini, C. (2005). Predictive value of BAL cellular analysis in differentiating pulmonary tuberculosis and sarcoidosis. *Eur Respir J*, Vol.26, pp. 360-362, ISSN 0903-1936

Greening, A.P.; Nunn, P., Dobson, N.; Rudolf, M. & Rees, A.D. (1985). Pulmonary sarcoidosis: alterations in bronchoalveolar lymphocytes and T cell subsets. *Thorax*, Vol.40, pp. 278-283, ISSN 0040-6376

Grunewald, J. & Eklund, A. (2007). Role of CD4+ T cells in sarcoidosis. *Proc Am Thorac Soc*, Vol.4, pp. 461-464, ISSN 1546-3222

Grutters, J.C.; Drent, M. & van den Bosch, J.M.M. (2009). Sarcoidosis. *Eur Respir Mon, Vol.* 46, pp. 126-154, ISSN 1025-448x

Hammoud, Z.T.; Anderson, R.C.; Meyers, B.F.; Guthrie, T.J.; Roper, C.L.; Cooper, J.D. & Patterson G.A. (1999). The current role of mediastinoscopy in the evaluation of thoracic disease. *J Thorac Cardiovasc Surg*, Vol.118, pp. 894-899, ISSN 0022-5223

Harber, P. (1981). The optimal number of trans-bronchoscopic biopsies for diagnosing sarcoidosis. *Chest, Vol.*79, pp. 1 124-125, ISSN 0012-3692

Hendricks, M.V.; Crosby, J.H. & Davis, W.B. (1999). Bronchoalveolar lavage fluid granulomas in a case of severe sarcoidosis. *Am J Respir Crit Care Med,* Vol.160, pp. 730-731, ISSN 1073-449X

Heo, J-N.; Choi, Y.W.; Jeon, S.C. & Park, C.K. (2005). Pulmonary tuberculosis: another disease showing clusters of small nodules. *Am J Roentgenol,* Vol.184, pp. 639-642, ISSN 1546-3141

Herth, F.J.F.; Rabe, K.F.; Gasparini, S. & Annema, J.T. (2006).Transbronchial and transoesophageal (ultrasound-guided) needle aspirations for the analysis of mediastinal lesions. *Eur Respir J,* Vol.28, pp. 1264-1275, ISSN 0903-1936

Hoogsteden, H.C.; van Dongen, J.J.; Adriaansen, H.J.; Hooijkaas, H.; Delahaye, M.; Hop, W & Hilvering, C. (1988). Bronchoalveolar lavage in extrapulmonary sarcoidosis. *Chest, Vol.*94, pp. 1 115-118, ISSN 0012-3692

Hosoda, Y.; Sasagawa, S. & Yasuda, N. (2002). Epidemiology of sarcoidosis: new frontiers to explore. *Curr Opin Pulm Med,* Vol.8, pp. 424-428, ISSN 1070-5287

Hunninghake, G.W.; Costabel, U.; Ando, M.; Baughman, R.; Cordier, J.F.; Du Bois, R.; Eklund, A.; Kitaichi, M.; Lynch, J.; Rizzato, G.; Rose, C.; Selroos, O.; Semenzato, G. & Sharma, O.P. (1999). ATS/ERS/WASOG statement on sarcoidosis. *Am J Respir Crit Care Med,* Vol.160, pp. 736-755, ISSN 1073-449X

Iannuzzi, M.C.; Rybicki, B.A. & Teirstein, A.S. (2007). Sarcoidosis. *N Engl J Med,* Vol.357, pp. 2153-2165, ISSN 0028-4793

Kaira, K.; Oriuchi, N.; Otani, Y.; Yanagitani, N.; Sunaga, N.; Hisada, T.; Ishizuka, T.; Endo, K. & Mori, M. (2007). Diagnostic usefulness of fluorine - 18-methyltyrosine positron emission tomography in combination with 18f-fluorodeoxyglucose in sarcoidosis patients. *Chest,* Vol.131, pp. 1019-1027, ISSN 0012-3692

Kantrow, S.P.; Meyer, K.C.; Kidd, P. & Raghu, G. The CD4/CD8 ratio in BAL fluid is highly variable in sarcoidosis. *Eur Respir J,* Vol.10, pp. 2716-2721, ISSN 0903-1936

Karfis, E.A.; Roustanis, E.; Beis, J. & Kakadellis J. (2008). Video-assisted cervical mediastinoscopy: our seven-year experience. *Interact CardioVasc Thorac Surg,* Vol.7, pp. 1015-1018, ISSN 1569-9293

Klech, H. & Pohl, W. (1989). Technical recommendations and guidelines for bronchoalveolar lavage (BAL). *Eur Respir J,* Vol.2, pp. 561-585, ISSN 0903-1936

Klech, H.; Pohl, W. & Hutter C. (1992). Safety and side-effects of bronchoalveolar lavage. *Eur Respir Rev,* Vol.2, pp. 54-57, ISSN 0905-9180

Koyama, T.; Ueda, H.; Togashi, K.; Umeoka, S.; Kataoka, M. & Nagai, S. (2004). Radiologic manifestations of sarcoidosis in various organs. *Radiographics,* Vol.24, pp. 87-104, ISSN 0271-5333

Kvale, P.A. (2003). Is it difficult to diagnose sarcoidosis? *Chest,* Vol.123, pp. 330-332, ISSN 0012-3692

Laurberg, P. (1975). Sarcoid reactions in pulmonary neoplasms. *Scand J Respir Dis,* Vol.56, pp. 20-27, ISSN 0903-1936

Lavergne, F. ; Clerici, C, ; Sadoun, D.; Brauner, M.; Battesti, J-P.; & Valeyre, D. (1999). Airway obstruction in bronchial sarcoidosis: outcome with treatment. *Chest, Vol.*116, pp. 5 1194-1199, ISSN 0012-3692

Laviolette, M.; Forge, J.L.; Tennina, S. & Boulet, L.P. (1991). Prognostic value of bronchoalveolar lavage lymphocyte count in recently diagnosed pulmonary sarcoidosis. *Chest, Vol.*100, pp. 2 380-384, ISSN 0012-3692

Lemaire, A.; Nikolic, I.; Petersen, T.; Haney, J.C.; Toloza, E.M.; Harpole Jr, D.H.; D'Amico, T.A. & Burfeind, W.R. (2006). Nine-year single center experience with cervical mediastinoscopy: complications and false negative rate. *Ann Thorac Surg*, Vol.82, pp. 1185-1190, ISSN 0003- 4975

Leonard, C.; Tormey, V.J.; O'Keane, C. & Burke, C.M. Bronchoscopic diagnosis of sarcoidosis. (1997). *Eur Respir J, Vol.*10, pp. 2722-2724, ISSN 0903-1936

Leonard, C.; Tormey, V.J.; Lennon, A. & Burke, C.M. (1997). Utility of Wang transbronchial needle biopsy in sarcoidosis. *Irish J Med Sci,* Vol.166, pp. 41-43,

Leslie, K.O.; Helmers, R.A.; Lanza, L.A. & Colby, T.V. (2000). Processing and evaluation of lung biopsy specimens. *Eur Respir Mon,* Vol.14, pp. 55-62, ISSN 1025-448x

Lin, Y.H.; Haslam, P.L. & Turner-Warwick, M. (1985). Chronic pulmonary sarcoidosis: relationship between lung lavage cell counts, chest radiograph, and results of standard lung function tests. *Thorax, Vol.40, pp.* 501-507, ISSN 0040-6376

Maxeiner, H. (2001). Lethal hemoptysis caused by biopsy injury of an abnormal bronchial artery. *Chest, Vol.*119, pp. 5 1612-1615, ISSN 0012-3692

McDougall, J.C. & Cortese, D.A. (1997). Bronchoscopic lung biopsy, In: *Bronchoscopy,* U.B.S. Prakash, (Ed.), 141-146, Lippincott-Raven Publ., ISBN 0-7817-0095-7, Philadelphia, USA

Midthun, D.E. & Cortese, D.A. (1997). Bronchoscopic needle aspiration and biopsy, *Bronchoscopy,* U.B.S. Prakash, (Ed.), 147-154, Lippincott-Raven Publ., ISBN 0-7817-0095-7, Philadelphia, USA

Mitchell, D.M.; Mitchell, D.N.; Collins, J.V. & Emerson, C.J. (1980). Transbronchial lung biopsy through fibreoptic bronchoscope in diagnosis of sarcoidosis. *Br Med J,* Vol.280, pp. 679-681,

Müller-Quernheim, J. (1998). Sarcoidosis: clinical manifestations, staging and therapy (part II). *Respir Med,* Vol.92, pp. 140-149, ISSN 0954-6111

Müller-Quernheim, J. (1998). Sarcoidosis: immunopathogenetic concepts and their clinical application. *Eur Respir J,* Vol.12, pp. 716-738, ISSN 0903-1936

Nunes, H.; Soler, P. & Valeyre, D. (2005). Pulmonary sarcoidosis. *Allergy,* Vol.60, pp. 565-582,

Ohara, K.; Okubo, A.; Kamata, K.; Sasaki, H.; Kobayashi, J. & Kitamura, S. (1993). Transbronchial lung biopsy in the diagnosis of suspected ocular sarcoidosis. *Arch Ophthalmol,* Vol.111, pp. 642-644,

Oki, M.; Saka, H.; Kitagawa C.; Tanaka, S.; Shimokata, T.; Kawata, Y.; Mori, K.; Kajikawa, S.; Ichihara, S. & Moritani, S. (2007). Real-time endobronchial ultrasound-guided transbronchial needle aspiration is useful for diagnosing sarcoidosis. *Respirology,* Vol.12, pp. 863-868,

Polychronopoulos, V.S. & Prakash, U.B.S. (2009). Airway involvement in sarcoidosis. *Chest, Vol.*136, pp. 5 1371-1380, ISSN 0012-3692

Popper, H.H. (1999). Epithelioid cell granulomatosis of the lung: new insights and concepts. *Sarcoidosis Vasc Diffuse Lung Dis,* Vol.16, pp. 32-46, ISSN 1460-2725

Porte, H.; Roumilhac, D.; Eraldi, L.; Cordonnier, C.; Puech, P. & Wurtz, A. (1998). The role of mediastinoscopy in the diagnosis of mediastinal lymphadenopathy. *Eur J Cardiothorac Surg*, Vol.13, pp. 196-199, ISSN 1010-7940

Poulter, L.W.; Rossi, G.A.; Bjermer, L.; Costabel, U.; Israel-Biet, D.; Klech, H.; Pohl, W. & Semenzato, G. (1992). The value of bronchoalveolar lavage in the diagnosis and prognosis of sarcoidosis. *Eur Respir Rev*, Vol.2, pp. 75-82, ISSN 0905-9180

Puar, H.S.; Young Jr, R.C. & Armstrong, E.M. (1985). Bronchial and transbronchial lung biopsy without fluoroscopy in sarcoidosis. *Chest, Vol.*87, pp. 3 303-306, ISSN 0012-3692

Reich, J.M.; Brouns, M.C.; O'Connor, E.A. & Edwards, M.J. *(*1998*)* Mediastinoscopy in patients with presumptive stage I sarcoidosis: a risk/benefit, cost/benefit analysis. *Chest, Vol.*113, pp. 147-153, ISSN 0012-3692

Reich, J.M. (2010). Endobronchial ultrasonography-guided transbronchial needle aspiration in patients with suspected sarcoidosis. *Chest, Vol.*137, pp. 1 235-236, ISSN 0012-3692

Remy-Jardin, M.; Beuscart, R.; Sault, M.C.; Marquette, C.H. & Remy, J. (1990). Subpleural micronodules in diffuse infiltrative lung diseases: evaluation with thin-section CT scans. *Radiology*, Vol.177, pp. 133-139, ISSN 0033-8419

Rennard, S.I.; Bauer, W. & Eckert H. (1992). Bronchoalveolar lavage: ethical considerations. *Eur Respir Rev*, Vol.2, pp. 125-127, ISSN 0905-9180

Reynolds, H.Y. (1992). Bronchoalveolar lavage has extended the usefulness of bronchoscopy. *Eur Respir Rev*, Vol.2, pp. 48-53, ISSN 0905-9180

Roethe, R.A.; Fuller, P.B.; Byrd, R.B. & Hafermann, D.R. (1980). Transbronchoscopic lung biopsy in sarcoidosis. Optimal number and sites for diagnosis. *Chest, Vol.*77, pp. 3 400-402, ISSN 0012-3692

Rosen, Y.; Amorosa, J.K.; Moon, S.; Cohen, J. & Lyons, H.A. (1977). Occurrence of lung granulomas in patients with stage I sarcoidosis. *Am J Roentgenol*, Vol.129, pp. 1083-1085, ISSN 1546-3141

Rosen, Y.; Athanassiades, T.J.; Moon, S. & Lyons, H.A. (1978). Nongranulomatous interstitial pneumonitis in sarcoidosis. *Chest*, Vol.74, pp. 122-125, ISSN 0012-3692

Rothkrantz-Kos, S.; van Dieijen-Visser, M.P.; Mulder, P.G.H. & Drent, M. (2003). Potential usefulness of inflammatory markers to monitor respiratory functional impairment in sarcoidosis. *Clin Chem*, Vol.49, pp. 1510-1517, ISSN 0009-9147

Schulte, W. & Costabel, U. (1998). Biopsies and bronchoalveolar lavage in interstitial lung diseases. *Eur Respir Mon*, Vol.9, pp. 171-180, ISSN 1025-448x

Segawa, Y.; Takigawa, N.; Okahara, M.; Maeda, Y.; Takata, I.; Fujii, M.; Mogami, H.; Mandai, K. & Kataoka, M. (1996). Primary lung cancer associated with diffuse granulomatous lesions in the pulmonary parenchyma. *Inter Med*, Vol.35, pp. 728-731, ISSN 0918-2918

Semenzato, G.; Bortoli, M.; Brunetta, E. & Agostini, C. (2005). Immunology and pathophysiology. *Eur Respir Mon, Vol.*32, pp. 49-63, ISSN 1025-448x

Shorr A.F.; Torrington, K.G. & Hnatiuk, O.W. (2001). Endobronchial biopsy for sarcoidosis: a prospective study. *Chest*, Vol.120, pp. 109-114, ISSN 0012-3692

Shorr A.F.; Torrington, K.G. & Hnatiuk, O.W. (2001). Endobronchial involvement and airway hyperreactivity in patients with sarcoidosis. *Chest*, Vol.120, pp. 3 881-886, ISSN 0012-3692

Sibille, A.; van Bleyenbergh, P.; Lagrou, K.; Verstraeten, A. & Wuyts, W. (2011). Three colleagues with sarcoidosis? *Eur Respir J*, Vol.37, pp. 962-964, ISSN 0903-1936

Spagnolo, P.; Richeldi, L. & Raghu G. (2009). The role of bronchoalveolar lavage cellular analysis in the diagnosis of interstitial lung diseases. *Eur Respir Mon, Vol.*46, pp. 36-46, ISSN 1025-448x

Stoopen, E.; Baquera-Heredia, J.; Cortes, D. & Green, L. (2001). Dieulafoy's disease of the bronchus in association with a paravertebral neurilemoma. *Chest*, Vol.119, pp. 1 292-294, ISSN 0012-3692

Sweerts, M.; Nicholson, A.G.; Goldstraw, P. & Corrin, B. (1995). Dieulafoy's disease of the bronchus. *Thorax, Vol.*50, pp. 697-698, ISSN 0040-6376

Takahashi, T.; Azuma, A.; Abe, S.; Kawanami, O.; Ohara, K. & Kudoh, S. (2001). Significance of lymphocytosis in bronchoalveolar lavage in suspected ocular sarcoidosis. *Eur Respir J*, Vol.18, pp. 515-521, ISSN 0903-1936

Thomas, A. & Lenox, R. (2008). Pulmonary lymphangitic carcinomatosis as a primary manifestation of colon cancer in a young adult. *CMAJ*, Vol.179, pp. 338-339, ISSN 0820-3946

Thomas, K.W. & Hunninghake, G.W. (2003). Sarcoidosis. *JAMA*, Vol.289, pp. 3300–3303, ISSN 0098-7484

Thomeer, M. & Demedts, M. (1997). Predictive value of CD4/CD8 ratio in bronchoalveolar lavage in the diagnosis of sarcoidosis. (abstract). *Sarcoidosis Vasc Diffuse Lung Dis*, Vol.14 (Suppl. 1), p. 36, ISSN 1460-2725

Tomimaru, Y.; Higashiyama, M.; Okami, J.; Oda, K.; Takami, K.; Kodama, K. & Tsukamoto, Y. (2007). Surgical results of lung cancer with sarcoid reaction in regional lymph nodes. *Jpn J Clin Oncol*, Vol.37, pp. 90-95, ISSN 0368-2811

Tournoy, K.G.; Bolly, A.; Aerts, J.G.; Pierard, P.; De Pauw, R.; Leduc, D.; Leloup, A.; Pieters, T.; Slabbynck, H.; Janssens, A.; Carron, K.; Schrevens, L.; Pat, K.; De Keukeleire, T. & Dooms, C. (2010). The value of endoscopic ultrasound after bronchoscopy to diagnose thoracic sarcoidosis. *Eur Respir J, Vol.*35, pp. 1329-1335, ISSN 0903-1936

Tremblay, A.; Stather, D.R.; MacEachern, P.; Khalil, M. & Field, S.K. (2009). A randomized controlled trial of standard vs endobronchial ultrasonography-guided transbronchial needle aspiration in patients with suspected sarcoidosis. *Chest, Vol.*136, pp. 2 340-346, ISSN 0012-3692

Trisolini, R.; Agli, L.L.; Cancellieri, A.; Poletti, V.; Tinelli, C.; Baruzzi, G. & Patelli, M. (2003). The value of flexible transbronchial needle aspiration in the diagnosis of stage I sarcoidosis *Chest, Vol.*124, pp. 6 2126-2130, ISSN 0012-3692

Trisolini, R.; Tinelli, C.; Cancellieri, A.; Paioli, D.; Alifano, M.; Boaron, M. & Patelli M. (2008). Transbronchial needle aspiration in sarcoidosis: Yield and predictors of a positive aspirate. *J Thorac Cardiovasc Surg*, Vol.135, pp. 837-842, ISSN 0022-5223

Valeyre, D.; Soler, P.; Clerici, C.; Pré, J.; Battesti, J.P.; Georges, R. & Hance A.J. (1988). Smoking and pulmonary sarcoidosis: effect of cigarette smoking on prevalence, clinical manifestations, alveolitis, and evolution of the disease. *Thorax, Vol.*43, pp.516-524, ISSN 0040-6376

van der Werf, T.S.; Timmer, A. & Zijlstra, J.G. (1999). Fatal haemorrhage from Dieulafoy's disease of the bronchus. *Thorax, Vol.*54, pp. 184-185, ISSN 0040-6376

Varela-Lema, L.; Fernández-Villar, A. & Ruano-Ravina, A. (2009). Effectiveness and safety of endobronchial ultrasound–transbronchial needle aspiration: a systematic review. *Eur Respir J, Vol.*33, pp. 1156-1164, ISSN 0903-1936

Venissac, N.; Alifano, M. & Mouroux, J. (2003). Video-assisted mediastinoscopy: experience from 240 consecutive cases. *Ann Thorac Surg*, Vol.76, pp. 208-212, ISSN 0003- 4975

Verstraeten, A.; Demedts, M.; Verwilghen, J.; van den Eeckhout, A .; Mariën, G.; Lacquet, L.M. & Ceuppens, J.L. (1990). Predictive value of bronchoalveolar lavage in pulmonary sarcoidosis. *Chest, Vol.*98, pp. 3 560-567, ISSN 0012-3692

Wang, K.P.; Fuenning, C.; Johns, C.J. & Terry P.B. (1989). Flexible transbronchial needle aspiration for the diagnosis of sarcoidosis. *Ann Otol Rhinol Laryngol*, Vol.98, pp. 298-300, ISSN 0096-8056

Ward, K.; O'Connor, C.; Odlum, C. & Fitzgerald, M.X. (1989). Prognostic value of bronchoalveolar lavage in sarcoidosis: the critical influence of disease presentation. *Thorax*, Vol.44, pp. 6-12, ISSN 0040-6376

Welker, L.; Jorres, R.A.; Costabel, U. & Magnussen, H. (2004). Predictive value of BAL cell differentials in the diagnosis of interstitial lung diseases. *Eur Respir J*, Vol.24, pp. 1000-1006, ISSN 0903-1936

Wells, A.U. & Hirani, N. (2008). Interstitial lung disease guideline: the British Thoracic society in collaboration with Thoracic society of Australia and New Zealand and the Irish Thoracic society. *Thorax*, Vol.63 (Suppl. 5), pp. 1-58, ISSN 0040-6376

Wildi, S.M.; Judson, M.A.; Fraig, M.; Fickling, W.E.; Schmulewitz, N.; Varadarajulu, S.; Roberts, S.S.; Prasad, P.; Hawes, R.H.; Wallace, M.B. & Hoffman, B.J. (2004). Is endosonography guided fine needle aspiration (EUS-FNA) for sarcoidosis as good as we think? *Thorax, Vol.*59, pp. 794-799, ISSN 0040-6376

Williams, W.J. & Williams, D. (1967). 'Residual bodies' in sarcoid and sarcoid-like granulomas. *J Clin Pathol*, Vol.20, pp. 574-577, ISSN 0021-9746

Winterbauer, R.H.; Lammert, J.; Selland, M.; Wu, R.; Corley, D. & Springmeyer, S.C. (1993). Bronchoalveolar lavage cell populations in the diagnosis of sarcoidosis. *Chest*, Vol.104, pp. 352-361, ISSN 0012-3692

Winterbauer, R.H.; Wu, R. & Springmeyer, S.C. (1993). Fractional analysis of the 120-ml bronchoalveolar lavage. Determination of the best specimen for diagnosis of sarcoidosis. *Chest, Vol.*104, pp. 2 344-351, ISSN 0012-3692

Wong, M.; Yasufuku, K.; Nakajima, T.; Herth, F.J.F.; Sekine, Y.; Shibuya, K.; Iizasa, T.; Hiroshima, K.; Lam, W.K. & rFujisawa T. (2007). Endobronchial ultrasound: new insight for the diagnosis of sarcoidosis. *Eur Respir J*, Vol.29, pp. 1182-1186, ISSN 0903-1936

Zavala, DC. (1978). Transbronchial biopsy in diffuse lung disease. *Chest*, Vol.73 (Suppl. 5), pp. 727-733, ISSN 0012-3692

Ziegenhagen, M.W.; Rothe, M.E.; Schlaak, M. & Müller-Quernheim, J. (2003). Bronchoalveolar and serological parameters reflecting the severity of sarcoidosis. *Eur Respir J*, Vol.21, pp. 407-413, ISSN 0903-1936

Ziora, M.; Grzanka, P.; Mazur, B.; Niepsuj, G.; Dworniczak, S.; Oklek, K. & Shani, J. (2001). Evaluation of alveolitis by bronchoalveolar lavage and high-resolution computed tomography in patients with sarcoidosis. *J Bronchol*. Vol.8, pp. 260–266, ISSN 1944-6586

Zissel, G. & Müller-Quernheim, J. (1998). Sarcoidosis: historical perspective and immunopathogenesis (part I). *Respir Med*. Vol.92, pp. 126-139, ISSN 0954-6111

Part 3

Management

7

Updated Guidelines for the Treatment of Pulmonary Sarcoidosis

Luis Jara-Palomares, Candela Caballero-Eraso,
Alicia Díaz-Baquero and Jose Antonio Rodríguez-Portal
Medical-Surgical Unit of Respiratory Diseases,
University Hospital Virgen del Rocio,
Spain

1. Introduction

Sarcoidosis is a systemic granulomatous disease that affects the lungs in 90% of cases. The stage of the disease is determined by the level of pulmonary damage as assessed by a chest x-ray. This pulmonary damage varies widely between stages I, when lymph node damage has no repercussions on lung functioning, and stage IV, in which interstitial pulmonary damage and the development of fibrosis has clear repercussions on lung functioning.

Systemic corticosteroids are the drugs of choice for the treatment of sarcoidosis, although no clear consensus exists regarding when to start treatment, the correct doses, or how long treatment should be maintained. We must keep in mind that the progression of this disease is often unpredictable, with frequent cases of spontaneous remission, above all in stage I patients. However, systemic steroids have side effects and the decision to start treatment is determined by the intensity of the symptoms, especially exercise-induced dyspnoea, and the level of lung functioning deterioration.

Sarcoidosis can affect both the upper and lower airways. Endobronchial damage occurs in 40% of stage I patients and approximately 70% of stage III and IV patients. Endobronchial granulomas have been described along with stenosis of the airway due to peribronchial damage. Clinically relevant airway stenosis is uncommon but difficult to treat. In the upper airway, granulomas can appear in the submucosa of the larynx, pharynx, and paranasal sinuses. Sleep apnoea has been described as a result of involvement of the epiglottis. This damage to the airway is occasionally manifested as the presence of persistent cough, with no findings in the pulmonary parenchyma. In up to 50% of cases, spirometry reveals obstructive phenomena, especially in patients with endobronchial damage due to the sarcoidosis.

The treatment of choice for pulmonary sarcoidosis is oral corticosteroids. Other alternative treatments have been described, such as immunosuppressive agents (methotrexate, azathioprine, cyclophosphamide, leflunomide, cyclosporine, and chlorambucil), cytokine inhibitors (thalidomide and pentoxifylline), and immunomodulatory agents (TNF-alpha antagonists, infliximab, adalimumab, and antimalarial agents such as chloroquine) (Table 1). Currently, no clear evidence exists showing the usefulness of these drugs, and they are only indicated when the sarcoidosis does not respond to conventional treatment with oral

corticosteroids, in patients with intolerance to corticosteroids (poorly controlled diabetes, myopathy, osteoporosis), or in order to reduce the dosage of corticosteroids (King, 2010). However, these drugs require close monitoring as they can cause severe adverse effects.
Here, we will review the different treatment options for patients with pulmonary sarcoidosis.

INHALED CORTICOSTEROIDS
ORAL CORTICOSTEROIDS
IMMUNOSUPPRESSIVE AGENTS a. Methotrexate b. Azathioprine c. Cyclophosphamide d. Chlorambucil e. Cyclosporine f. Leflunomide
IMMUNOMODULATORY AGENTS a. Tumour necrosis factor (TNF) antagonists • Etanercept b. Monoclonal antibodies • Infliximab • Adalimumab c. Thalidomide d. Pentoxifylline
ANTIMALARIAL AGENTS a. Chloroquine and hydroxychloroquine

Table 1. Drugs used for the treatment of sarcoidosis

2. Treatment options in patients with pulmonary sarcoidosis

2.1 Inhaled corticosteroids

The mild ocular and cutaneous manifestations of sarcoidosis can be treated using topical corticosteroids. For the treatment of pulmonary damage, an alternative to the use of systemic corticosteroids is inhaled corticosteroids, which can be useful in selected groups of patients. This treatment has been used in two types of patients: a) those with an affected airway, with chronic coughing as the primary symptom, and b) as a treatment used for suspending or at least reducing the need for systemic corticosteroids.
Several randomised studies have compared the efficacy of inhaled corticosteroids with that of a placebo. The characteristics of both patient groups were similar with regard to radiological findings, lung function (FEV1), DLCO (%), and symptoms. Alberts et al (Albert et al., 1995) compared the administration of 1.2mg budesonide with a placebo in a group of stage I-III sarcoidosis patients during 6 months of treatment and another 6 months of follow-

up. DuBois et al (DuBois et al., 1999) compared the administration of 2mg/day of fluticasone with a placebo in stage II-III sarcoidosis patients for 6 months, with no follow-up. Erkkila et al (Erkkila et al., 1988) compared the treatment of stage I-II sarcoidosis patients with 0.8mg budesonide twice/ day with a placebo for 10 weeks. None of these studies demonstrated improvement in lung function or radiological parameters in the treatment group compared to the placebo group. Only the study by Alberts et al (Albert et al., 1995) found that the group treated with budesonide at high doses improved in the global clinical index, including symptoms. In all other studies regarding treatment with inhaled corticosteroids, symptoms were not improved when compared to the placebo group. One study did demonstrate that inhaled fluticasone could help to reduce coughing in cases of acute sarcoidosis (Baughman et al., 2002).

It has been reported that treatment with inhaled steroids may reduce the need for systemic steroids, and thus considerably reduce the adverse effects from this type of treatment. Milman et al (Milman et al., 1994) studied the use of budesonide at 1.2-2mg/day and oral steroids in 8 patients with stage I-II sarcoidosis. The study lasted 12 months, with 18 months of follow-up. They found no beneficial effect from the use of inhaled budesonide. Pietinalho et al (Pietinalho et al., 1999) compared a group of patients initially treated with 10-20mg prednisolone during 3 months, followed by inhaled budesonide at 1.6mg/day during 15 months, with a control group that received a placebo. After 3 months of treatment, a radiological improvement was observed in the treatment group compared to the control group. At 6 months of treatment, these differences were still significant, but from that time on, there were no differences between the two groups. In patients that started the study in stage I of the disease, neither FVC nor DLCO changed during the study, since they were at normal levels at the start of the treatment. In patients that started the study in stage II, FVC did not change during the treatment period. In this group, those patients that were treated for 18 months did show significant differences in FVC and DLCO. These difference were greater in patients with initial values of FVC<80% and DLCO<75%. The authors concluded that, in stage II sarcoidosis patients, treatment change from initial oral steroids to inhaled steroids is a good option to avoid the long-term administration of oral corticosteroids. However, based on the information that is currently available (Paramothayan & Lasserson, 2008), we can conclude that insufficient evidence exists based on randomised clinical trials that could establish the efficacy and/or usefulness of inhaled corticosteroids in the treatment of sarcoidosis.

2.2 Oral corticosteroids

2.2.1 Introduction

The US guidelines and the recently updated BTS guidelines substantially updated the treatment options for pulmonary sarcoidosis (American Thoracic Society [ATS], 1999; Bradley et al., 2008). Dempsey OJ et al. later summarised and published a treatment update based on both guidelines (Dempsey et al., 2009). One of the main recommendations that they made was to carefully assess the decision to start treatment with corticosteroids (the most frequently used treatment), comparing the benefits with potential risks. In general, treatment should be considered when organ function is affected. The primary conclusions obtained from conferences and consensus documents developed by experts are summarised in Table 2 (Bradley et al., 2008).

• Many patients do not require treatment and the disease can regress spontaneously.
• Erythema nodosum can be painful, and treatment should be paracetamol or NSAID on a short-term, on-demand basis.
• Treatment is not indicated in: • Asymptomatic stage I disease • Stable stage II asymptomatic disease • Stage III disease with slightly altered lung function
• Oral steroids can benefit patients: • In stage II or III with moderate, severe, or progressive symptoms • With changes observed in chest x-rays
• Absolute indications for oral steroids include: • Hypercalcaemia • Neurological involvement • Cardiac involvement • Ocular involvement (only when topical treatment fails)

Table 2. Primary conclusions obtained from conferences and consensus documents developed by experts (Baughman et al. 2003)

2.2.2 Treatment plan

The UK guidelines indicate that treatment should start with prednisolone at 0.5mg/kg/day for 4 weeks (Bradley et al., 2008). The dosage should then be gradually reduced over the next 6 months, with an ideal dose of ≤10mg/day. In order to avoid bone loss caused by the corticosteroids, patients must also start treatment with oral biphosphonates along with bone densitometry tests. The duration of treatment can vary, but frequently ranges between 6 months and 2 years. Some patients need more than 10mg/day of prednisolone in order to control the disease. In these circumstances, another drug may be added in order to further decrease the dosage of corticosteroids (steroid-sparing), thus achieving a final dosage of ≤10mg/day of prednisone.

A systematic review of randomised placebo-controlled clinical trials on patients with pulmonary damage that started treatment with oral or inhaled corticosteroids concluded that oral corticosteroids improved chest x-ray results and overall score in symptoms, spirometry, and radiological tests between 3 and 24 months of treatment. However, little evidence pointed towards improved lung function, and data were scarce regarding the impact of oral corticosteroids in the long-term progression of the disease (Paramothayan et al., 2000).

However, there are no clear guidelines for the initiation of corticosteroid treatment, when to decide that treatment has failed or consider a therapeutic alternative for pulmonary sarcoidosis. As such, the use of corticosteroids in pulmonary sarcoidosis continues to be discussed, and a final conclusion has yet to be made regarding the optimal duration of treatment. With the medical literature currently available, we do not know if oral corticosteroids can alter the final result of this disease. However, the benefits of this type of treatment do now outweigh the side effects. Some retrospective studies have suggested that patients with sarcoidosis and do not take corticosteroids (Gottlieb et al., 1997) or only at low doses (Rizzato et al., 1998) have a lower rate of relapse. These data suggest that, when making a decision to treat acute pulmonary sarcoidosis with oral corticosteroids, the lowest dosage possible must be used.

In this respect, McKinzie et al. (McKinzie et al., 2010) performed a retrospective study of patients with pulmonary sarcoidosis that were treated with ≤20mg of oral prednisone during exacerbations, and clinical evolution and changes in spirometry values were assessed after two weeks. This study demonstrated that these patients improved in clinical symptoms and spirometry values, although it did have some limitations: 1) the study was retrospective, implying a patient selection bias; 2) it did not follow up on long-term patient progression, and therefore, we cannot comment on the evolution of the disease; 3) the study was not designed specifically to measure the adverse effects of corticosteroid treatment; 4) it lacked a control group; 5) the two-week follow-up period was not maintained in all patients (median: 21 days). Even so, it did show that the treatment of acute exacerbations of pulmonary sarcoidosis using 20mg of prednisone for a median 21 days significantly improves symptoms and lung function test results. This low dosage with a short duration of treatment has the potential to minimise the side effects of corticosteroids. This study opened the possibility of performing prospective studies that compare long- and short-term treatment plans, low and high doses, and the side effects and recurrence of the disease for each method of treatment.

Even so, it is clear that there is no standardisation in the treatment of pulmonary sarcoidosis, and this is due to the lack of clinical trials. The majority of published studies are not blinded, randomised, or controlled, and involve a very small number of patients, using different doses or lengths of treatment and different endpoints (McKinzie et al., 2010).

For these reasons, Schutt et al. (Schutt et al., 2010) used the Delphi research technique. The Delphi method uses an expert panel with a voting system in order to reach a consensus in special situations in which insufficient data exists in order to come to an objective conclusion. The aim of this study was to gather a panel of experts in the treatment of pulmonary sarcoidosis to formulate a consensus whenever possible, using rigorous Delphi methods including interactive questions and feedback for previous responses. The conclusions from this study of expert opinions were the following: 1) oral corticosteroids are the initial treatment recommended for pulmonary sarcoidosis; 2) it is not recommended to start concomitant treatment using inhaled corticosteroids as a general practice; 3) treating pulmonary sarcoidosis with dosages >40mg of prednisolone or equivalent does not provide any additional benefit; 4) regarding the treatment of chronic pulmonary sarcoidosis, the dosage should be decreased to a minimum maintenance dose of 10mg of prednisone or equivalent. The final conclusion was that methotrexate was the preferred agent for replacing or reducing the dosage of corticosteroids. Several different controversies arose in various subjects that could aid in developing future studies, as no consensus was reached 1) regarding the dosage of corticosteroids to be administered in *de novo* pulmonary sarcoidosis; 2) regarding the decision to treat or observe patients with mild sarcoidosis based on symptoms, lung function, and chest x-ray results.

This study also had several limitations. First, the use of multiple-choice questions can limit or potentially affect the responses. Second, there were experts that did not answer all questions. Third, it was not established whether all participants in the study were in fact pulmonary sarcoidosis experts. Fourth, the majority of experts worked in the USA.

2.3 Immunosuppressive agents

2.3.1 Methotrexate

Mechanism of action: Methotrexate is an immunosuppressive and anti-inflammatory agent. After corticosteroids, this is the most commonly used drug for the treatment of sarcoidosis. It is also used in other pathologies such as rheumatoid arthritis, Crohn's disease, and psoriasis.

Several studies have evaluated the efficacy of this treatment in systemic sarcoidosis (cutaneous, ocular, pulmonary, and neurological sarcoidosis) (Baughman & Lower, 1999;

Lacher, 1968; Lower & Baughman, 1990, 1995). In 2000, Baughman focused on the efficacy of methotrexate as a corticosteroid saver, performing a prospective randomised study in which one group of patients took prednisone with methotrexate and the control group took a placebo. This study demonstrated that patients treated with methotrexate required smaller amounts of prednisone after 6 months than those that took the placebo (Baughman et al., 2000).

Administration route and dosage: This medication can be administered orally or intramuscularly, using the second option as an alternative in the case of oral intolerance or a lack of response after 3-6 months of treatment. The initial dosage is 7.5mg once per week, with progressive increases until reaching 10-15mg per week. In order to decrease the level of myelosuppression associated with methotrexate, folic acid must also be administered, and liver function must be periodically checked. This drug is contraindicated in patients with chronic liver disease or chronic infection by HBV or HCV, creatinine clearance <30ml/h, or alcoholism (Saag et al., 2008)

Side effects: The most frequent side effects are leukopaenia, hepatic fibrosis, and interstitial pneumonitis (Baughman et al., 2008). In a study of 100 liver biopsies from 68 patients with sarcoidosis, 14 had changes from the use of methotrexate (Baughman et al., 2003). Other, less frequent side effects have also been described, such as baldness, cutaneous rashes, and lymphoproliferative syndrome that occasionally regresses after treatment suspension (Hoshida et al., 2007; Niitsu et al., 2010).

2.3.2 Azathioprine

Mechanism of action: Azathioprine acts on RNA synthesis from DNA and inhibits the proliferation of lymphocytes, but its mechanism of action in sarcoidosis is unclear.

Second-line drug. In 1985, Pacheco assessed the efficacy of azathioprine in 10 patients with sarcoidosis refractory to corticosteroids. Patients were treated for 6 months with 150mg azathioprine per day, and 70% of cases had clinical and radiological improvements (Pacheco et al., 1985). Currently, this drug is primarily indicated in association with corticosteroids (Baughman, 2004; Bradley et al., 2008). In a study involving 11 patients with chronic sarcoidosis, the efficacy of treatment using azathioprine as a corticosteroid saver was evaluated. Patients underwent a combined treatment for 20 months with 0.1mg/kg prednisolone along with 2mg/kg azathioprine per day, producing clinical and radiological improvements with no evidence of relevant adverse effects (abdominal pain + transitory increase in lipase levels in 1 case) (Mueller-Quernheim et al., 1999).

Administration route and dosage: Orally administered, 25mg/day, with progressive increase until reaching 2mg/kg (maximum: 200mg/day). The toxicity of azathioprine is linked to the existence of thiopurine-S-methyltransferase polymorphisms (Bakker et al., 2007).

Adverse effects: The most frequent adverse effects are: gastrointestinal discomfort, cutaneous rash, and fever. Another less frequent but more serious side effect is pancytopaenia (difficult to distinguish from suppressed bone marrow, which can occur in sarcoidosis). The patient's blood cell levels must be checked weekly while the dosage is being increased, and every 8-12 weeks during the first few months of treatment. The frequency can be decreased for long-term treatment in patients with normal levels from previous measurements.

2.3.3 Cyclophosphamide

Mechanism of action: Cyclophosphamide acts by reducing the number and function of lymphocytes, with an added anti-inflammatory effect.

This third-line drug is not frequently used as a corticosteroid saver in the treatment of sarcoidosis due to its adverse effects (Salomon et al., 1975).
Administration route and dosage: Treatment with this drug starts at 25mg-50mg/day orally, with a progressive increase until reaching white blood cell counts of 4000mm^3-7000mm^3, with twice-weekly monitoring during the first 3 months, and once per month afterwards. It has been rarely administered intravenously.
Adverse effects: The most important adverse effect is the appearance of pancytopaenia, which requires an immediate adjustment of the dosage. Other side effects are: gastrointestinal discomfort, infertility, haemorrhagic cystitis, and it has even been related to the appearance of bladder carcinomas.

2.3.4 Chlorambucil

The use of chlorambucil is very limited in the treatment of pulmonary sarcoidosis. Its mechanism of action is similar to that of cyclophosphamide, as inhibits the immune response by reducing the number of lymphocytes and other bone marrow cells. Given the relative efficacy of this drug as a corticosteroid saver (Kataria, 1980) and the important side effects (Sahgal & Sharma, 1984), it is not commonly recommended in the treatment of this disease.

2.3.5 Cyclosporine

Cyclosporine is an immunosuppressive drug that is widely used in organ transplants in order to reduce the risk of rejection. It is also used in diseases that involve T-cells, such as uveitis and rheumatoid arthritis. Its use is very limited in pulmonary sarcoidosis due to the lack of experience and its severe side effects (Wyser et al., 1997).

2.3.6 Leflunomide

Mechanism of action: Leflunomide is a cytotoxic agent used alone or in combination with methotrexate for the treatment of rheumatoid arthritis, but little experience has been gained in its use for treating pulmonary sarcoidosis. In a study published in 2004 (Baughman & Lower, 2004) that treated 32 patients using leflunomide (15 of them also were administered methotrexate), good tolerance was observed to leflunomide with a response at least as efficient as methotrexate and with lower toxicity. Its use was then recommended in patients with chronic sarcoidosis and intolerance to methotrexate, or in combination with methotrexate in patients with chronic pulmonary sarcoidosis refractory to other second-line drugs (Baughman et al., 2001).
Administration route and dosage: 20mg/day orally, starting with 10mg and increasing dosage in the presence of good tolerance.
Adverse effects: Gastrointestinal symptoms, rash, peripheral neuropathy, and hepatotoxicity (Emery et al., 2000; Savage et al., 2006; Utz et al., 2003), which increases in the case of previous hepatopathy or concomitant treatment with hepatotoxic treatments.

2.4 Immunomodulatory agents

2.4.1 Tumour necrosis factor (TNF) antagonists

- Etanercept

Utz et al started a clinical trial in which etanercept was used for the treatment of stage II-II sarcoidosis. This study was suspended due to a lack of results from the treatment, defined as progression of the disease, need for other immunosuppressive agents, or intolerance to treatment (Utz et al., 2003). Its use is not currently indicated in the treatment of sarcoidosis.

2.4.2 Monoclonal antibodies

- Infliximab

Infliximab is a monoclonal antibody with important anti-inflammatory activity. Several different studies have proven its efficacy in the treatment of pulmonary and extrapulmonary sarcoidosis refractory to corticosteroids (Baughman et al., 2006; Pritchard & Nadarajah, 2004). In a double-blind study which divided 138 patients with chronic pulmonary sarcoidosis into three groups: one treated with low doses of infliximab, other treated with placebo, and the third treated with high doses of infliximab at the start of treatment and at weeks 2, 6, 12, and 24, forced vital capacity improved during weeks 24-54, compared to initial values . There were no significant differences regarding the adverse effects produced in the three groups (Baughman et al., 2006). According to a study published in 2010 (Crouser et al., 2010), patients with decreased CD4+ T-cell count and resistance to conventional immunosuppressive treatment have a better response to this drug.

Although its long-term toxicity is still unclear, some severe complications have been associated with its use, such as the appearance of tuberculosis (Kean et al., 2001).

- Adalimumab

The experience with this drug has been limited to extrapulmonary chronic sarcoidosis (Heffernan & Smith, 2006; Patel, 2009).

2.4.3 Thalidomide

Just as in the case of the previous drug, the use of thalidomide has only been described in the treatment of extrapulmonary sarcoidosis, mainly the cutaneous form (Baughman et al., 2002). Its use in pulmonary sarcoidosis appears to provide no benefit, as was observed in a study by Judson et al. published in 2006, in which no clinical improvements were documented, and dosage had to be reduced in 9 out of the 10 patients due to adverse effects produced, including excessive somnolence and peripheral neuropathy (Judson et al., 2006).

2.4.4 Pentoxifylline

In a clinical trial by Zabel et al., they observed a positive response to treatment with pentoxifylline in patients with acute pulmonary sarcoidosis (Zabel et al., 1997) although no studies currently exist testing its use in chronic sarcoidosis.

2.5 Antimalarial agents

2.5.1 Chloroquine and hydroxychloroquine

These drugs have been used for the treatment of chronic sarcoidosis for many years (British Tuberculosis Association, 1967). They have a low level of toxicity, and have proven effective in treating cutaneous sarcoidosis (Siltzbach & Teirstein, 1964). Some studies also exist in which these drugs have been used to treat pulmonary sarcoidosis (Chloroquine in pulmonary sarcoidosis, 1968). Bazan et al. (Baltzan et al., 1999) studied the use of chloroquine to treat chronic sarcoidosis. After treating 18 patients for 6 months, treatment was continued with a group of patients with a slower decrease in FEV1 and diffusion capacity, but no changes in forced vital capacity were registered, although important adverse effects were produced in 13% of cases.

Administration route and dosage: The commonly used dosage is 250mg-750mg/day, taken orally for 6 months or 9 months.

Side effects: The most severe side effect is irreversible retinopathy and blindness, therefore, ophthalmologic follow-up is necessary at the start of treatment and after 6 months.

2.6 Conclusions

In patients with chronic pulmonary sarcoidosis in which treatment with corticosteroids has not been sufficient, or when the patient has intolerance to the drug or it is causing severe adverse effects, intensification of the therapy is indicated using methotrexate, azathioprine, or leflunomide (stage IIB). The first choice drug is methotrexate due to the greater experience gained in the treatment of pulmonary sarcoidosis using this drug. If the patient has intolerance or it does not produce a positive response, the use of leflunomide or azathioprine is recommended, and can occasionally lead to a reduced need or even cessation of treatment with corticosteroids.

Given that all of the previously mentioned drugs imply severe side effects such as myelosuppression with predisposition to opportunistic infections and hepatotoxicity, their use must be evaluated on an individual basis. Before starting treatment with methotrexate, azathioprine, and leflunomide, the patient must undergo liver function, haemogram, and creatinine tests. Also, hepatitis B and C tests must be performed before starting treatment with methotrexate and leflunomide.

In patients in which treatment with immunosuppressive agents with or without corticosteroids is insufficient, two different second-line drugs may be combined, or administered along with a TNF antagonist, which should be decided upon according to patient characteristics.

Before starting treatment with a TNF antagonist, the patient must also be screened for tuberculosis, hepatitis B, and hepatitis C.

Because of their mechanisms of action, many of the drugs proposed for the treatment of chronic sarcoidosis are not commonly used due to their secondary side effects (colchicine, chlorambucil, cyclophosphamide, cyclosporine, and pentoxifylline).

3. Follow-up

Patients with sarcoidosis must have a periodical follow-up regimen with a specialist. The lung is the primary organ affected by the disease, and so a pneumologist must be involved in the follow-up process. The BTS recommends a multi-disciplinary follow-up by clinics that specialise in interstitial lung diseases (Bradley et al., 2008). Check-ups must be performed initially every 3-6 months, or more frequently if drug treatment is started. Patients with clinically stable disease can be seen less frequently. Patients with stage II-IV must continue with an indefinite follow-up period, whereas patients with mild levels of the disease (stage 0 or I) can be discharged from the follow-up after 2 years. In these check-ups, the patient should undergo clinical (signs and symptoms), radiological (chest x-ray as the primary tool), and functional (respiratory function) tests. The follow-up protocol may also require laboratory analyses (especially if the patient had a previous case of hypercalcaemia, renal or liver involvement, or if tests show some type of alteration in serum angiotensin-converting enzyme). Patients rarely develop progressive pulmonary sarcoidosis with failed pharmacological treatment. In this case, the next step would be a lung transplant.

4. References

Alberts C, Van der Mark TW, & Jansen HM. (1995). Inhaled budesonide in pulmonary sarcoidosis: a double-blind, placebo-controlled study. *Eur Respir J*, Vol. 8, pp. 682–68, ISSN 7656936

American Thoracic Society. Statement on sarcoidosis. (1999). *Am J Resp Crit Care Med,* Vol. 160, pp. 736-755.

Bakker JA, Drent M, & Bierau J. (2007). Relevance of pharmacogenetic aspects of mercaptopurine metabolism in the treatment of interstitial lung disease. *Curr Opin Pulm Med.,* Vol. 13, No. 5, pp. 458-463, ISSN 17940494

Baltzan M, Mehta S, Kirkham TH, Cosio MG. (1999). Randomized trial of prolonged chloroquine therapy in advanced pulmonary sarcoidosis. *Am J Respir Crit Care Med,* Vol. 160, pp. 192–197, ISSN 10390399

Baughman RP, & Lower EE. (1999). A clinical approach to the use of methotrexate for sarcoidosis. *Thorax,* Vol. 54, pp. 742-6, ISSN 10413729

Baughman RP, Winget DB, & Lower EE. (2000). Methotrexate is steroid sparing in acute sarcoidosis: results of a double blind, randomized trial. *Sarcoidosis Vasc Diffuse Lung Dis,* Vol. 17, pp. 60-66, ISSN 10746262

Baughman RP, Ohmichi M, & Lower EE. (2001). Combination therapy for sarcoidosis. *Sarcoidosis Vasc Diffuse Lung Dis.,* Vol. 18, No 2, pp. 133-137, ISSN 11436533

Baughman RP, Iannuzzi MC, Lower EE, Moller DR, Balkissoon RC, Winget DB, & Judson MA. (2002). Use of fluticasone in acute symptomatic pulmonary sarcoidosis. Sarcoidosis Vasc Diffuse Lung Dis., Vol. 19, No. 3, pp. 198-204, ISSN 12405489

Baughman RP, Judson MA, Teirstein AS, Moller DR, & Lower EE. (2002). Thalidomide for chronic sarcoidosis. *Chest.,* Vol. 122, No. 1, pp. 227-232, ISSN 12114363

Baughman RP, Koehler A, Bejarano PA, Lower EE, & Weber FL Jr. (2003). Role of liver function tests in detecting methotrexate-induced liver damage in sarcoidosis. *Arch Intern Med.,* Vol. 163, pp. 615–620, ISSN 12622609

Baughman RP. (2004). Pulmonary sarcoidosis. *Clin Chest Med.,* Vol. 25; 521–530, ISSN 15331189

Baughman RP, & Lower EE. (2004). Leflunomide for chronic sarcoidosis. *Sarcoidosis Vasc Diffuse Lung Dis.,* Vol. 21, No. 1, pp. 43-48, ISSN 15127974

Baughman RP, Drent M, Kavuru M, Judson MA, Costabel U, du Bois R, Albera C, Brutsche M, Davis G, Donohue JF, Müller-Quernheim J, Schlenker-Herceg R, Flavin S, Lo KH, Oemar B, & Barnathan ES; Sarcoidosis Investigators. (2006). Infliximab Therapy in Patients with Chronic Sarcoidosis and Pulmonary Involvement. *Am J Resp Crit Care Med.,* Vol. 174, pp. 795-802, ISSN 16840744

Baughman R, Costabel U, & Bois R. (2008). Treatment of Sarcoidosis. *Clinics in Chest Medicine,* Vol. 29, No. 3, pp. 533-548, ISSN 18539243

Bradley B, Branley HM, Egan JJ, Greaves MS, Hansell DM, Harrison NK, Hirani N, Hubbard R, Lake F, Millar AB, Wallace WA, Wells AU, Whyte MK, & Wilsher ML; British Thoracic Society Interstitial Lung Disease Guideline Group, British Thoracic Society Standards of Care Committee; Thoracic Society of Australia; New Zealand Thoracic Society; Irish Thoracic Society. (2008). Interstitial lung disease guideline: the British Thoracic Society in collaboration with the Thoracic Society of Australia and New Zealand and the Irish Thoracic Society. *Thorax,* Vol. 63, Suppl. 5, pp. 1-58, ISSN 18757459

British Tuberculosis Association: Chloroquine in the treatment of sarcoidosis. (1967). *Tubercle,* Vol. 48, pp. 257–272, ISSN 4872114

Chloroquine in pulmonary sarcoidosis. (1968). *Lancet;* Vol. 1, pp. 736, ISSN 4170972

Crouser ED, Lozanski G, Fox CC, Hauswirth DW, Raveendran R, & Julian MW. (2010). The CD4+ lymphopenic sarcoidosis phenotype is highly responsive to anti-tumor necrosis factor-{alpha} therapy. *Chest.,* Vol. 137, No. 6, pp. 1432-1435, ISSN 20525654

Dempsey OJ, Paterson EW, Kerr KM, & Denison AR. (2009). Sarcoidosis. *BMJ* , Vol. 339, pp. 3206, ISSN 20534676

DuBois RM, Greenhalgh PM, Southcott AM, Johnson NM, & Harris TA. (1999). Randomized trial of inhaled fluticasone proprionate in chronic stable pulmonary sarcoidosis: a pilot study. *Eur Respir J.*, Vol. 13, pp. 1345–1350, ISSN 10445610

Emery P, Breedveld FC, Lemmel EM, Kaltwasser JP, Dawes PT, & Gömör B. (2000). A comparison of the efficacy and safety of leflunomide and methotrexate for the treatment of rheumatoid arthritis. *Rheumatology.*, Vol. 39, pp. 655-665, ISSN 10888712

Erkkila S, Froseth B, Hellstrom PE, Kaltiokallio K, Taskinen E, Viljanen A, Viljanen B, & Selroos O. (1988). Inhaled budesonide influences cellular and biochemical abnormalities in pulmonary sarcoidosis. *Sarcoidosis*, Vol. 5, pp. 106–110, ISSN 2852389

Gottlieb JE, Israel HL, Steiner RM, Triolo J, & Patrick H. (1997). Outcome in sarcoidosis. The relationship of relapse to corticosteroid therapy. *Chest*, Vol. 111, pp. 623–631, ISSN 9118698

Heffernan MP, & Smith DI. (2006). Adalimumab for Treatment of Cutaneous Sarcoidosis. *Arch Dermatol.*, Vol. 142, pp. 17-19, ISSN 16415380

Hoshida Y, Xu JX, Fujita S, Nakamichi I, Ikeda J, Tomita Y, Nakatsuka S, Tamaru J, Iizuka A, Takeuchi T, & Aozasa K. (2007). Lymphoproliferative disorders in rheumatoid arthritis: clinicopathological analysis of 76 cases in relation to methotrexate medication. *J Rheumatol.*, Vol. 34, No. 2, pp. 322-331, ISSN 17117491

Judson MA, Silvestri J, Hartung C, Byars T, & Cox CE. (2006). The effect of thalidomide on corticosteroid-dependent pulmonary sarcoidosis. *Sarcoidosis Vasc Diffuse Lung Dis.*, Vol 23, No. 1, pp. 51-57. ISSN 16933470

Kataria YP. (1980). Chlorambucil in sarcoidosis. *Chest*, Vol. 78, No. 1, pp. 36-43, ISSN 7471842

Kean J, Gershon S, Wise RP, Mirabile-Levens E, Kasznica J, Schwieterman WD, Siegel JN, & Braun MM. (2001). Tuberculosis associated with infliximab, a tumor necrosis factor-alpha neutralizing agent. *N Engl J Med*, Vol. 345, pp. 1098–1104, ISSN 11596589

King TE. (2010). Treatment of pulmonary sarcoidosis with alternatives to glucocorticoids. *Up To Date.*

Lacher MJ. (1968). Spontaneous remission response to methotrexate in sarcoidosis. *Ann Intern Med.*, Vol. 69, pp. 1247–1248, ISSN 5725738

Lower EE, & Baughman RP. (1990). The use of low dose methotrexate in refractory sarcoidosis. *Am J Med Sci.*, Vol. 299, pp. 153–157, ISSN 2316559

Lower EE, & Baughman RP. (1995). Prolonged use of methotrexate for sarcoidosis. *Arch Intern Med.*; Vol. 155, pp. 846–851. ISSN 7717793

McKinzie BP, Bullington WM, Mazur JE, & Judson MA. (2010). Efficacy of short-course, low-dose corticosteroid therapy for acute pulmonary sarcoidosis exacerbations. *Am J Med Sci.*, Vol. 339, No. 1, pp. 1-4, ISSN 19996733

Milman N, Graudal N, Grode G, & Munch E. (1994). No effect of high-dose inhaled corticosteroids in pulmonary sarcoidosis: a doubleblind, placebo- controlled study. *J Intern Med*, Vol. 236, pp. 285–290, ISSN 8077885

Mueller-Quernheim J, Kienast K, Held M, Pfeifer S, & Costabel U. (1999). Treatment of chronic sarcoidosis with an azathioprine/prednisolone regimen. *Eur Respir J.*, Vol. 14, pp. 1117-1122. ISSN 10596700

Niitsu N, Okamoto M, Nakamine H, & Hirano M. (2010). Clinicopathologic correlations of diffuse large B-cell lymphoma in rheumatoid arthritis patients treated with methotrexate. *Cancer Sci.*, Vol. 101, No. 5, pp. 1309-1313, ISSN 20210795

Pacheco Y, Marechal C, Marechal F, Biot N, & Perrin Fayolle M. (1985). Azathioprine treatment of chronic pulmonary sarcoidosis. *Sarcoidosis.*, Vol. 2, No.2, pp. 107-113, ISSN 3031790

Paramothayan NS, Lasserson TJ, & Jones PW. (2005). Corticosteroids for pulmonary sarcoidosis. *Cochrane Database Syst Rev.*, Vol. 2, CD001114

Paramothayan S, & Lasserson T. (2008). Treatments for pulmonary sarcoidosis. *Respiratory Medicine*, Vol. 102, pp. 1-9, ISSN 17954027

Patel SR. (2009). Systemic sarcoidosis with bone marrow involvement responding to therapy with adalimumab: a case report. *Journal of Medical*, Vol. 3, pp. 8573. ISSN 19830230

Pietinalho A, Tukiainen P, Haahtela T, Persson T, & Selroos O. (1999). Oral prednisolone followed by inhaled budesonide in newly diagnosed pulmonary sarcoidosis. A double-blind, placebo-controlled multicentre study. *Chest*, Vol. 116, pp. 424–431, ISSN 10453872

Pritchard C, & Nadarajah K. (2004). Tumour necrosis factor a inhibitor treatment for sarcoidosis refractory to conventional treatments: a report of five patients. *Ann Rheum Dis*, Vol. 63, pp. 318–320, ISSN 14962969

Rizzato G, Montemurro L, & Colombo P. (1998). The late follow-up of chronic sarcoid patients previously treated with corticosteroids. *Sarcoidosis Vasc Diffuse Lung Dis.*; Vol. 15, pp. 52–58. ISSN 9572002

Saag KG, Teng GC, Patkar NM, Anuntiyo J, Finney C, Curtis JR, Paulus HE, Mudano A, Pisu M, Elkins-Melton M, Outman R, Allison JJ, Suarez Almazor M, Bridges SL Jr, Chatham WW, Hochberg M, MacLean C, Mikuls T, Moreland LW, O'Dell J, Turkiewicz AM, & Furst DE; American College of Rheumatology. (2008). American College of Rheumatology 2008 recommendations for the use of non-biologic and biologic disease-modifying anti-rheumatic drugs in rheumatoid arthritis. *Arthritis Rheum.*, Vol. 59, pp. 762, ISSN 18512708

Sahgal SM, & Sharma OP. (1984). Fatal herpes simplex infection during chlorambucil therapy for sarcoidosis. *J R Soc Med*, Vol. 77, No. 2, pp. 144–146, ISSN 6737398

Salomon MI, Poon TP, Hsu KC, King EJ, & Tchertkoff V. (1975). Membranous glomerulopathy in a patient with sarcoidosis. *Arch Pathol.,*; Vol. 99, No. 9, pp. 479-483, ISSN 1100020

Savage RL, Highton J, Boyd IW, & Chapman P. (2006). Pneumonitis associated with leflunomide: a profile of New Zealand and Australian reports. *Internal Medicine Journal.*, Vol. 36, pp. 162–169, ISSN 16503951

Siltzbach LE, & Teirstein AS. (1964). Chloroquine therapy in 43 patients with intrathoracic and cutaneous sarcoidosis. *Acta Medica Scandinavica*; Vol. 176, pp. 302-308, ISSN 5884512

Schutt AC, Bullington WM, & Judson MA. (2010). Pharmacotherapy for pulmonary sarcoidosis: a Delphi consensus study. Respir Med., Vol. 104, No. 5, pp. 717-723, ISSN

Utz JP, Limper AH, Sanjay Kalra, et al. (2003). Etanercept for the Treatment of Stage II and III Progressive Pulmonary Sarcoidosis. *Chest*, Vol. 124, pp. 177-185, ISSN 20089389

Wyser CP, Schalwyk EM, Berthold A, Bardin PG, & Joubert JR. (1997). Treatment of Progressive Pulmonary Sarcoidosis with Cyclosporin A. *Am. J. Respir. Crit. Care Med.*, Vol. 156, No. 5, pp. 1371-1376, ISSN 9372647

Zabel P, Entzian P, Dalhoff K, & Schlaak M. (1997). Pentoxifylline in treatment of sarcoidosis. *Am J Respir Crit Care Med.*, Vol. 155, pp. 1665–1669, ISSN 9154873

8

Prognostic Factors in Sarcoidosis

Wojciech J. Piotrowski
Division of Pneumology and Allergy, Department of Internal Medicine, Medical University of Lodz, Poland

1. Introduction

Sarcoidosis is a multisystem disorder of unknown etiology. Inflammation mediated by lymphocytes of Th1 phenotype leads to formation of non-caseating granulomas, consisting of epithelioid and multinucleated giant cells. In the majority of patients it affects intrathoracic lymph nodes and lungs, but all organs may be involved (ATS, ERS, WASOG Statement on Sarcoidosis). The overall prognosis is good, and in about 60 % of all cases the disease regresses spontaneously. In the rest of patients, sarcoidosis is a chronic disease, sometimes showing up with relapses, which often follow withdrawal or dose reduction of steroids (Gottlieb et al., 1997; Neville et al., 1983; Scadding, 1961). In about 10-15 % it slowly progresses to lung fibrosis, which is the major cause of death, affecting less than 1 % of patients in Europe and up to 5% in North America. The immunopathological concepts on sarcoidosis describe mechanisms leading to induction of granuloma formation, mechanisms responsible for prolongation and sustaining of inflammation, and mechanisms responsible for fibrosis (the latter are the worse recognized). Although the etiology of sarcoidosis is unknown, it is generally acknowledged that the disease develops in genetically predisposed subjects who were exposed to unidentified (presumably inhaled) antigen(s). This unidentified "sarcoid factor" has the ability to persist in the intracellular milieu of macrophages, which results in the production of cytokines responsible for transformation of Th0 to Th1 cells. In response, lymphocytes produce a variety of cytokines which conversely stimulate macrophages and induce their transformation to granuloma cells. There is premise to speculate that the ability to eliminate the antigen from the intracellular environment is *sine qua non* of complete and definitive remission (Grunewald, 2002). Although mechanisms regulating these processes are not known, this knowledge seems to be critical for understanding the pathogenesis of persistent and progressive sarcoidosis.

Selection of patients at higher risk of lung fibrosis or other unfavorable outcomes at the early stages of disease is a hard task for a physician. There are no objective tests which would be helpful in this matter. Some prognostic factors important for a certain ethnic group may be useless in another. The most important question is whom to treat, and how to treat to achieve the best final cost/effect ratio.

Statement on Sarcoidosis, a document published by ATS, ERS and WASOG in 1999, lists a number of clinical factors of prognostic significance. These factors include: lupus pernio, chronic uveitis, age of onset >40 yr, chronic hypercalcemia, nephrocalcinosis, black race, progressive pulmonary sarcoidosis, nasal mucosal involvement, cystic bone lesions, neurosarcoidosis, myocardial involvement and chronic respiratory insufficiency. Different prognostic factors of real or potential clinical relevance will be discussed in this chapter.

2. Radiology

2.1 Chest X-ray

In the 50's, two radiologists, Nitter and Wurm (DeRemee, 1983; Nitter, 1953; Wurm et al, 1958) proposed a three-stage classification system based on chest X-ray (1-enlarged lymph-nodes alone; 2- enlarged lymph-nodes plus parenchymal changes; 3- parenchymal changes without signs of intrathoracic lymph-nodes involvement). Today, a five-stage radiological classification is in use. It is ascribed to Scadding, who added stage 0 (for patients with normal chest X-ray) and stage IV (for patients with signs of irreversible lung fibrosis) (Scadding, 1961).

Scadding was one of the first to report on the influence of radiological stage on the long-term prognosis. He found that after > 5-years follow-up, 84% of patients with initial radiological stage I experienced complete radiological remission and even in the situation when hilar enlargement persisted, patients presented only with mild symptoms or were asymptomatic. In stage II, radiological remissions were observed in 58% of patients, and in stage III (clearly separated from stage IV) this percentage was as high as 43% (in later studies the chance of spontaneous remission in this stage was estimated at 10-20%). Of note, there were no remissions in the group with radiological signs of fibrosis (stage IV), and only in this group did sarcoidosis-related deaths occur. Many authors further confirmed the adverse relationship between III/IV radiological stage and worse long-term prognosis. Reich, in his meta-analysis (Reich, 2002), estimated that sarcoidosis mortality is 4.8% in referral centers and 0.5% in population-based settings, and is attributed to stage III/IV radiological stage. Viskum and Vestbo (1993) reported on their results of a 27-year follow-up study of 254 sarcoidosis patients, showing that radiological stage III was related to excess mortality. The authors also proved that early clearance of chest X-ray is a good prognostic factor.

Staging based on the chest X-ray remains the main clinico-radiological classification of sarcoidosis, but limitations are evident, and include: low sensitivity in determining small lymph nodes and tiny parenchymal shadows, problems with differentiation between parenchymal granulomatous infiltrations from signs of fibrosis, and relatively low levels of agreement between examiners (Baughman et al, 2009). Advantages of chest X-ray-based classification are: low costs, low radiation dose per one examination, general availability of a chest X-ray, and paradoxically, low sensitivity (what allows a clinician a first-glance diagnosis).

2.2 Computed tomography

Contrast-enhanced CT scans may be helpful in diagnosis of hilar/mediastinal lymphadenopathy, differentiating lymph nodes from vessels, and in all cases where there is a threat of malignancy. However, the presence of adenopathy, in contrast to parenchymal changes, is not an adverse risk factor for unfavorable outcome. Therefore, high resolution computed tomography (HRCT), which enables a precise estimation of the extent of pulmonary involvement and a detailed qualitative description of parenchymal changes, may be more useful as a tool for disease severity evaluation. Drent et al (2003) proposed a simple classification of HRCT signs based on the presence and extent of the most frequent findings in sarcoidosis patients: thickening or irregularity of the bronchovascular bundle, intra-parenchymal nodules, septal and nonseptal lines, and parenchymal consolidation, including ground-glass opacifications. The authors found that patients with higher total

HRCT scores were more likely to have worse lung function parameters and abnormal gas exchange. They found HRCT superior to chest X-ray in depicting respiratory disability. Thickening of bronchovascular bundle and septal/nonseptal lines were especially linked to worse spirometric values and gas exchange parameters. Interestingly, "clear" lung parenchyma did not rule out abnormal gas exchange. Other authors confirmed that patients with extensive bronchovascular bundle thickening are at increased risk of developing irreversible bronchial obstruction (Handa et al., 2006). Another group of authors evaluated HRCT initially and after a mean follow-up period of 7.4 years in 40 patients and concluded that predominant small and multiple large nodules in the majority of cases disappeared or decreased in size, whereas ground-glass opacities and consolidations evolved into honeycombing. In addition, significant functional and respiratory impairment accompanied this evolution (Akira et al, 2005). Abehsera et al (2000) defined three CT signs of definitive lung fibrosis in patients suffering from stage IV disease: bronchial distortion, honeycombing and linear patterns. Emphysematous pattern is rare, but should be added to the list of possible irreversible radiologic changes in stage IV sarcoidosis (Akira et al, 2005). These and other reports (Malaisamy et al, 2009) indicate that small disseminated nodules (the most frequent finding in lung parenchyma of sarcoidosis patients) and also confluent nodes are potentially reversible, whereas others may represent fibrosis at different stages of evolution. Therefore, HRCT scans may be useful in predicting the outcomes of patients with pulmonary sarcoidosis.

3. Lung function tests and other measures of functional disability

3.1 Lung function tests

The risk of lung function impairment is greater in patients with a more advanced radiological stage. However, the disparity between radiological signs of parenchymal involvement and lung function tests results is quite common in sarcoidosis. It has been estimated that normal spirometry (vital capacity) may be seen in up to 80% of patients with stage I and 35% of patients with stage II and III (Winterbauer & Hutchinson, 1980]. A restrictive pattern of ventilatory impairment occurs in about 30-50% of all sarcoidosis patients. Atypical to other interstitial lung diseases, a significant proportion of patients present with bronchial obstruction. In one series from Japan, the percentage of patients with FEV_1/FVC <70% was 8.8, and was associated with radiographic stage IV, higher age, smoking, and thickened bronchovascular bundles on CT (Handa et al., 2006). Other authors reported a much higher incidence of bronchial obstruction (Kieszko et al., 2004; Sharma & Johnson, 1988). Harrison et al. estimated that bronchial obstruction at different levels of the bronchial tree is the most common functional abnormality in sarcoidosis (Harrison et al., 1999). Bronchial obstruction may be independent of the parenchymal involvement, and results from the predilection to peribronchial and endobronchial formation of granulomas (Kieszko et al., 2004; Sharma & Johnson, 1988). Its frequency increases with the increasing radiological stage (Lamberto, 1985).

Initial lung function impairment has an obvious impact on long-term prognosis. In one study (Viscum & Vestbo, 1993) patients with FEV_1 <50% of predicted had an increased mortality risk of 4.2, compared to patients with FEV_1 >80%. Bronchial obstruction (FEV_1/FVC<70%) increased the mortality risk to 1.9. Also, patients with lung restriction defined as TLC<80% of predicted value had an increased mortality risk (RR=2.6). Other authors in a long-term follow-up study (Mañá et al., 1996) found that initial FVC<80% of predicted value is a strong predictor of persistent disease (RR=2.17).

Regardless of the evident negative prognostic value of impaired lung function test results at the initial evaluation, it was shown by many authors that in some patients these abnormalities are potentially reversible after long term observation. Approximately 80% of subjects had an improved or stable FVC and FEV_1 after two years follow-up. Interestingly, changes in FVC alone were found unreliable as descriptors of pulmonary status, as they did not fully correspond to radiological changes or symptoms (Judson et al., 2003). Although bronchial obstruction (FEV_1/FVC <70%) is a strong predictor of unfavorable outcome, it was shown that when it is attributed merely to bronchial sarcoid granulomas, it may be completely or partially reversible with immunosuppressive treatment in >70% of patients (Lavergne et al., 1999). Bronchial obstruction related to other mechanisms like bronchial scarring, airway distortion secondary to interstitial fibrosis, or other mechanisms may be burdened with a much worse prognosis.

3.2 Diffusion capacity

Diffusion capacity for carbon monoxide (DLCO) is a measure frequently used to estimate the severity of lung parenchymal involvement. DLCO disturbances may result from deprivation of gas exchange area, increase of barrier thickness or ventilation-perfusion mismatching. According to general understanding, DLCO is a very sensitive marker and its decrease may herald the development of irreversible fibrosis. It may be especially useful in monitoring of disease progression or regression (spontaneous or resulting from treatment). It was shown to be a good predictor of gas exchange abnormalities at exercise; moreover, from the two components of DLCO (alveolar membrane diffusing capacity and pulmonary capillary blood volume), the effect was rather related to the "membrane" component (Lamberto, 1985). However, the vascular component may also be important, as DLCO<60% predicted was proven to be a strong predictor of pulmonary hypertension in sarcoidosis (Bourbonnais & Samavati., 2008). Unfortunately, DLCO also has some limitations. DLCO may represent transient gas transfer impairment, especially in patients with stage I or II with low grade parenchymal lung disease, where gas exchange may be altered by reversible mechanisms. Dunn et al. reported that DLCO of idiopathic pulmonary fibrosis (IPF) patients was significantly lower comparing to sarcoidosis patients; regardless the comparison was performed in patients with the same level of lung volume impairment. This observation suggests that diffusing capacity may not be a sensitive indicator of pulmonary pathology in sarcoidosis since lung volume can be altered independently of abnormalities in the diffusing capacity (Dunn et al., 1988).

3.3 Six-minute walk test

The six-minute walk test (6MWT) is a simple test used to assess the exercise capacity in patients suffering from different respiratory and heart diseases. Changes in exercise capacity may be due to such factors as lung function, cardiac status, respiratory and skeletal muscle strength. Its role in the clinical assessment of sarcoidosis is still growing. In one series of patients, six-minute walk distance (6MWD) <400 m was documented in >50% of patients (Baughman et al., 2007). Several factors were associated with reduced results of the test, including FVC, oxygen saturation with exercise and self-reported respiratory health (Baughman et al., 2007). Some authors suggest that distance-saturation product (DSP), which is a result of the 6MWD multiplied by the lowest oxygen saturation, better reflects the functional status in patients with sarcoidosis, and it was shown to correlate with female gender, pulmonary function parameters (especially FEV_1), partial pressure of oxygen, Borg dyspnea score, lung fibrosis on HRCT, pulmonary hypertension and systemic therapy (Alhamad et al., 2010). The impaired exercise tolerance in sarcoidosis may be explained at least in part by reduced peripheral muscle strength (Marcellis et al., 2011). Patients with sarcoidosis-associated pulmonary hypertension walk shorter distances and desaturate during the 6MWT. Desaturation <90% during the test was shown to be a very strong predictor of sarcoidosis-associated pulmonary hypertension (Bourbonnais & Samavati, 2008).

Alveolar-arterial oxygen pressure gradient ($P(A-a)O_2$) during exercise may be useful in selection of patients demanding immunosuppressive treatment. Of note, impaired gas exchange during exercise also occurred in some patients with normal spirometry and DLCO. Good correlation was observed with radiological staging (Kollert et al., 2011).

4. Bronchoalveolar lavage (BAL) cells

The typical finding in sarcoidosis is an increase of BAL lymphocyte count, displayed by 80-90% of patients at the time of initial diagnosis. The lymphocyte percentage is an activity marker, and an average increase in active disease reaches 30-60%, but higher percentages are also observed. About 60% of patients have a CD4/CD8 ratio above 3.5, which is highly specific for sarcoidosis. Sensitivity of both high BAL lymphocyte percentage and CD4/CD8 ratio is however, unacceptably low (Costabel, 1998).

It was shown that lymphocytic alveolitis is an unstable feature, because in 75% of initial high intensity alveolitis the lymphocyte BAL content spontaneously dropped and in 12% of patients with initial low-grade alveolitis it spontaneously reverted to high intensity alveolitis after approximately 6-month follow-up observation. In the latter case, the increase of BAL lymphocyte percentage was frequently followed by the deterioration in at least one lung function parameter at the next 6-month follow-up examination (Keogh et al., 1983). According to the majority of authors, high BAL lymphocytes are not connected with worse long-term prognosis, and may even determine a subpopulation of patients with evidently better prognosis (Tahanovich et al., 2003). BAL lymphocytes >35 % predicted a good response to treatment, as indicated by an increase in FVC value in >90% of patients, whereas patients with low-intensity alveolitis deteriorated in 50% of cases, regardless of the treatment (Hollinger et al., 1985). Many authors did not find any differences in BAL lymphocytes content between subgroups of different prognosis as defined by radiological stage, chronicity or other factors (Vidal Serrano et al., 2005; Ziegenhagen et al., 2003); whereas some authors report higher intensity alveolitis in patients with stage I comparing to stage III (Danila et al., 2008; Verstraeten et al., 1990). Follow-up studies clearly show the lack of negative prognostic value of high lymphocyte content in BAL. The recovery of lymphocytes in lavage fluid had no prognostic value for persistent disease in the over two-year follow-up studies (Bjermer et al., 1988; Verstraeten et al., 1990).

High content of CD4 lymphocytes or high CD4/CD8 ratio in BAL are more relevant markers of activity comparing to total lymphocyte BAL percentage (Costabel, 1998). Patients who improved radiologically had higher numbers of CD4 cells and higher CD4/CD8 ratio comparing to patients who deteriorated or remained unchanged (Verstraeten et al., 1990). Also, patients with higher CD4/CD8 at initial diagnosis responded better to treatment (Baughman et al., 1984; Płodziszewska et al., 2000).

The detailed characterization of BAL lymphocyte subpopulations by flow cytometry may be promising in description of patients with worse prognosis. For instance, lymphocytes with higher expression of CD95, an apoptotic molecule (Fas), were found in unexpectedly high amount on the surface of BAL lymphocytes from patients with progressive sarcoidosis (Ozdemir et al., 2007). Increased number of Th17 cells may be predictive for progressive sarcoidosis and may help in selecting patients under increased risk of lung fibrosis (Facco et al., 2011). As yet, lymphocytes subpopulations other than CD4 and CD8 are not in everyday use in clinical practice.

Several authors report on the possible prognostic value of BAL neutrophils. Patients with stage 3 had higher concentrations of BAL neutrophil elastase than patients with stage 1 or 2 (Danila et al., 2008; Peros-Golubcić et al., 2001). The length of disease duration correlated with the lung lavage neutrophil counts (Peros-Golubcić et al., 2001). It was shown that patients with lower neutrophil count in BAL have a greater chance to recover spontaneously (Drent et al., 1999). Ziegenhagen et al reported on significantly elevated percentage of BALF neutrophils in patients with progressive disease, and found that increased percentage of neutrophils in BAL >3% may predict the future necessity of treatment (Ziegenhagen et al., 2003).

Some authors reported on possible prognostic value of increased BALF eosinophils (Danila et al., 2008; Ziegenhagen et al., 2003) and mast cells (Bjermer et al., 1988). Patients with high percentage of neutrophils and eosinophils in BAL fluid more frequently have gas exchange impairment on exercise (Kollert et al., 2011).

5. Laboratory markers

A huge number of biochemical and immunological markers have been evaluated so far in the context of diagnosis, estimation of activity or prognosis. The most frequently used biological materials are serum and BAL fluid, but some new possibilities emerged recently, for instance, exhaled breath condensate (EBC) analysis (Piotrowski et al., 2007; Psathakis et al., 2004). These markers include substances that are directly produced by granuloma cells (angiotensin converting enzyme, ACE) or that result from their metabolic activity (increased serum and urinary calcium due to increased rate of hydroxylation of vitamin D), or acute phase reactants (CRP), or various immunological markers involved in initiation and propagation of granulomatous inflammation (cytokines, soluble receptors, lipid peroxidation products, other mediators).

5.1 Angiotensin converting enzyme (ACE)

Angiotensin converting enzyme is a product of active granuloma cells. It has been the most widely used laboratory marker in sarcoidosis, as it was shown to correlate with the total volume of granulomas within an organism. Unfortunately, it is neither specific nor sensitive. Its serum concentration is elevated only in about 60% of patients with active sarcoidosis (Gupta et al., 1979), and high concentrations were reported in patients with lung diseases other than sarcoidosis (Farber et al., 1980; Studdy et al., 1978). Moreover, its levels may be influenced by polymorphism of the ACE gene (Arbustini et al., 1996). SACE concentrations were proven to correlate with the extent of lung parenchymal infiltrations (Studdy et al., 1980). It was also shown to normalize in response to treatment and to follow spontaneous remissions (Pietinalho et al., 1999; Planck et al., 2003; Studdy et al., 1978; Studdy et al., 1980). It correlates with BAL lymphocytes, although it was shown to be inferior comparing to BAL lymphocyte count in differentiating active from inactive disease (Rossman et al., 1982). Patients with stage I sarcoidosis and low SACE levels seem to have better prognosis than patients with the same radiological stage and elevated SACE concentrations (DeRemee & Rohrbach, 1984; Krychniak-Soszka & Kuś, 2002). According to some authors, SACE may help to differentiate patients with stable and persistent or progressive disease (Mañá et al., 1996), but other authors do not confirm this observation (Rust et al., 1985; Ziegenhagen et al., 2003). Therefore, it may be concluded that the role of SACE in predicting the course of sarcoidosis is limited.

5.2 Altered calcium metabolism

25-hydroxyvitamin D undergoes 1α-hydroxylation to form more active 1,25 dihydroxyvitamin D, and granuloma cells possess high amounts of 25-hydroxyvitamin D-1α-hydroxylase, responsible for this conversion (Bell et al., 1979). Elevated serum calcium concentrations may be found in about 11% of patients with sarcoidosis, abnormal urinary calcium loss in about 40 % of patients, and nephrocalcinosis in about 10 % [Ianuzzi et al., 2007]. Severe abnormalities in calcium metabolism, like persistent hypercalcemia, may bear serious and sometimes life-threatening consequences and constitute an independent indication to treatment (ATS, ERS, WASOG Statement on Sarcoidosis, 1999). Therefore, hypercalcemia *per se* is a factor which may potentially worsen the prognosis. Altered calcium metabolism is more frequent in patients with more advanced and chronic lung sarcoidosis and in those with extrapulmonary disease (Neville et al., 1983). Also, chronic nephrocalcinosis in the course of sarcoidosis is usually linked to a chronic course and often an unfavorable outcome (Neville et al., 1983).

5.3 Acute phase reactants

Serum C-reactive protein (CRP) is elevated in almost all patients with Löfgren syndrome and is frequently normal in asymptomatic patients and those with more advanced disease (Rothkrantz-Kos et al., 2003; Mert et al., 2007). Therefore it may not be linked to worse prognosis in the crude population of sarcoidosis patients. In chronic sarcoidosis, however, elevated CRP may identify a subpopulation of patients with more extensive and severe disease. It may also be helpful in identifying patients with better response to treatment with the anti-TNF agent, infliximab (Sweiss et al., 2010).

Serum amyloid A (SAA) is another acute phase reactant which is related to HDL-cholesterol. Its diagnostic value in sarcoidosis is similar to CRP (Rothkrantz-Kos et al., 2003), but recent data show its potential role in the pathogenesis of sarcoidosis, as it was shown to be deposited in granuloma cells. This molecule is capable of triggering the release of cytokines through an interaction with toll-like receptor 2 (Chen et al., 2010). This may be one of mechanisms responsible for chronicity of inflammation, but the clinical value of SAA in predicting the chronic course of sarcoidosis is unknown. Patients suffering from sarcoidosis-related fatigue did not have higher concentrations of CRP and SAA in serum (de Vries et al., 2004).

The level of immunoglobulins is elevated in serum (and BAL) in above 50 % of patients (Bergmann et al., 1997). Circulating immune complement binding complexes are detected in 67% of patients (Schoenfeld et al. 1994). Hyperglobulinemia was shown to influence the persistence of activity over time in one study (Maña et al., 1996).

5.4 Other immunological markers

Neopterin is a product of macrophages, and its serum concentration may reflect the level of macrophage stimulation. The exact biological role of this pro-inflammatory mediator is unclear. Among others, it was shown to induce intercellular adhesion molecule (ICAM-1) in type 2 pneumocytes, and it may contribute to prolongation of the inflammatory response (Hoffman et al., 1999). Serum neopterin level is higher in patients with progressive sarcoidosis compared to patients with stable disease or Löfgren syndrome (Ziegenhagen et al., 2003). In patients who experienced spontaneous regression, the concentration of neopterin decreased with time (Planck et al., 2003).

Soluble receptor of IL-2 (sIL2R) is a marker of T-cell activation, and is a reliable activity marker in sarcoidosis. Similarly to neopterin, it was elevated in progressive rather than in stable disease or patients with Löfgren syndrome (Ziegenhagen et al., 2003). It was shown to be the most reliable activity marker when compared with hsCRP (hs for high sensitivity), SACE and SAA (Rothkrantz-Kos et al., 2003). The same authors reported that only 7 of 31 untreated patients with low sIL2R values, but 8 of 11 with high sIL2R values needed treatment in follow-up observation (meaning that 73 % of patients with high values, but only 23% of patients with low sIL2R had less favorable outcome). Both sIL2R and neopterin were increased in sera of patients who needed treatment in a follow-up, and this effect was especially strongly pronounced in a subgroup of patients with acute symptoms, indicating a rare subpopulation of severe acute sarcoidosis at high risk of progression (Prasse et al., 2008).

Another product of inflammatory cells is a mucin-like high molecular weight glycoprotein KL-6. It was shown to be superior to other markers, such as SAA, sIL2R, lysozyme, and SACE in predicting chronic course. It was the best to reflect the level of lymphocytic alveolitis and was the only marker which predicted a progressive parenchymal disease (Miyoshi et al., 2010). In another study, KL-6 in serum inversely correlated with lung function parameters and DLCO, and highest concentrations were associated with persistence and progression of parenchymal infiltrates (Janssen et al., 2003).

A huge number of other immunological markers were evaluated in the context of prognosis and outcome in sarcoidosis. Tumor necrosis factor (TNF)-α is produced spontaneously by lung macrophages and T cells at the site of inflammation, whereas peripheral cells are quiescent (Müller-Quernheim et al., 1998; Rastogi et al., 2011). It is one of the key cytokines for granuloma formation, and its importance was documented by the effectiveness of anti-TNF agents in the treatment of refractory sarcoidosis. In one study, low TNF-α levels in BAL fluid were shown to better predict poor outcome, rather than high concentrations. In this context, TNF-α seems to behave like an acute phase reactant, as the highest concentrations were detected in patients with Löfgren syndrome, and were accompanied by high concentrations of IL-6 and higher percentage of lymphocytes in BAL (Tahanovich et al., 2003). Other authors do not confirm such a relationship. Ziegenhagen et al. (2002) found exaggerated release of TNF-α from BAL macrophages in corticosteroid-resistant sarcoidosis. Other authors have recently shown reduced expression of Th1 cytokines, including TNF-α, in HLA-DRB1*0301 positive patients characterized by excellent prognosis (Idali et al., 2006).

Interferon (IFN)-γ is another Th1 related cytokine, indispensible for granuloma formation (Müller-Quernheim et al., 1998). It is a key cytokine in sarcoid inflammation. Treatment with interferons may induce sarcoidosis (Papaioannides et al., 2004). Its BAL concentrations are correlated to CD4/CD8 ratio (Kopiński et al., 2007). BAL levels of IFN- γ and IL-12 (a strong stimulant of IFN production) were significantly higher in sarcoidosis patients comparing to systemic sclerosis or IPF, diseases of much worse prognosis (Meloni et al., 2004). A group of IFN-inducible chemokines may be responsible for sustaining the inflammation. These cytokines are called CXCR3 ligands due to a common affinity to

CXCR3 receptor, include monokines induced by IFN-γ - MIG (CXCL9), IFN-γ-inducible protein 10 - IP-10 (CXCL10) and IFN-γ-inducible T-cell α chemoattractant - ITAC (CXCL11). These chemokines may be elevated in BAL or serum of sarcoidosis patients, and the trend towards higher concentrations in patients with more advanced radiological stage in opposition to patients with Löfgren syndrome was noticed (Busuttil et al., 2009; Nishioka et al., 2007). Potential usefulness of these cytokines as prognostic markers merit further study.

Interleukin (IL)-18 is a monocyte/macrophage derived cytokine, playing an important role in induction of Th1 response. It is a very strong IFN-γ inducing factor. IL-18 level was the highest in plasma of patients with disease progression, in patients with lung interstitial changes and patients with extrapulmonary manifestation of the disease (Kieszko et al., 2007). Chitotriosidase, an enzyme secreted by activated macrophages and involved in defense against chitin-containing pathogens, was shown to correlate with the extent of lung changes, as assessed by radiological staging (Grosso et al., 2004). Higher serum vascular endothelial growth factor (VEGF) concentrations were found in patients with severe sarcoidosis who deserved treatment and in patients with extrapulmonary sarcoidosis (Sekiya et al., 2003).

Another example of a biological marker of potential prognostic value is tryptase, which was elevated in serum of sarcoidosis patients, and the highest values were detected in subjects with progressive disease (Bargagli et al., 2009). In another study, it was found that patients with positive collagenase activity in BAL are more likely to require therapy, and had worse pulmonary function tests at initial evaluation (Ward et al., 1990).

8-Isoprostane, a product of non-enzymatic peroxidation of arachidonic acid, is elevated in BAL (Montuschi et al., 1998) and exhaled breath condensate (EBC) of patients with sarcoidosis, and a trend towards higher levels was noticed in patients with parenchymal disease. Patients with low concentrations of 8-isoprostane in EBC were more likely to recover early (Piotrowski et al., 2010). These observations, however, have experimental rather than practical value.

The list of agents involved in the pathogenesis of sarcoidosis is very long and almost all may be measured in biological fluids of sarcoidosis patients. Some of them have been evaluated in clinical context as potential markers of activity and some of them have been shown to predict unfavorable outcome. In the majority of cases the knowledge on the potential prognostic value of these agents is based on single reports, and the studied groups were rather small. None of these markers, except for SACE, CRP and parameters of calcium metabolism are used in everyday clinical practice.

6. Extrapulmonary sarcoidosis

Intrathoracic lymph nodes and lungs are involved in above 90% of patients. The frequency of extrapulmonary sarcoidosis is estimated by different authors from few to above 80%, depending largely on geographical location or ethnic origin (ATS, ERS, WASOG, 1999; Ianuzzi et al., 2007). Multiorgan involvement is always connected with chronic and more severe course.

Some locations negatively influence the course due to potential serious disability or possible fatal outcome. Cardiac sarcoidosis and neurosarcoidosis are the best examples. Ocular sarcoidosis is a serious problem as it may insidiously lead to blindness. Rare examples of severe life-threatening extrapulmonary disease are renal and laryngeal sarcoidosis. A severe complication of sarcoidosis which may influence the outcome is sarcoidosis-related pulmonary hypertension.

Cardiac sarcoidosis is frequently unrecognized, as there is a great disproportion between clinical diagnosis and autopsy findings. This is a dangerous situation as unrecognized cardiac sarcoidosis may lead to sudden death (Reid, 1998). In Europe and North America cardiac sarcoidosis is the second cause of death in sarcoidosis patients. In Japan, where cardiac sarcoidosis is very frequent, it is a primary reason. Cardiac sarcoidosis is listed as one of the cardinal indications for treatment (ATS, ERS, WASOG, 1999). In one study, the survival in most patients with symptomatic cardiac disease was limited to approximately 2 years (Roberts et al., 1977), but may be much better when patients are diagnosed and treated early (Chapelon-Abric et al., 2004). New studies with use of modern diagnostic techniques (MRI, PET) provide evidence of very good prognosis in some asymptomatic patients with minimal changes in the heart (Yazaki et al., 2001).

Also, in the case of neurosarcoidosis, there is a discrepancy between clinical diagnosis and real involvement of the nervous system. Symptoms are frequently mild and unspecific and include headaches, dizziness, vertigo, etc. In about 10 % of cases, magnetic resonance images are normal (Zajicek et al., 1999). Similar to cardiac sarcoidosis, neurosarcoidosis is a cardinal indication for treatment. It is, however, important from the clinical point of view that among the various presentations of neurosarcoidosis, not all have an evidently bad prognosis. Facial nerve palsy, aseptic meningitis, isolated headache and vertigo resolve frequently without sequelae. Definitely worse prognosis is connected with spinal cord disease, optic nerve involvement, epilepsy and intracranial mass (Pawate et al., 2009; Zajicek et al., 1999).

There are several extrapulmonary locations that are not life-threatening but which are statistically associated with chronic and progressive course, and are therefore predictors of poor outcome. Examples are: lupus pernio, chronic uveitis, chronic hypercalcemia, nephrocalcinosis, nasal mucosal involvement and cystic bone lesions (Neville et al., 1983; Panselinas et al., 2010; Stagaki et al., 2009).

7. Symptoms

Löfgren syndrome, which is more frequent in younger patients, consists of arthritis, fever, erythema nodosum in a patient with hilar lymphadenopathy and forecasts a good prognosis. In about 80-90 % of these patients symptoms vanish within 2-8 weeks, and radiological changes disappear within 2 years at the latest (Maña et al., 1996). Recurrent Löfgren syndrome may occur many years after the first episode, but further episodes do not seem to worsen the prognosis (Maña et al., 2003). Erythema nodosum is a good prognostic sign, both for stage I and stage II patients (Krychniak-Soszka & Kuś, 2002). Acute symptoms at the beginning do not, however, guarantee an excellent prognosis, as about 16% of patients presenting with erythema nodosum pursued a chronic course (Neville et al., 1983).

Respiratory symptoms related to severe functional dysfunction have obvious negative prognostic value. But patients with chronic sarcoidosis frequently report non-respiratory and respiratory symptoms not necessarily connected with lung function impairment or other evident causes. The most frequent are fatigue, breathlessness, reduced exercise capacity and arthralgia, and they significantly influence the patients' quality of life (Michielsen et al., 2007). Fatigue is reported by more than 80% of patients with sarcoidosis.

Reduced exercise tolerance and fatigue are also frequent and may be unrelated to radiological stage and the degree of functional impairment (Marcellis et al., 2011).
In patients with chronic sarcoidosis, an asymptomatic course usually occurs in less severely ill patients. For instance, fatigue is more severe in patients with both pulmonary and extrapulmonary disease than in patients with only pulmonary involvement (Gvozdenovic et al., 2008) .
Other chronic symptoms, like loss of weight, sweating, or elevated body temperature, are more frequent in patients with liver involvement, but prognostic value of these symptoms is unknown.

8. Age and gender

8.1 Age

Typically, sarcoidosis is a disease of young adults, with an incidence peak between 20-29 years, and a second "smaller" peak, at least in Caucasians, in patients over 50. The disease is rare in the elderly, and very rare in children. African American patients are usually older at onset. A worse outcome in patients with disease onset >40 years was reported (Romer, 1982, as cited in ATS, ERS, WASOG, 1999). It should be taken into consideration that sarcoidosis spotted in an elderly patient is frequently the result of an asymptomatic disease which had lasted for many years. Co-morbidities, frequent in this age group (including neoplasms), may influence the general prognosis. Self-limiting disease with an acute clinical presentation more typical of younger patients may also be observed in patients over 60. On the other hand, sarcoidosis in children may be systemic, chronic, progressive and recurrent (Baculard et al., 2001; Kendig & Brummer, 1976). Lenner et al. (2002) compared clinical features of patients with disease onset < 50 and > 50 year of age, and did not find significant differences. In conclusion, although older patients deserve more thorough clinical monitoring, the influence of mere age on the course of sarcoidosis is uncertain.

8.2 Gender

Female sex is slightly overrepresented in patients suffering from sarcoidosis. Gender may also influence the clinical presentation of symptoms. For instance, in patients with acute sarcoidosis, erythema nodosum is more frequent in women, while periarticular inflammation of the ankles or ankle arthritis is more prevalent in men (Grunewald & Eklund, 2007). Women suffering from sarcoidosis experience more symptoms, lower quality of life and greater degree of functional impairment (Alhamad et al., 2010; Bourbonnais et al., 2010; De Vries et al., 1999). Women of African-American origin may have greater risk of co-morbities (Westney et al., 2007). Female gender is also associated with higher incidence of coexisting autoimmune disorders (Antonelli et al., 2006). Women with sarcoidosis are over 2 times more frequently treated in hospital than men, however this effect may be limited to black race (Foreman et al., 2006). The analysis of sarcoidosis-related mortality in the US over a period of 20 years revealed an increase in mortality related to an increase in non-Hispanic black females (Swigris et al., 2011). But gender did not predict the need for therapy at 18-24 month follow-up (Baughman et al., 2006). In a large series of patients from Finland and Japan, gender did not influence the rate of spontaneous remissions (Pietinalho et al., 2000). Also in Arabs and Asians, gender did not influence the long-term prognosis (Behbehani et al., 2006). From the cited studies it may be concluded that female gender may be linked to a worse prognosis, but this effect seems to be influenced by patients' ethnic origin, and is the most visible among African American women.

9. Genetics

The role of genetics in the pathogenesis of sarcoidosis is well acknowledged. It has been supported by occurrence of familial sarcoidosis, differences in the disease incidence between different ethnic groups and race-specific clinical features. It has been well documented that the incidence of sarcoidosis is four times higher among African Americans than among Americans of Caucasian origin. African Americans suffer from more severe disease. Higher incidence of extrapulmonary sarcoidosis, progressive sarcoidosis and sarcoidosis related deaths were reported in this population (Israel et al., 1986, ATS, ERS, WASOG, 1999). Black race is therefore a risk factor of chronic and progressive course (ATS, ERS, WASOG, 1999). In Japanese patients, the extraordinarily high frequency of cardiac and ocular sarcoidosis was reported, but the rate of spontaneous radiological remissions is much higher in this population than in Finnish patients (Pietinalho et al., 2000).

The last two decades has yielded a number of genetic studies in sarcoidosis in the context of disease susceptibility and prognosis. Polymorphisms in HLA class I and II have been the most extensively studied. The interplay between antigen, HLA class II molecules and T cell receptors seem to be critical in the initiation of the sarcoid reaction (Baughman et al., 2011). Other non HLA polymorphisms suspected to play a role in the pathogenesis of sarcoidosis include genes encoding TNF-α (Kieszko et al,.2010), TGF-β1 (Jonth et al., 2007), BTNL2 (Rybicki et al., 2005), other proinflammatory cytokines, receptors (Fridlender et al., 2010; Schürmann et al., 2008) and other agents (Salobir et al., 2007). Results of these studies do not have universal value. Some results found in a defined ethnic group may not be confirmed in another. It may be concluded, however, that HLA-DRB1 and HLA-DQB1 alleles determine the susceptibility, phenotype and outcome in different populations (Rossman et al., 2003, Rybicki et al., 2003). From a vast armamentarium of different studied HLA class II polymorphisms, some evidently influence the course and outcome of sarcoidosis. The carriage of DR17 (DRB1*0301) in Swedish sarcoidosis patients is strongly linked to the development of Löfgren syndrome, rapid resolution of radiological changes and good overall prognosis, whereas patients with DR15 and DR16 genotypes are more likely to have chronic disease (Berlin et al., 1997). HLA DR17 patients were shown to accumulate T-lymphocytes in bronchoalveolar lavage fluid expressing the T-cell receptor V gene segment AV2S3 at disease onset (suggesting stimulation with a specific antigen), and the population of these cells normalized in recovered patients (Planck et al., 2003). The latter indirectly proves that this genotype may predispose to easier elimination of an unknown antigen from macrophages, which results in a rapid remission. The better prognosis in HLA-DRB1*0301 patients may be related to reduced Th1 response in the lung (Idali et al., 2006). In one of the latest studies, the same group of authors found that in a population of Swedes suffering from sarcoidosis, HLA alleles DRB1*01 and HLA DRB1*03 protected against non-resolving disease in non-Löfgren patients, and HLA DRB1*07, DRB1*14 and DRB1*15 were more frequently associated with chronic disease (Grunewald et al., 2010). The protective influence of HLA DRB1*01 was also shown in other populations of patients coming from United Kingdom, Poland, Czech Republic, and the Netherlands (Foley et al.., 2001; Sato et al., 2010a). Interestingly, HLA DRB1*0301 is absent among Japanese patients (Sato et al., 2010). A predominant occurrence of HLA DRB1*14 and its linked DQ alleles in patients with insidious onset, chronic course, more advanced radiographic stage, and frequent relapses was also shown in Asian Indians (Sharma et al., 2003).

Interesting results are also delivered by studies on non-HLA polymorphisms. For instance, -765G>C promoter polymorphism in prostaglandin-endoperoxide synthase 2 gene, encoding a key regulatory enzyme in the synthesis of anifibrotic prostaglandin E2, may identify patients at increased risk of lung fibrosis (Hill et al., 2006). Other data suggest that the haplotype containing the -509C and codon 10T in the TGF-β1 gene predispose to more severe sarcoidosis, whereas -509T and codon 10C are protective (Jonth et al., 2007). CARD15/NOD 2 polymorphisms in the caspase recruitment domain and receptor for CC chemokine genes, which is common both in sarcoidosis and Crohn disease patients, may be responsible for severe courses of sarcoidosis (Sato et al. , 2010b). Other examples are increased risk of chronic or systemic sarcoidosis in patients with functional polymorphisms in COX-2 gene (Lopez-Campos et al., 2008), ACE gene (Tahir et al., 2007) or TNF-α gene (Kieszko et al., 2011; Sehan et al., 2008). The strong linkage was found between the -308G>A TNF-α (of positive prognostic value) and HLA DRB1*03 genes (Wijnen et al., 2010). Authors suggest that genotyping of one simple and less expensive TNF-alpha single nucleotide polymorphism can be used to predict the prognosis of pulmonary sarcoidosis in clinical practice. So far, genetic polymorphisms have not been used in clinical practice to predict the prognosis.

10. Clinical phenotypes

A variety of clinical and radiological presentations and different prognoses in patients suffering from sarcoidosis imposed the need of defining clinical phenotypes. It has been clear since the first description of acute sarcoidosis by Swedish pulmonologist Swen Löfgren that this complex of specific symptoms comprises a separate entity (Löfgren & Lundback, 1952). Patients with Löfgren syndrome are distinguished by an excellent prognosis. As described in the chapter on genetics, the susceptibility to acute sarcoidosis is determined by the carriage of a certain HLA DRB1 haplotype. In one study performed on a population of Swedish patients with acute onset of sarcoidosis, almost all patients positive for DRB1*0301/DQB1*0201 had resolving disease, whereas about half of DRB1*0301/DQB1*0201-negative patients presented with non-resolving sarcoidosis (Grunewald & Eklund, 2007). Therefore, even in so strictly defined phenotype the outcome within the group is also genetically determined.

At the other end of the spectrum of clinical presentations there is a non-resolving/progressive sarcoidosis, which is frequently accompanied by multiorgan involvement (systemic sarcoidosis). Genetic linkage analysis with clinical phenotypes revealed that genes influencing clinical presentation of sarcoidosis are likely to be different from those that underlie disease susceptibility (Rybicki et al., 2007).

Although there is no doubt that genetics play a crucial role in determining the chronicity, the type of exposure may also contribute to clinical presentation. For instance, agricultural organic dusts and wood burning was associated with significantly less likelihood of having extrapulmonary disease (Kreider et al., 2005). The "chronic" phenotype is much more poorly defined than an "acute," self-resolving phenotype. Besides, there is a variety of "intermediate" presentations in between which slip away from the definitions of these two main phenotypes. For scientific use, patients are frequently divided to "Löfgren" and "non-

Löfgren" subgroups, which reflects the obvious differences in prognosis. A novel protocol of phenotyping sarcoidosis was proposed based on these three criteria: 1. the type of onset (acute vs non-acute); 2. the need of treatment; 3. the need of long-term treatment (Prasse et al., 2008). According to these criteria, patients are further classified into 6 classes (table 1).

CLASS	DEFINITION
1	Acute onset, no need for immunosuppressive therapy
2	Acute onset, one period of treatment, not lasting longer than 1 year
3	Acute onset, need for several periods of immunosuppressive therapy or long-lasting treatment (>12 months)
4	Subacute onset, no need for immunosuppressive therapy
5	Subacute onset, one period of immunosuppressive treatment, not lasting longer than 1 year
6	Subacute onset, need for several periods of immunosuppressive treatment or long-lasting treatment (>12 mo)

Table 1. Protocol for clinical classification of sarcoidosis, proposd by Prasse et al . (2008).

The disadvantage of this classification is the need for long-term observation and lack of possibility to classify the patient to an appropriate category at the first visit. Table 2 shows clinical and laboratory features of "acute" and "chronic" phenotypes.

SELF-LIMITING DISEASE	CHRONIC DISEASE
Acute symptoms at onset	Subacute or subsidious onset
Radiological stage I and II	Radiological stage II, III, IV
Usually younger age at onset	Usually older age at onset
Acute phase reaction frequently present	Sporadic acute phase reaction
Frequent intensive lymphocytic alveolitis	Less frequent lymphocytic alveolitis, possible increased number of neutrophils and eosinophils in BAL
Systemic sarcoidosis unlikely	Systemic sarcoidosis likely
Rare altered calcium metabolism, especially rare hypercalcemia	More frequent altered calcium metabolism and nephrolithiasis

Table 2. Most important clinical features characterizing self-limiting and chronic phenotypes.

11. Conclusions

Several clinical and laboratory indices are used in everyday practice in order to estimate future prognosis in patients suffering from sarcoidosis. The most recognized are based on radiological classification and lung function test results. Patients with lung parenchymal involvement at presentation (radiological stage II and III) have worse prognosis comparing to patients with enlarged hilar/mediastinal lymhnodes only (stage I), although even in stage III spontaneous remissions are possible. The prognosis in patients with radiological signs of irreversible fibrosis (stage IV) is the worst, and these patients are at increased risk of respiratory insufficiency, death, and are potential candidates for lung transplantation. Impaired lung function at initial presentation or progressive impairment has obvious negative prognostic value. Therefore, patients presenting with progressive lung infiltrates, especially when lung function impairment coexists, are candidates for long term treatment with steroids, other immunosuppressive drugs, or alternative therapy. Both restriction, best defined as decrease of TLC , and bronchial obstruction defined as decrease of FEV_1/FVC <70%, increase the risk of unfavorable outcome, i.e. risk of death, chronic course or need of chronic treatment. Decreased diffusion capacity for CO is a sensitive and useful marker of gas transfer impairment and may predict progression of sarcoidosis-related interstitial lung disease or indicate the need for screening towards pulmonary hypertension. The six-minute walk test is a simple exercise test which allows for selection of patients at increased risk of lung fibrosis and pulmonary hypertension. Different laboratory markers have been proposed, but none has been proven to be sensitive, specific and reliable enough to become a routine clinical test. Two laboratory markers are in clinical usage: serum angiotensin converting enzyme (SACE) and indices of calcium metabolic status (serum calcium concentration and 24 hrs urinary calcium loss). SACE has limited prognostic value, but altered calcium metabolism and nephrolithiasis may indicate the risk of chronic course. Increased number and percentage of lymphocytes in bronchoalveolar fluid (BALF) is not linked to worse prognosis, but increased content of neutrophils and eosinophils may have negative value.

There is a need for better defining sarcoidosis clinical phenotypes. It is clearly visible that patients with Löfgren syndrome constitute a different entity, not only in terms of different clinical course, but also in terms of evidently better prognosis. At the other end of this clinical spectrum are patients with chronic and progressive disease and involvement of multiple organs. There is no doubt, that these phenotypes are genetically determined, and especially some HLA DRB1 and DQB1 polymorphic alleles are responsible. Future studies will probably bring new genetic methods helpful in determining self-limiting and chronic phenotypes in everyday practice. They may be a promising new tool to select patients at highest need for therapy, and those who need more attention during clinical monitoring.

12. Acknowledgements

Many thank to David Fam, a student of Medical University of Lodz, for linguistic corrections.

13. References

Abehsera, M.; Valeyre, D.; Grenier, P.; Jaillet, H..; Battesti, J.P. & Brauner, M.W. (2000). Sarcoidosis with pulmonary fibrosis: CT patterns and correlation with pulmonary function. *American Journal of Roentgenology,* Vol. 174, No. 6, (June 2000), pp. 1751-1757, ISSN 0361-803X

Akira, M.; Kozuka, T.; Inoue, Y. & Sakatani, M. (2005). Long-term follow-up CT scan evaluation in patients with pulmonary sarcoidosis. *Chest,* Vol. 127, No. 1, (January 2005), pp. 185-191, ISSN 1931-3543

Alhamad, E.H.; Shaik, S.A.; Idrees, M.M.; Alanezi, M.O. & Isnani, A.C. (2010). Outcome measures of the 6 minute walk test: relationship with physiologic and computed tomography findings in patients with sarcoidosis. *BMC Pulmonary Medicine,* Vol. 10, (August 2010), p. 42, ISSN 1471-2466

American Thoracic Society: European Respiratory Society: World Association of Sarcoidosis and Other Granulomatous Disorders. (1999). Statement on sarcoidosis. *American Journal of Respiratory and Critical Care Medicine,* Vol. 160, No. 2, (August 1999), pp. 736-55, ISSN 1073-449X

Antonelli, A.; Fazzi, P.; Fallahi, P.; Ferrari, S.M. & Ferrannini, E. (2006). Prevalence of hypothyroidism and Graves disease in sarcoidosis. *Chest,* Vol. 130, No. 2, (February 2006), ISSN 1931-3543

Arbustini, E.; Graso, M.; Leo, G.; Tinelli, C.; Fasani, R.; Diegoli, M.; Banchieri, N.; Cipriani, A.; Gorrini, M.; Semenzato, G. & Luisetti M. (1996). Polymorphism of angiotensin-converting enzyme gene in sarcoidosis. *American Journal of Respiratory and Critical Care Medicine* , Vol. 153, No. 2, (February 1996), pp. 851-854, ISSN 1073-449X

Baculard, A.; Blanc, N.; Boulé, M. ; Fauroux, B. ; Chadelat, K. ; Boccon-Gibod, L. ; Tournier, G. & Clement, A. Pulmonary sarcoidosis in children : a follow-up study. *European Respiratory Journal,* Vol. 17, No. 4, (April 2001), pp. 628-635, ISSN 1399-3003

Bargagli, E.; Mazzi, A.; Mezzasalma, F.; Perrone, A.; Olivieri, C.; Prasse, A.; Bianchi, N.; Pieroni, M.G. & Rottoli, P. (2009). The analysis of trypatse in serum of sarcoidosis patients. *Inflammation* , Vol. 32, No. 5, (October 2009), pp. 310-314, ISSN 0360-3997

Baughman, R.P.; Fernandez, M.; Boskeb, C.H.; Mantil, J. & Hurtubise, P. (1984). Comparison of gallium-67 scanning, bronchoalveolar lavage, and serum angiotensin-converting enzyme levels in pulmonary sarcoidosis. Predicting response to therapy. *American Review of Respiratory Disease,* Vol. 129, No. 5, (May 1984), pp. 676-681, ISSN 003-0805

Baughman , R.P.; Judson, M.A.; Teirstein, A.; Yeager, H.; Rossman, M.; Knatterud, G.L. & Thompson, B. (2006). Presenting characteristics as predictors of duration of treatment in sarcoidosis. *Quarterly Journal of Medicine,* Vol. 99, No. 5, (May 2006), pp. 307-315, ISSN 0033-5622

Baughman, R.P.; Shipley, R.; Desai, S.; Drent, M.; Judson, M.A.; Costabel, U.; du Bois, R.M.; Kavuru, M.; Schlenker-Herceg, R.; Flavin, S.; Hung Lo, K. & Barnathan, E.S. on behalf of the Sarcoidosis Investigators. (2009). Changes in chest roentgenogram of sarcoidosis patients during a clinical trial of infliximab therapy. *Chest,* Vol. 136, No. 2, (August 2009), pp. 526-535, ISSN 1931-3543

Baughman, R.P.; Sparkman, B.K. & Lower, E.E. (2007). Six-minute walk test and health status assessment in sarcoidosis. *Chest,* Vol. 132, No. 1, (July 2007), pp. 207-213, ISSN 1931-3543

Baughmann, R.P.; Culver, D.A. & Judson, M.A. (2011). A concise review of pulmonary sarcoidosis. *American Journal of Respiratory and Critical Care Medicine,* Vol. 183, No. 4, (February 2011), pp. 573-581, ISSN 1073-449X

Bell, N.H.; Stern, P.H.; Pantzer, E.; Sinha, T.K. & DeLuca, H.F. (1979). Evidence that increased circulating 1a,25-dihydroxyvitamin D is the probable cause for abnormal calcium metabolism in sarcoidosis. *Journal of Clinical Investigation,* Vol. 64, No. 1, (July 1979), pp. 218-225, ISSN 0021-9738

Bergmann, M.; Jonasson, S.; Klause, N,; Engler, F.; Kirsten, D. & Barth, J. (1997). Analysis of immunoglobulins in sarcoidosis. *Sarcoidosis Vasculitis and Diffuse Lung Diseases,* Vol. 14, No. (1997); pp. 139-145, ISSN 1124-0490

Berlin, M.; Fogdell-Hahn, A.; Olerup, O.; Eklund, A. & Grunewald, J. (1997). HLA-DR predicts the prognosis in Scandinavian patients with pulmonary sarcoidosis.

American Journal of Respiratory and Critical Care Medicine, Vol. 156, No. 5, (November 1997), pp. 1601-1605, ISSN 1073-449X

Bjermer, L.; Rosenhall, L.; Ångström, T. & Hällgren, R. (1988). Predictive value of bronchoalveolar lavage cell analysis in sarcoidosis. *Thorax,* Vol. 43, No. 4, (April 1988), pp. 284-288, ISSN 1468-3296

Bourbonnais, J.M. & Samavati, L. (2008). Clinical predictors of pulmonary hypertension in sarcoidosis. *European Respiratory Journal,* Vol. 32, No. 2, (August 2008), pp. 296-302, ISSN 1399-3003

Bourbonnais, J.M. & Samavati, L. (2010). Effect of gender on health related quality of life in sarcoidosis. *Sarcoidosis Vasculitis and Diffuse Lung Diseases,* Vol. 27, No.2, (2010); pp. 96-102, ISSN 1124-0490

Busuttil, A.; Weigt, S.S.; Keane, M.P.; Xue, Y.Y.; Palchevskiy, V.; Burdick, M.D.; Huang, C.; Zisman, D.A.; Fishbein, M.; Lynch III, J.P.; Strieter, R.M.; Elashoff, R.M. & Belpeiro, J.A. (2009). CXCR3 ligands are augmented during the pathogenesis of pulmonary sarcoidosis. *European Respiratory Journal,* Vol. 34, No. 3, (September 2009), pp. 676-86, ISSN 1399-3003

Chapelon-Abric, C.; de Zuttere, D.; Duhaut, P.; Veyssier, P.; Wechsler, B.; Huong, D.L.; de Gennes, C.; Papo, T.; Blétry, O.; Godeau, P. & Piette, J.C. (2004). Cardiac sarcoidosis: a retrospective study of 41 cases. *Medicine (Baltimore),* Vol. 83, No. 6, (November 2004), pp. 315-334, ISSN 0025-7974

Chen, E.S.; Song, Z.; Willett, M.H.; Heine, S.; Yung, R.C.; Liu, M.C.; Groshong, S.D.; Zhang, Y.; Tuder, R.M. & Moller, D.R. (2010). Serum amyloid A regulates grnaulomatous inflammation in sarcoidosis through Toll-like receptor-2. *American Journal of Respiratory and Critical Care Medicine* , Vol. 181, No. 4, (February 2010), pp. 360-373, ISSN 1073-449X

Costabel, U. (1998). *Atlas of bronchoalveolar lavage.* Chapman and Hall Medical, ISBN 0-412-79270-2, London, UK.

Danila, E.; Jurgauskiené, L. & Malickaité, R. (2008). BAL fluid cells and pulmonary funcion in different radiographic stages of newly diagnosed sarcoidosis. *Advances in Medical Sciences,* Vol. 53, No. 2, (December 2008), pp. 228-233, ISSN 1898-4002

De Vries, J.; Rothkrantz-Kos, S.; van Dieijen-Visser, M.P. & Drent, M. (2004). The relationship between fatigue and clinical parameters in pulmonary sarcoidosis. *Sarcoidosis Vasculitis and Diffuse Lung Diseases,* Vol. 21, No. (2004), pp. 127-136, ISSN 1124-0490

De Vries, J.; Van Heck, G.L. & Drent, M. Gender differences in sarcoidosis: symptoms, quality of life, and medical consumption. *Women & Health,* Vol.. 30, No. 2, (March 1999), pp. 99-114. ISSN 0363-0242

DeRemee, R.A. & Rohrbach, M.S. (1984). Normal serum angiotensin converting enzyme activity in patients with newly diagnosed sarcoidosis. *Chest,* Vol. 85, No.1, (January 1984), pp. 45-48, ISSN 1931-3543

DeRemee, R.A. (1983). The roentgenographic staging of sarcoidosis. Historic and contemporary perspectives. *Chest,* Vol. 83, No. 1, (January 1983), pp. 128-133, ISSN 1931-3543

Drent, M.; De Vries, J.; Lenters, M.; Lamers, R.J.S.; Rothkranz-Kos, S.; Wouters, E.F.M.; van Dieijen-Visser, M.P. & Verschakelen, J.A. (1999). Sarcoidosis: assessment of disease severity using HRCT. *European Radiology*, Vol. 13, No. 11, (November 2003), pp. 2462-2471, ISSN 1432-1084

Drent, M.; Jacobs, J.A.; de Vries, J.; Lamers, R.J.S.; Liem, I.H. & Wouters, E.F.M. (1999). Does the cellular bronchoalveolar lavage fluid profile reflect the severity of sarcoidosis? *European Respiratory Journal*, Vol. 13, No. 6, (June 1999), pp. 1338-1344, ISSN 1399-3003

Drent, M.; Wirnsberger, R.M.; de Vries, J.; van Dieijen-Visser, M.P.; Wouters, E.F. & Schols, A.M. (1999). Association of fatigue with an acute phase response in sarcoidosis. *European Respiratory Journal*, Vol. 13, No. 4, (April 1999), pp. 718-722, ISSN 1399-3003

Dunn, T.L.; Watters, L.C.; Hendrix, C.; Cherniack, R.M.; Schwartz, M.I. & King, T.E. Jr. (1988). Gas exchange at a given degree of volume restriction is different in sarcoidosis and idiopathic pulmonary fibrosis. *American Journal of Medicine* , Vol. 85, No. 2, (August 1988), pp. 221-224, ISSN 1555-7162

Facco, M.; Cabrelle, A.; Teramo, A.; Olivieri, V.; Gnoato, M.; Teolato, S.; Ave, E.; Gattazzo, C.; Fadini, G.P.; Calabrese, F.; Semenzato, G. & Agostini, C. (2011). Sarcoidosis is a Th1/Th17 multisystem disorder. *Thorax*, Vol. 66, No. 2, (February 2011), pp.144-150, ISSN 1468-3296

Farber, H.W.; Mathers, J.A. Jr. & Glauser, F.L. (1980). Gallium scans and serum angiotensin converting enzyme levels in talc granulomatosis and lymphocytic interstitial pneumonitis. *Southern Medical Journal*, Vol. 73, No. 12, (December 1980), pp. 1663-1667, ISSN 0038-4348

Foley, P.J.; McGrath, D.S.; Puścińska, E.; Petrek, M.; Kolek, V.; Drabek, J.; Lympany, P.A.; Pantelidis, P.; Welsh, K.I,; Zieliński, J. & Du Bois, R.M. (2001). Human leukocyte antigen-DRB1 position residues are a common protective marker for sarcoidosis. *American Journal of Respiratory Cell and Molecular Biology*, Vol. 25, No. 3, (September 2001), pp. 272-277, ISSN 1044-1549

Foreman, M.G.; Mannino, D.M.; Kamugisha, L & Westney, G.E. (2006). Hospitalization for patients with sarcoidosis: 1979-2000. *Sarcoidosis Vasculitis and Diffuse Lung Diseases*, Vol. 23, No. 2, (June 2006), pp. 124-129, ISSN 1124-0490

Fridlender, Z.G.; Schwartz, A.; Kohan, M.; Amir, G.; Glazer, M. & Berkman, N. (2010). Association between CD14 gene polymorphisms and disease phenotype in sarcoidosis. *Respiratory Medicine*, Vol. 104, No. 9, (September 2010), pp. 1336-1343, ISSN 0954-6111

Gottlieb, J.E.; Israel, H.L.; Steiner, R.M.; Triolo, J. & Patrick, H. (1997). Outcome in sarcoidosis. The relationship of relapse to corticosteroid therapy. *Chest*, Vol. 111, No. 3, (March 1997), pp. 623-631, ISSN 1931-3543

Grosso, S.; Margollicci, M.A.; Bargagli, E.; Buccoliero, Q.R.; Perrone, A.; Galimberti, D.; Morgese, G.; Balestri, P. & Rottoli, P. (2004). Serum levels of chitotriosidase as a marker of disease activity and clinical stage in sarcoidosis. *Scandinavian Journal of Clinical and Laboratory Investigation*, Vol. 64, No. 1(January 2004), pp. 57-62, ISSN 0036-5513

Grunewald, J.; Brynedal, B.; Darlington, P.; Nisell, M.; Cederlund, K.; Hillert, J. & Eklund, A. (2010). Different HLA-DRB1 allele distribution in distinct clinical subgroups of sarcoidosis patients. *Respiratory Research*, Vol. 11, No. 2 (February 2010), p. 25, ISSN 1465-9921

Grunewald, J. & Eklund, A. (2007). Sex-specific manifestations of Löfgren syndrome. *American Journal of Respiratory and Critical Care Medicine,* Vol. 175, No. 1 (January 2007), pp. 40-44, ISSN 1073-449X

Grunewald, J.; Wahlström, J.; Berlin, M.; Wigzell, H.; Eklund, A. & Olerup, O. (2002). Lung restricted T cell receptor AV2S3+ CD4+ T cell expansions in sarcoidosis patients with a shared HLA-DRβ chain conformation. *Thorax,* Vol. 57, No. 4, (April 2002), pp. 348-352, ISSN 1468-3296

Gupta, R.G.; Oparil, S.; Szidon, J. & Daise, M. (1979). Clinical significance of serum angiotensin-converting enzyme levels in sarcoidosis. *Journal of Laboratory and Clinical Medicine,* Vol. 93, No. 6, (June 1979), pp. 940-949, ISSN 0022-2143

Gvozdenovic, B.S.; Mihailovic-Vucinic, V.; Ilic-Dudvarski, A.; Zugic, V. & Judson, M.A. (2008). Differences in symptom severity and health status impairment between patients with pulmonary and pulmonary plus extrapulmonary sarcoidosis. *Respiratory Medicine,* Vol. 102, No. 11, (November 2008). pp. 1636-1642, ISSN 0954-6111

Handa, T.; Nagai, S.; Fushimi, Y. Miki, S.; Ohta, K.; Niimi, A.; Mishima, M. & Izumi, T. (2006). Clinical and radiographic indices associated with airflow limitation in patients with sarcoidosis. *Chest,* Vol. 130, No. 6, (December 2006), pp. 1851-1856, ISSN 1931-3543

Harrison, B.D.; Shaylor, J.M.; Stokes, T.C. & Wilkes, A.R. Airflow limitation in sarcoidosis: a study of pulmonary function in 107 patients with newly diagnosed disease. (1991). *Respiratory Medicine,* Vol. 85, No. 1, (January 1991), pp. 59-64, ISSN 0954-6111

Hill, M.R.; Papafili, A.; Booth, H.; Lawson, P.; Hubner, M.; Beynon, H.; Read, C.; Lindahl, G.; Marshall, R.P.; McAnulty, R.J. & Laurent, G.J. (2006). Functional prostaglandin-endoperoxide synthase 2 polymorphism predicts poor outcome in sarcoidosis. *American Journal of Respiratory and Critical Care Medicine,* Vol. 174, No. 8, (October 2006); pp. 915-922, ISSN 1073-449X

Hoffmann, G.; Rieder, J.; Smolny, M.; Seibel, M.; Wirleitner, B.; Fuchs, D. & Schobersberger, W. (1999). Neopterin-induced expression of intercellular adhesion molecule-1 (ICAM-1) in type II-like alveolar epithelial cells. *Clinical and Experimental Immunology,* Vol. 118, No. 3 (December 1999), pp. 435-440, ISSN 1365-2249

Hollinger, W.M.; Staton, G.W. Jr.; Fajman, W.A.; Gilman, M.J.; Pine, J.R. & Check, I.J. (1985). *American Review of Respiratory Disease,* Vol. 132, No. 1, (July 1985); pp. 65-69, ISSN 003-0805

Iannuzzi, M.C.; Rybicki, B.A. & Teirstein, A.S. (2006). Medical progress. Sarcoidosis. *New England Journal of Medicine,* Vol. 357, No 21, (November 2007), pp. 2153-2165, ISSN 1533-4406

Idali, F.; Wiken, M.; Wahlström, J.; Mallstedt, H.,; Eklund, A.; Rabbeni, H. & Grunewald, J. (2006). Reduced Th1 response in the lung of HLA-DRB1*0301 patients with pulmonary sarcoidosis. *European Respiratory Journal,* Vol. 27, No. 3, (March 2006), pp. 451-459, ISSN 1399-3003

Israel, H.L.; Karlin, P.; Menduke, H. & DeLisser, O.G. (1986). Factors affecting outcome of sarcoidosis. Influence of race, extrathoracic involvement, and initial radiologic lung lesions. *Annals of the New York Academy of Sciences,* Vol. 465, No. 6, (June 1986), pp. 609-618, ISSN 1749-6632

Janssen, R.; Sato, H.; Grutters, J.C.; Bernard, A.; van Velzen-Blad, H.; du Bois, R.M. & van den Bosch, J.M. (2003). Sudy of Clara cell 16, KL-6, and surfactant protein-D in serum as disease markers in pulmonary sarcoidosis. *Chest*, Vol. 124, No. 6, (December 2003), pp. 2119-2125, ISSN 1931-3543

Jonth, A.C.; Silveira, L.; Fingerlin, T.E.; Sato, H.; Luby, J.C.; Welsh, K.I.; Rose, C.S.; Newman, L.S.; du Bois, R.M. & Maier, L.A. and the ACCESS Group. (2007). TGF-β1 variants in chronic beryllium disease and sarcoidosis. *Journal of Immunology*, Vol. 179, No. 7, (October 2007), pp. 4255-4262, ISSN 1550-6606

Judson, M.A.; Baughman, R.P.; Thompson, B.W.; Teirstein, A.S.; Terrin, ML.; Rossman, M.D.; Yeager, H. Jr.; McLennan, G.; Bresnitz, E.A.; DePalo, D.L.; Hunninghake, G.; Ianuzzi, M.C.; Johns, C.J.; Moller, D.R.; Newman, L.S.; Rabin, D.L.; Rose, C.; Rybicki, B.A.; Weinberger, S.E.; Knatterud, G.L.; Cherniak, R. & ACCESS Research Group. (2003). Two year prognosis of sarcoidosis: the ACCESS experience. *Sarcoidosis Vasculitis and Diffuse Lung Diseases*, Vol. 20, No. 3, (October 2003), pp. 204-211, ISSN 1124-0490

Kendig, E.L. & Brummer, D.L. The prognosis of sarcoidosis in children. *Chest*, Vol. 70, No. 3, (September 1976), pp. 351-353, ISSN 1931-3543

Keogh, B.A.; Hunninghake, G.W.; Line, B.R. & Crystal, R.G. (1983). The alveolitis of pulmonary sarcoidosis. Evaluation of natural history and alveolitis-dependent changes in lung function. *American Review of Respiratory Disease*, Vol. 128, No 2, (August 1983), pp. 256-265, ISSN 003-0805

Kieszko, R.; Krawczyk, P.; Chocholska, S.; Dmoszyńska, A. & Milanowski, J. (2010). TNF-alpha and TNF-beta gene polymorphisms in Polish patients with sarcoidosis. Connection with the susceptibility and prognosis. *Sarcoidosis Vasculitis and Diffuse Lung Diseases*, Vol. 27, No. 2, (July 2010), pp. 131-137, ISSN 1124-0490

Kieszko, R.; Krawczyk, P.; Jankowska, O.; Chocholska, S.; Król, A. & Milanowski, J. (2007). The clinical significance of interleukin 18 assessment in sarcoidosis patients. *Respiratory Medicine*, Vol 101, No. 4, (April 2007), pp. 722-728, ISSN 0954-6111

Kieszko, R.; Krawczyk, P.; Michna, M.; Chocholska, S. & Milanowski, J. (2004). The yield of endobronchial biopsy in pulmonary sarcoidosis: Connection between spirometric impairment and lymphocyte subpopulations in bronchoalveolar lavage fluid. *Respiration*, Vol. 71, No. 1, (January-February 2004), pp. 72-76, ISSN 0025-7931

Kollert, F.; Geck, B.; Suchy, R.; Jörres, R.A.; Arzt, M.; Heidinger, D.; Hamer, O.W.; Prasse, A.; Müller-Quernheim, J.; Pfeifer, M. & Budweiser, S. (2011). The impact of gas exchange measurement during exercise in pulmonary sarcoidosis. *Respiratory Medicine*, Vol. 105, No. 1, (January 2011), pp. 122-129, ISSN 0954-6111

Kopiński, P.; Przybylski, G.; Jarzemska, A.; Sładek, K.; Soja, J.; Iwaniec, T.; Balicka-Slusarczyk, B.; Pinis, G.; Dyczek, A.; Szabłowska, K.; Golińska, J.; Jankowski, M. & Szczeklik, J. (2007). Interferon gamma (IFN-gamma) level in broncholaveolar lavage (BAL) fluid is positively correlated with CD4/CD8 ratio in selected interstitial lung diseases. *Polski Merkuriusz Lekarski*, Vol. 23, No. 133, (July 2007), pp. 15-21, ISSN 1426-9686

Kreider, M.E.; Christie, J.D.; Thompson, B.; Newman, L.; Rose, C.; Barnard, J.; Bresnitz, E.; Judson, M.A.; Lackland, D.T.; Rossman, M.D. & ACCESS Research Group. Relationship of environmental exposures to the clinical phenotype of sarcoidosis. *Chest*, Vol. 128, No. 1, (July 2005), pp. 207-215, ISSN 1931-3543

Krychniak-Soszka, A. & Kuś, J. (2002). Prognostic value of some clinical, radiological, laboratory and functional parameters in sarcoidosis. *Pneumonologia i Alergologia Polska*, Vol 70, No. 11-12, (December 2002), pp. 573-582, ISSN 0867-7707

Lamberto, C.; Nunes, H.; Le Toumelin, P.; Duperron, F.; Valeyre, D. & Clerici, C. (2004). Membrane and capillary blood components of diffusion capacity of the lung for carbon monoxide in pulmonary sarcoidosis: relation to exercise gas exchange. *Chest*, Vol. 125, No. 6, (June 2004), pp. 2061-2068, ISSN 1931-3543

Lamberto, C.; Saumon, G. ; Loiseau, P. ; Battesti, J.P. & Georges, R. (1985). Respiratory function in recent pulmonary sarcoidosis with special reference to small airways. *Bulletin Europeén Physiopathologie Respiratorie*, Vol. 21, No. 4, (July-August 1985), pp. 309-315, ISSN 0395-3890

Lavergne, F.; Clerici, C.; Sadoun, D.; Brauner, M.; Battesti, J.P. & Valeyre, D. (1999). Aiway obstruction in bronchial sarcoidosis. Outcome with treatment. *Chest*, Vol. 116, No. 5, (November 1999), pp. 1194-1199, ISSN 1931-3543

Lenner, R.; Schilero, G.J.; Padilla, M.L. & Teirstein, A.S. (2002). Sarcoidosis presenting in patients older than 50 years. *Sarcoidosis Vasculitis and Diffuse Lung Diseases*, Vol. 19, No. 2, (June 2002), ISSN 1124-0490

Löfgren, S. & Lundback, H. (1952). The bilateral hilar lymphoma syndrome; a study of the relation to tuberculosis and sarcoidosis in 212 cases. *Acta Medica Scandinavica*, Vol. 142, No. 4, (March 1952), pp. 259-264, ISSN 0001-6101

Lopez-Campos, J.L.; Rodriguez-Rodriguez, D.; Rodriguez-Becerra, E.; Michavila, I.A.; Guerra, J.F.; Hernandez, F.J.; Casanova, A.; de Córdoba Gamero, J.F.; Ortiz, A.R.; Arellano-Orden, E. & Montes-Worboya, A. (2008). Association of the 3050G>C polymorphism in the cyclooxygenase 2 gene with systemic sarcoidosis. *Archives of Medical Research*, Vol. 39, No. 5, (July 2008), pp. 525-530, ISSN 0188-4409

Malaisamy, S.; Dalal, B.; Bimenyuy, C. & Soubani, A.O. (2009). The clinical and radiologic features of nodular pulmonary sarcoidosis. *Lung*, Vol. 187, No 1, (January-February 2009); pp. 9-15, ISSN 0341-2040

Mañá, J.; Montero, A.; Vidal, M.; Marcoval, J. &, Pujol, R. (2003). Recurrent sarcoidosis: a study of 17 patients with 24 episodes of recurrence. *Sarcoidosis Vasculitis and Diffuse Lung Diseases*, Vol. 20, No. 3, (October 2003), pp. 212-221, ISSN 1124-0490

Mañá, J.; Salazar, A.; Pujol, R. & Manresa, F. (1996). Are the pulmonary function tests and the markers of activity helpful to establish the prognosis of sarcoidosis. *Respiration*, Vol. 63, No. 5, (1996), pp. 298-303, ISSN 0025-7931

Marcellis, R.G.J.; Lenssen, A.F.; Elfferich, M.D.P.; De Vries, J.; Kassim, S.; Foerster, K. & Drent, M. (2011). Exercise capacity, muscle strength and fatigue in sarcoidosis. *European Respiratory Journal* (April 2011) (doi: 10.1183/09031936.00117710), ISSN 1399-3003

Meloni, F.; Caporali, R.; Marone Bianco, A.; Paschetto, E.; Morosini, M.; Fietta, A.M.; Patrizio, V.; Bobbio-Pallavicini, F.; Pozzi, E. & Montecucco, C. (2004). BAL cytokine profile in different interstitial lung diseases: a focus on systemic sclerosis. *Sarcoidosis Vasculitis and Diffuse Lung Diseases*, Vol. 21, No. 2, (June 2004), pp. 111-118, ISSN 1124-0490

Mert, A.; Kumbasar, H.; Ozaras, R.; Erten, S.; Tasli, L.; Tabak, F. & Ozturk, R. (2007). Erythema nodosum: an evaluation of 100 cases. *Clinical and Experimental Rheumatology*, Vol. 25, No. 4, (July-August 2007), pp. 563-570, ISSN 0392-856X

Michielsen, H.J.; Peros-Golubicic, T.; Drent, M. & De Vries, J. (2007). Relationship between symptoms and quality of life in a sarcoidosis population. *Respiration*, Vol. 74, No. 4, (2007), pp. 401-405, ISSN 0025-7931

Miyoshi, S.; Hamada, H.; Kadowaki, T.; Hamaguchi, N.; Ito, R.; Irifune, K. & Higaki, J. (2010), Comparative evaluation of serum markers in pulmonary sarcoidosis. *Chest*, Vol. 137, No. 6, (June 2010), pp. 1391-1397, ISSN 1931-3543

Montuschi, P.; Ciabattoni, G.; Paredi, P.; Pantelidis, P; du Bois, R.M.; Kharitonov, S.A. & Barnes, P.J. (1998). 8-isoprostane as a biomarker of oxidative stress in interstitial lung diseases. *American Journal of Respiratory and Critical Care Medicine*, Vol. 158, No. 5, (November 1998), pp. 1524-1527, ISSN 1073-449X

Neville, E.; Walker, A.N. & James, D.G. (1983) Prognostic factors predicting outcome of sarcoidosis: an analysis of 818 patients. *Quarterly Journal of Medicine*, Vol. 52, No. 208, (Autumn 1983), pp. 525-533, ISSN 0033-5622

Nishioka, Y.; Manabe, K.; Kishi, J.; Wang, W.; Inayama, M.; Azuma, M. & Sone, S. (2007). CXCL9 and 11 in patients with pulmonary sarcoidosis: a role of alveolar macrophages. *Clinical and Experimental Immunology*, Vol. 149, No. 2, (August 2007), pp. 317-326, ISSN 1365-2249

Nitter, L. (1953). Changes in the chest roentgenogram in Boeck's sarcoid of the lungs. *Acta Radiologica* [Suppl](Stockh) , Vol. 105, (1953), pp. 7-29, ISSN 0567-8056

Ozdemir, O.K.; Celik, G.; Dalva, K.; Ulger, F.; Elhan, A. & Beksac, M. (2007). High CD95 expression of BAL lypocytes predicts chronic course in patients with sarcoidosis. *Respirology*, Vol. 12, No. 6, (November 2007), pp. 869-873, ISSN 1323-7799

Panselinas, E.; Halstead, L.; Schlosser, R.J. & Judson, M.A. (2010). Clinical manifestations, radiographic findings, treatment options, and outcome in sarcoidosis patients with upper respiratory tract involvement. *Southern Medical Journal*, Vol. 103, No. 9, (September 2010), pp. 870-875, ISSN 0038-4348

Papaioannides, D.; Fotinou, M.; Korantzopoulos, P.; Latsi, P.; Sinapidis, D.; Akritidis, N. & Orphanidou, D. (2004). Sarcoidosis associated with interferon-α therapy for chronic hepatitis C. *Medical Science Monitor*, Vol. 10, No. 1, (January 2004), pp. CS5-7, ISSN 1234-1010

Pawate, S.; Moses, H. & Sriram, S. (2009). Presentations and outcomes of neurosarcoidosis: a study of 54 cases. *Quarterly Journal of Medicine*, Vol. 102, No. 7, (July 2009), pp. 449-460, ISSN 0033-5622

Peros-Golubcić, T.; Ivicević, A.; Bekić, A.; Alilović, M.; Tekavec-Trkanjec, J. & Smojver-Jezek, S. (2001). Lung lavage neutrophils, neutrophil elastase and albumin in the prognosis of pulmonary sarcoidosis. *Collegium Antropologicum*, Vol. 25, No. 1 (June 2001), pp. 349-355, ISSN 0350-6134

Pietinalho, A.; Ohmichi, M.; Löfroos, A.B.; Hiraga, Y. & Selroos, O. (2000). The prognosis of pulmonary sarcoidosis in Finland and Hokkaido, Japan. A comparative five-year study of biopsy-proven cases. *Sarcoidosis Vasculitis and Diffuse Lung Diseases*, Vol. 17, No. 2, (June 2000), pp. 158-166, ISSN 1124-0490

Pietnialho, A.; Tukiainen, P.; Haahtela, T.; Persson, T. & Selroos, O. (1999). Oral prednisolone followed by inhaled budesonide in newly diagnosed pulmonary sarcoidosis: a double-blind, placebo-controlled multicenter study. Finnish Pulmonary Sarcoidosis Study Group. *Chest*, Vol. 116, No. 2, (August 1999), pp. 424-431, ISSN 1931-3543

Piotrowski, W.J.; Antczak, A.; Marczak, J.; Nawrocka, A.; Kurmanowska, Z. & Górski, P. (2007). Eicosanoids in exhaled breath condensate and BAL fluid of patients with sarcoidosis. *Chest*, Vol. 132, No. 2, (August 2007), pp. 589-596, ISSN 1931-3543

Piotrowski, W.J.; Kurmanowska, Z.; Antczak, A.; Marczak, J. & Górski P. (2010). Exhaled 8-isoprostane as a prognostic marker in sarcoidosis. A short term follow-up. *BMC Pulmonary Medicine*, Vol. 10, No. 4, (April 2010), p. 23, ISSN 1471-2466

Planck, A.; Eklund, A. & Grunewald, J. (2003). Markers of activity in clinically recovered human leukocyte antigen-DR17-positive sarcoidosis patients. *European Respiratory Journal*, Vol. 21, No. 1, (January 2003); pp. 52-57, ISSN 1399-3003

Płodziszewska, M.; Chorostowska, J.; Polubiec-Kownacka, M.; Jaroń, B.; Lenarcik, D.; Marzinek, M.; Szopiński, J.; Wiatr, E.; Załęska, J.; Zych, J.; Skopińska-Różewska, E. & Rowińska-Zakrzewska, E. (2000). The relation between lymphocyte profile in BALF and the course of sarcoidosis based on short term observation. *Pneumonologia i Alergologia Polska*, Vol. 68, No. 11-12 (November 2000), pp. 557-565, ISSN 0867-7707

Prasse, A.; Katic, C.; Germann, M.; Buchwald, A.; Zissel, G. & Muller-Quernheim, J. (2008). Phenotyping sarcoidosis from a pulmonary perspective. *American Journal of Respiratory and Critical Care Medicine*, Vol. 177, No. 3, (February 2008), pp. 330-336, ISSN 1073-449X

Psathakis, K.; Papatheodorou, G.; Plataki, M.; Panagou, P.; Loukides, S.; Siafakas, N.M. & Bouros, D. (2004). 8-Isoprostane, a meraker of oxidative stress, is increased in the expired breath condensate of patients with pulmonary sarcoidosis. *Chest*, Vol. 125, No. 3, (March 2004), pp. 1005-1011, ISSN 1931-3543

Rastogi, R.; Du, W.; Ju, D.; Pirockinaite, G.; Liu, Y.; Nunez, G. & Samavati, L. (2011). Dysregulation of p38 and MKP-1 in response to NOD1/TLR4 stimulation in sarcoid bronchoalveolar cells. *American Journal of Respiratory and Critical Care Medicine*, Vol. 183, No 4, (February 2011), pp. 500-510, ISSN 1073-449X

Reich, J.M. (2002). Mortality of intrathoracic sarcoidosis in referral vs population-based settings. Influence of stage, ethnicity, and corticosteroid therapy. *Chest*, Vol. 121, No. 1, (January 2002), pp. 32-39, ISSN 1931-3543

Reid JD. (1998). Sarcoidosis in coroner's autopsies: a critical evaluation of diagnosis and prevalence from Cuyahoga County, Ohio. *Sarcoidosis Vasculitis and Diffuse Lung Diseases*, Vol. 15, No. 1, (January 1998), pp. 44-51, ISSN 1124-0490

Roberts, W.C.; McAllister, H.A. Jr. & Ferrans, V.J. (1977). Sarcoidosis of the heart. A clinicopathologic study of 35 necropsy patients (group 1) and review of 78 previously described necropsy patients (group 11). *American Journal of Medicine*, Vol. 63, No. 1, (July 1977), pp. 86-108, ISSN 1555-7162

Rossman, M.D.; Dauber, J.H.; Cardillo, M.E. & Daniele, R.P. (1982). Pulmonary sarcoidosis: correlation of serum angiotensin-converting enzyme with blood and bronchoalveolar lymohocytes. *American Review of Respiratory Disease*, Vol. 125, No. 3, (March 1982), pp. 366-369, ISSN 003-0805

Rossman, M.D.; Thompson, B.; Frederick, M.; Maliarik, M.; Iannuzzi, M.C.; Rybicki, B.A.; Pandey, J.P.; Newman, L.S.; Magira, E.; Beznik-Cizman, B.; Monos, D. & ACCESSS group (2003). HLA-DRB1*1101: a significant risk factor for sarcoidosis in blacks and whites. *American Journal of Human Genetics*, Vol. 73, No. 4, (October 2003), pp. 720-735, ISSN 1537-6605

Rothkrantz-Kos, S.; van Dieijen-Visser, M.P.; Mulder, P.G.H. & Drent, M. (2003). Potential usefulness of inflammatory markers to monitor respiratory functional impairment in sarcoidosis. *Clinical Chemistry*, Vol. 49, No. 9, (September 2003); pp. 1510-1517, ISSN 1530-8561

Rust, M.; Bergmann, L.; Kuhn, T.; Tuengerthal, S.; Bartmann, K.; Mitrou, P.S. & Meier-Sydow, J. (1985). Prognostic value of chest radiograph, serum-angiotensin-converting enzyme and T helper cell count in blood and in broncholaveolar lavage of patients with pulmonary sarcoidosis. *Respiration*, Vol. 48, No. 3, (1985), pp. 231-236, ISSN 0025-7931

Rybicki, B.A.; Maliarik, M.J.; Poisson, L.M.; Sheffer, R.; Chen, K.M.; Major, M.; Chase, G.A. & Ianuzzi, M.C. (2003). The major histocompatibility complex gene region and sarcoidosis susceptibility in African Americans. *American Journal of Respiratory Critical Care Medicine*, Vol. 167, No. 3, (February 2003), pp. 444-449, ISSN 1073-449X

Rybicki, B.A.; Sinha, R.; Iyengar, S.; Gray-McGuire, C.; Elston, R.C. & Iannuzzi, M.C. & SAGA Study Consortium. (2007). Genetic linkage analysis of sarcoidosis phenotypes: the sarcoidosis genetic analysis (SAGA) study. *Genes and Immunity*, Vol. 8, No. 5, (July 2007), pp. 379-386, ISSN 1466-4879

Rybicki, B.A.; Walewski, J.L.; Maliarik, M.J.; Kian, H.; Iannuzzi, M.C. & ACCESS Research Group. The BTNL2 gene and sarcoidosis susceptibility in African Americans and Whites. *American Journal of Human Genetics*, Vol. 77, No. 3, (September 2005), pp. 491-499, ISSN 0002-9297

Salobir, B.; Medica, I.; Tercelj, M.; Kastrin, A.; Sabovic, M. & Peterlin, B. (2007). Association of angiotensin-converting enzyme/DD genotype with sarcoidosis susceptibility in Slovenian patients. *Medical Science Monitor*, Vol. 13, No. 12, (December 2007), pp. CR538-542, ISSN 1234-1010

Sato, H.; Williams, H.R.; Spagnolo, P.; Abdallah, A.; Ahmad, T.; Orchard, T.R.; Copley, S.J.; Desai, S.R.; Wells, A.U.; du Bois, R.M. & Welsh, K.I. (2010b). CARD15/NOD2 polymorphisms are associated with severe pulmonary sarcoidosis. *European Respiratory Journal*, Vol. 35, No. 2, (February 2010), pp. 324-330, ISSN 1399-3003

Sato, H.; Woodhead, F.A.; Ahmad, T.; Grutters, J.C.; Spagnolo, P.; van den Bosch, J.M.; Maier, L.A.; Newman, L.S.; Nagai, S.; Izumi, T.; Wells, A.U.; du Bois, R.M. & Welsh, K.I. (2010a). Sarcoidosis HLA class II genotyping distinguishes differences of clinical phenotype across ethnic groups. *Human Molecular Genetics*, Vol.19, No. 20, (October 2010); pp. 4100-4111, ISSN 0964-6906.

Scadding, J. (1961). Prognosis of intrathoracic sarcoidosis in England. A review of 136 patients after 5 years' observations. *British Medical Journal*, Vol. 2, No. 5261 (November 1961); pp. 1165-1172, ISSN 0267-0631

Schoenfeld, N.; Schmolke, B.; Schmitt, M.; Remy, N.; Ellensohn, P.; Wahn, U. & Loddenkemper, R. (1994). Specification and quantitation of circulating immune complexes in the serum of patients with active pulmonary sarcoidosis. *Thorax*, Vol. 49, No. 7, (July 1994), pp. 688-691, ISSN 1468-3296

Schürmann, M.; Kwiatkowski, R.; Albrecht, M.; Fischer, A.; Hampe, J.; Müller-Quernheim, J.; Schwinger, E. & Schreiber, S. (2008). Study of toll-like receptor gene loci in sarcoidosis. *Clinical and Experimental Immunology*, Vol. 152, No. 3, (June 2008), pp. 423-431, ISSN 1365-2249

Sekiya, M.; Ohwada, A.; Miura, K.; Takahashi, S. & Fukuchi, Y. (2003). Serum vascular endothelial growth factor as a possible prognostic indicator in sarcoidosis. *Lung*, Vol. 181, No. 5, (May 2003), pp. 259-265, ISSN 0341-2040

Seyhan, E.C.; Cetinkaya, E.; Altin, S.; Gunluoglu, Z.; Demir, A.; Koksal, V. & Issever, H. (2008). Tumor necrosis factor gene polymorphisms in Turkish patients with sarcoidosis. *Internal Medicine*, Vol. 47, No. 9, (2008), pp. 833-888, ISSN 0918-2918

Sharma, O.P. & Johnson, R. (1988). Airway obstruction in sarcoidosis: a study of 123 nonsmoking black American patients with sarcoidosis. *Chest*, Vol. 94, No. 2 (August 1988); 94: 343-346, ISSN 1931-3543

Sharma, S.K.; Balamurugan, A.; Pandey, R.M.; Kumar Saha, P. & Mehra, N.K. (2003). Human leukocyte antigen-DR alleles influence the clinical course of pulmonary sarcoidosis in Asian Indians. *American Journal of Respiratory Cell and Molecular Biology*, Vol. 29, No. 2, (August 2003), pp. 225-231, ISSN 1044-1549

Stagaki, E.; Mountford, W.K.; Lackland, D.T. & Judson, M.A. (2009). The treatment of lupus pernio: results of 116 treatment courses in 54 patients. *Chest*, Vol. 135, No. 2, (February 2009), pp. 468-476, ISSN 1931-3543

Studdy, P.; Bird, R. & James, D.G. (1978). Serum angiotensin-converting enzyme (SACE) in sarcoidosis and other granulomatous disorders. *Lancet*, Vol. 2, No. 8104-8105, (December 1978), pp. 1331-1334, ISSN 0099-5355

Studdy, P.R.; Bird, R.; Neville, E. & James, D.G. (1980). Biochemical findings in sarcoidosis. *Journal of Clinical Pathology*, Vol. 33, No. 6, (June 1980), pp. 528-533, ISSN 0021-9746

Sweiss, N.J.; Barnathan, E.S.; Lo, K.; Judson, M.A. & Baughman, R. (2010). T48 Investigators. C-reactive protein predicts response to infliximab in patients with chronic sarcoidosis. *Sarcoidosis Vascular and Diffuse Lung Diseases*, Vol. 27, No. 1, (July 2010), pp. 49-56, ISSN 1124-0490

Swigris, J.J.; Olson, A.L.; Huie, T.J.; Fernandez-Perez, E.R.; Solomon, J.; Sprunger, D. & Brown, K.K. Sarcoidosis-related mortality in the U.S. from 1988-2007. *American Journal of Respiratory and Critical Care Medicine*, (February 2011), [Epub ahead of print], ISSN 1073-449X

Tahanovich, A.D.; Katovich, I.L. & Baradzina, H.L. (2003). Evaluation of bronchoalveolarlavage fluid phospolipids and cytokine release by alveolar macrophages as prognostic markers in sarcoidosis. *Respiration*, Vol. 70, No. 4, (July-August 2003), pp. 376-381, ISSN 0025-7931

Tahir, M.; Sharma, S.K.; Ashraf, S. & Mishra, H.K. (2007). Angiotensin converting enzyme genotype affects development and course of sarcoidosis in Asian Indians. *Sarcoidosis Vascular and Diffuse Lung Diseases*, Vol. 24, No. 2, (September 2007), pp. 106-112, ISSN 1124-0490

Verstraeten, A.; Demedts, M.; Verwilghen, J.; van den Eeckhout, A.; Mariën, G.; Lacquet, L.M. & Ceuppens, J.L. (1990). Predictive value of bronchoalveolar lavage in pulmonary sarcoidosis. *Chest*, Vol. 98, No. 3, (March 1990), pp. 560-567, ISSN 1931-3543

Vidal Serrano, S.; Martín Juan, J.; Gómez Izquierdo, L.; Sánchez Rodríguez, I.; Rodríguez Becerra, E. & Rodríguez Panadero, F. (2005). Radiographic staging and bronchoalveolar lavage cell counts in sarcoidosis. *Archivos Bronconeumologia*, Vol . 41, No. 8, (August 2005), pp. 425-429, ISSN 0300-2896

Viscum, K. & Vestbo, J. (1993). Vital prognosis in intrathoracic sarcoidosis with special reference to pulmonary function and radiological stage. *European Respiratory Journal*, Vol. 6, No. 6, (March 1993), pp. 349-353, ISSN 1399-3003

Ward, K.; O'Connor, C.M.; Odlum, C.; Power, C. &, Fitzgerald, M.X. (1990). Pulmonary disease progress in sarcoid patients with and without bronchoalveolar lavage collagenase. *American Review and Respiratory Disease*, Vol. 142, No. 3, (September 1990), pp. 636-641, ISSN 003-0805

Westney, G.E.; Habib, S. & Quarshie, A. (2007). Comorbid illnesses and chest radiographic severity in African-American sarcoidosis patients. *Lung*, Vol. 185, No. 3, (May-June 2007), ISSN 0341-2040

Wijnen, P.A.; Nelemans, P.J.; Verschakelen, J.A.; Bekers, O.; Voorter, C.E. & Drent, M. (2010). The role of tumor necrosis factor alpha G-308A polymorphisms in the course of pulmonary sarcoidosis. *Tissue Antigens*, Vol. 75, No. 3, (March 2010), pp. 262-268, ISSN 0001-2815

Winterbauer, R.H. & Hutchinson, J.F. (1980). Use of pulmonary function tests in the management of sarcoidosis. *Chest*, Vol. 78, No. 5, (May 1980), pp. 640-647, ISSN 1931-3543

Wurm, K.; Reindell, H. &, Heilmeyer, L. (1958). Der Lungenboeck in Rontgenbild. Thieme, Stuttgart (1958), Germany

Yazaki, Y.; Isobe, M.; Hiroe, M.; Morimoto, S.; Hiramitsu, S.; Nakano, T.; Izumi, T. & Sekiguchi, M. (2001). Central Japan Heart Study Group. Prognostic determinants of long-term survival in Japanese patients with cardiac sarcoidosis treated with prednisone. *American Journal of Cardiology*, Vol. 88, No. 9, (November 2001), pp. 1006-1010, ISSN 0002-9149

Zajicek, J.P.; Scolding, N.J.; Foster, O.; Rovaris, M.; Evanson, J.; Moseley, I.F.; Scadding, J.W.; Thompson, E.J.; Chamoun, V.; Miller, D.H.; McDonald, W.I. & Mitchell, D. (1999). Central nervous system sarcoidosis--diagnosis and management. *Quarterly Journal of Medicine*, Vol. 92, No. 2 (February 1999), pp. 103-117, ISSN 0033-5622

Ziegenhagen, M.W.; Rothe, M.E.; Schlaak, M. & Müller-Quernheim, J. (2003). Bronchoalveolar and serological parameters reflecting the severity of sarcoidosis. *European Respiratory Journal*, Vol. 21, No. 3, (March 2003), pp. 407-413, ISSN 1399-3003

Ziegenhagen, M.W.; Rothe, M.E.; Zissel, G. & Müller-Quernheim, J. (2002). Exaggerated TNFalpha release of alveolar macrophages in corticosteroid resistant sarcoidosis. *Sarcoidosis Vascular and Diffuse Lung Diseases*, Vol. 19, No. 3, (October 2002), pp. 185-190, ISSN 1124-0490

9

Lung Transplantation for Pulmonary Sarcoidosis

Dominic T. Keating
Allergy, Immunology and Respiratory Medicine, Alfred Hospital Melbourne, Australia

1. Introduction

Sarcoidosis, a multisystem disorder, results in the production of multiple non-caseating granulomas capable of affecting all organs of the body. It usually occurs in patients between the ages of 10 and 40 years of age in 90% of cases. The prevalence has been reported to be 10-20 per 100,000 in the general population however the annual incidence is 107 per 100,000 (Rybicki, Major et al. 1997). There also appears to be a variation in the racial prevalence of the disease with Caucasians having a 0.85% lifetime risk for the disease while the lifetime risk for Black Americans is 2.5% (Rybicki, Major et al. 1997). The racial implications of the disease are not just confined to prevalence, evidence suggests that along with the increased prevalence of Sarcoidosis Black American patients also have a more acute and severe process in contrast to the usually slow insidious symptoms commonly seen in Caucasian patients (Newman, Rose et al. 1997). Familial clustering has also been identified in linkage studies and this has identified the short arm of chromosome 6 as the area of most interest (Baughman, Lower et al. 2003).

Despite intense study an exact etiology for Sarcoidosis has remained elusive for investigators, leaving many to speculate as to the pathogenesis of the disease. Most commonly the respiratory system is the primary target of the disease, in addition to this the skin and eyes are regularly affected leading researchers to believe that an environmental cause was the most likely cause. Many associations have been suggested ranging from wood burning stoves to inorganic particles, insecticides and moulds (Bresnitz and Strom 1983; Newman, Rose et al. 2004; Rybicki, Amend et al. 2004). The recent advancement in technology and the use of polymerase chain reaction to amplify the genetic products of sampled tissue resulted in the discovery of mycobacterial antigens in serum samples taken from patients with Sarcoidosis (Song, Marzilli et al. 2005). Most investigators however favour an immune response abnormality and that the antigen in question is of lesser significance. Evidence for this was seen with the association between human leukocyte antigen variants and Sarcoidosis, especially the good correlation between HLA-DQB1*0201 and acute disease with a good prognosis (Sato, Grutters et al. 2002).

The majority of Sarcoidosis affected individuals do not develop progressive fibrotic disease; indeed, two thirds of patients will have a remission with half achieving this within three years. The response once achieved is also favourable with less than 5% of patients achieving remission in one year subsequently having a relapse. In essence this results in one third of patients developing progressive disease in addition to the 5% of patients who have a relapse. While the numbers with significant disease are less than the potential that might be affected, with 90% of patients presenting with respiratory impairment, the implications for surgery could be significant.

In Mississippi, over 47years ago, the first human lung transplant was performed on a patient with emphysema and lung carcinoma of the left main bronchus (Hardy, Webb et al. 1963). The patient survived for 18 days; 20 years later surgeons in Toronto performed another procedure with the use of coronary bypass technology and since then it has developed into a significant part of the clinical armamentarium used to treat a number of end stage lung diseases including Sarcoidosis. Improved outcome from lung transplantation has been attributed to better use of immunosuppression, surgical techniques and better donor selection. Recipients have also been scrutinised for acceptability with some believing that a multisystem disease such as Sarcoidosis might result in increased deaths postoperatively. This turned out to be unfounded as long as the individual patients fulfilled the routine testing requirements outlined below.

In order to assist in making the process of transplantation more transparent and equitable the method by which lungs are distributed in the United States has recently been updated. Diseases are given a number calculated from clinical parameters which is weighted based on the likelihood of surviving one year before transplantation and one year after transplantation. The calculated number, referred to as the LAS (lung allocation score), is based on historical data and is to be reviewed on a regular basis to maintain its accuracy(Egan, Murray et al. 2006). Sarcoidosis figures are therefore based on previous outcomes and survival data, and due to the low numbers of transplants performed historically for Sarcoidosis, patients may benefit when the reviews are performed. Outside the United States many units rely on clinical parameters and regular outpatient reviews to decide on urgency both for listing and organ allocation. This review will detail when patients should be referred and listed for lung transplantation and the complications that can be encountered during the process.

2. Diagnosis

To accurately diagnose Sarcoidosis three criteria are required. These include consistent clinical and radiographical features, supporting histology classically described as non-caseating epithelioid cell granulomas, and the exclusion of other causes of granulomatous disorders. Unless patients present with a characteristic Lofgren's syndrome a biopsy of the affected organ is usually necessary, however, considering the multisystem nature of the disease the area easiest to access can be used, for example a cervical or axillary lymph node.

2.1 Clinical presentation

Up to 50% of patients with Sarcoidosis may be asymptomatic at the time of diagnosis. Many patients will in fact be suspected of having the disease based on findings during incidental radiological testing. If present the respiratory system is most commonly involved with symptoms reported in 40% of patients. These symptoms usually manifest as dyspnoea, cough which can be productive or non-productive of sputum, chest pain, or haemoptysis in decreasing order of frequency. Constitutional symptoms are also reported in up to 40%with patients reporting fatigue, malaise, weight loss, night sweats, chills and fever. These features are also more frequently reported in Black patients and patients from the Indian subcontinent.

Acute presentation with Lofgren's syndrome has been reported in 9-34% of cases comprising arthritis, erythema nodosum and bilateral hilar adenopathy (Siltzbach, James et al. 1974). Women may present differently with this syndrome affected predominantly with erythema nodosum, while men usually develop ankle periarticular inflammation and no erythema nodosum. The frequency of other organ involvement including liver, spleen, cardiac, ocular, central and peripheral nerve involvement is listed in Table 1.

Clinical Symptoms	Rate (%)
Asymptomatic	12-50%
Constitutional Symptoms	15-40%
Respiratory Symptoms	15-40%
Skin	10-35%
Eyes	10-25%
Joints	5-17%
Neurological	5%
Cardiac	5%

Table 1. Frequency of Clinical symptoms

2.2 Radiological features

As only 50% of patients have symptoms at diagnosis radiological features have become central to diagnosing and staging Sarcoidosis. Although there is a pantheon of modalities now available for radiological investigation not all have been assessed in Sarcoidosis. Chest X-Ray (CXR) remains the commonest first investigation to raise the suspicion of Sarcoidosis. As CXR has long been available the common abnormalities associated with Sarcoidosis are well described. These include bilateral hilar lymphadenopathy, with or without interstitial infiltration, nodular changes or fibrosis. This has resulted in the classification of Sarcoidosis into four stages based on the array of findings that might be present. Stage 1 is bilateral hilar lymphadenopathy without parenchymal infiltration, stage 2 is bilateral hilar lymphadenopathy with parenchymal infiltration, stage 3 is parenchymal infiltration without hilar enlargement, and stage 4 has hilar retraction, bullae, fibrotic banding, traction bronchiectasis and diaphragmatic tenting (Scadding 1961).

Computed tomography (CT) develops superior views of the thoracic cage and so has superseded the CXR for usefulness in the diagnostic algorithm. CT scanning can identify subtle changes in the parenchyma allowing staging to be more accurately applied to the patient. Identification of ground glass opacification in this way may also identify steroid responsive disease (Murdoch and Muller 1992). In addition parenchymal markings identified before bronchoscopy allows a targeted approach to transbronchial biopsies.

Although no longer part of routine assessment due to poor sensitivity Gadolinium 67 scanning has previously been used. If present a classical distribution of uptake involving the lung parenchyma, hilar nodes, parotid and lacrimal gland (the 'panda' sign) favours a diagnosis of Sarcoidosis (Sulavik, Spencer et al. 1990). It has been suggested however that Gadolinium may be useful in the diagnosis of cardiac Sarcoidosis in combination with other modalities (Niida, Isoda et al. 2009).
A recent report on positron emission tomography (PET) scanning suggests that using fluoro-alpha-methyltyrosine in combination with 18-F-fluorodeoxyglucose-PET may be beneficial in allowing a better distinction between malignancy and Sarcoidosis (Shulman, Latkany et al. 2009). Magnetic resonance imaging on the other hand has been extensively used in the diagnosis of systemic and especially cardiac Sarcoidosis (Mehta, Lubitz et al. 2008). Its use in parenchymal lung Sarcoidosis is limited; however, there is a role for its use to rule out the presence of mediastinal fibrosis as a cause of pulmonary artery impingement syndrome (Dhote, Vignaux et al. 2003).

2.3 Investigations and diagnostics

Historically the Kveim-Siltzbach test has been utilized for diagnosis and involves the intradermal injection of a homogenate of human Sarcoid tissue, this is followed up four weeks after the injection when a papule has formed at the site. The papule is then biopsied and assessed histologically for classical histological features of Sarcoidosis. Currently its use is limited by the lack of commercial antigen availability, current controls with regards the use of human tissue and new preparations requiring validation in vivo therefore it is reserved for use when lesions are not easily accessible, which in reality is uncommon (Iannuzzi, Rybicki et al. 2007).
Histological findings in Sarcoidosis are characteristic but by no means are they pathognomic. The classically described epithelioid granuloma may be found in any organ of the body and usually consists of distinct lesions with epithelioid cells and multinucleated giant cells at the centre. In the lung it usually involves the peri bronchial, interstitial and subpleural compartments. Associated vasculitis is not a common feature and when present other diagnoses should be considered in the differential. Indeed the granulomas themselves may be preceded by an interstitial pneumonitis with macrophage and lymphocyte infiltrates, although the exact relationship between the extent and severity of these activated macrophages and lymphocytes and the extent of granuloma formation subsequently is not well understood. The finding of non–caseating granulomas requires further evaluation in order to exclude other causes some of which are listed in Table 2.
Laboratory investigations have been poor in confirming the diagnosis of Sarcoidosis but helpful in ruling out other possible causes. Non-caseating granulomas associated with Sarcoidosis are known to produce angiotensin converting enzyme and research has shown it to be elevated in 75% of patients with Sarcoidosis (Studdy and Bird 1989). Its use as a diagnostic test, however, has been hindered because the level can be raised in many other diseases some of which are listed in Table 2. Bronchoalveolar lavage samples taken at bronchoscopy have found an associated imbalance in the CD4/CD8 ratio in Sarcoidosis. When this ratio is elevated to greater than 3.5 it has a specificity of 95%, unfortunately the specificity is low at 59% (Costabel, Bonella et al. 2010). Lavage samples also assist in ruling out many of the infective causes of granulomatous disease.

Inflammatory	Sarcoidosis Berylliosis Granulomatous Vasculitis Eosinophilic Granuloma Hypersensitivity Pneumonitis Crohn's Disease
Infection	Mycobacterial Infections Fugal infections Syphillis Leprosy Catscratch Disease Parasitic Infection
Neoplasia	Carcinoma Lymphoma

Table 2. Differential Diagnosis for Non Caseating Granulomas

Use of lung function testing may contribute to diagnosis if the pattern of spirometry is consistent. Usually however its use is reserved for follow up and assessment of treatment. Most patients have a restrictive deficit on spirometry but in 50% there is a coexisting obstruction as evidenced by a reduced ratio of forced expiration in one second to forced vital capacity. Interestingly, this obstruction has been shown in some patients to be reversible (Baughman, Teirstein et al. 2001; Shorr, Torrington et al. 2001). The advantage of lung function testing in Sarcoidosis is that it may highlight other disease for example in patients with a conspicuously low diffusion capacity for carbon monoxide out of proportion for the spirometric values might suggest a pulmonary vascular component is present. As a means of follow up in patients commenced on treatment lung function is useful with studies suggesting that abnormalities returns to normal in 80% of patients after two years (Judson, Baughman et al. 2003).

Acquiring tissue for histological assessment has also changed over the recent decades. While tests like the Kveim test had their place, the most commonly affected organ is the lung and as a result this has become the most commonly accessed site for most patients. Open or video-assisted thoracoscopic biopsy remains the gold standard as direct visualisation allows identification of granulomas in 90% of cases. Mediastinoscopy has also been performed and while it possesses a high sensitivity rate it is an invasive procedure with a morbidity rate that may render it unjustifiable in many cases.

Development of the fibreoptic bronchoscope has allowed targeted transbronchial biopsies to be performed whish has resulted in a high yield for lesions in a peribronchial distribution. A minimum of four transbronchial biopsies are needed to guarantee sufficient tissue for diagnosis, while reports using this method demonstrated a sensitivity of 90%(Gilman and Wang 1980). The development of endobronchial ultrasound has also advanced the diagnostic capabilities of bronchoscopy. The advantage of this approach is that not only can transbronchial lung biopsies be performed but enlarged mediastinal lymph nodes can also be targeted for tissue sampling. The use of endobronchial ultrasound in many centres have negated the need to perform mediastinoscopy, and in expert hands the sensitivities can approach 96% with specificities of 100% (Costabel, Bonella et al. 2010). The safety profile of linear endobronchial ultrasound is also superior to that of mediastinoscopy and in many centres where it is available it has become the investigation of choice.

It remains difficult to devise a severity index for Sarcoidosis although there have been some attempts. The six minute walk test has significant age and racial variability however lung function and diffusion capacity race, immunosuppression use and organ involvement have all been incorporated into an algorithm of severity however it remains to be validated (Wasfi, Rose et al. 2006; Alhamad 2009).

3. Treatment

Most patients with Sarcoidosis will recover spontaneously and don't require any pharmacological treatment, in those that do the most commonly used agents are corticosteroids. These are usually indicated when patients are significantly symptomatic, have decreasing lung function or diffusion capacity over a 3-6 month period, or have advancing radiological disease. Treatment is also indicated for extrapulmonary disease including neurological, ocular, renal calcification or hypercalcaemia (Baughman, Costabel et al. 2008). Other agents have also been assessed for use but these are usually reserved for those who have had a poor response to corticosteroids, have side effects or in patients who have coexistent adverse events and are intolerant of lower doses of corticosteroids (1999). Alternative therapies have included methotrexate, most commonly, but also azathioprine and leflunamide (Baughman, Costabel et al. 2008). These agents can be used either alone or in combination, however, if the response is still unsatisfactory Infliximab (tumour necrosis factor-alpha antagonist) can be considered as an alternative. While a number of other agents have been considered useful their use has delivered unsatisfactory results. Some of the agents trialled include colchicine, cyclophosphamide, mycophenylate mofetil, pentoxyphylline and non-steroidal anti-inflammatory agents (Fazzi 2003).

3.1 Timing of transplantation

Referral for transplantation has always been the Achilles heal of Sarcoidosis treatment. Of particular concern in Sarcoidosis is the difficulty gauging the extent of organ involvement, identifying which patients will respond to treatment, and which test is the best prognostic indicator. Factors that need to be considered when deciding about the timing of lung transplant referral include making sure all avenues of treatment have been exhausted leaving lung transplantation as the 'last option', prognosis needs to be within the transplantation window where the patient has a survival advantage from surgery, while the patient also needs to be in sufficient health to survive the procedure. Most transplantation centres accept a combination of factors to decide when patients should be accepted for transplant workup.

Extensive fibrocystic disease in stage 4 disease is more likely to derive benefit from lung transplantation. Other stages of disease also need to be observed closely in the outpatient setting to watch for worsening radiological changes and clinical status as this may be the onset of treatment failure. Arterial blood gases revealing a $PaCO_2$ > 6.7 kPa (50 mm Hg) or a PaO_2 < 7.3 kPa (55 mm Hg) are suggestive of more advanced disease, although, while they are evidence of more extensive disease they have not been found to be useful in terms of prognosis or identification of progressive disease. Lung function is also a useful indicator when following patients and a forced vital capacity between 40-50% with or without a declining diffusing capacity below 40% are likely to be symptomatic on exertion if not at rest and should be referred for consideration (Judson 1998). Another factor to take into consideration is the impact of disease on quality of life and the patient's ability to cope with the disease. If the patient satisfies some or all of these parameters then referral for transplant assessment is prudent.

Recently the development of pulmonary hypertension has been shown to be a good discriminator for future survival (Corte, Wells et al. 2010). Research has revealed that the likelihood of mortality on a lung transplant waiting list with a diagnosis of Sarcoidosis was equivalent to that for patients with idiopathic pulmonary fibrosis although Sarcoidosis patients were less likely to receive a transplant. For Sarcoidosis patients pulmonary hypertension had more impact on the disease than for those with idiopathic pulmonary fibrosis and may have contributed to the Sarcoidosis deaths (Shorr, Davies et al. 2002). Evidence of clinical decline with or without a decline in lung function or diffusion capacity should prompt investigation with an echocardiogram, if there is evidence of onset of pulmonary hypertension referral for consideration of lung transplantation should be considered.

3.2 Lung transplantation workup

Screening is used in order select the most appropriate patients for the process of lung transplantation. The process ensures not only the appropriate choice of recipient but also ensures that the donor families can see that due diligence is performed with respect to the ultimate allocation the donor organs. Recent data shows that for all deceased donor lung transplants the 1, 5, and 10 year survival is 83, 54 and 29 percent respectively (OPTN/SRTR 2009). Patients with a 20-30% one year survival should be considered appropriate for lung transplant work up (Christie, Edwards et al. 2008).

There are a number of tests that are performed as part of transplant workup that are in no way particular to one or other of the many diseases that are considered suitable for lung transplant. These are investigations required to assist in guiding the patient successfully through the process and are listed in table 3. Sarcoidosis is a multisystem disorder and therefore potentially represents a higher risk to transplant recipients in terms of post-operative complications. A number of other organs may be involved and so diligent pretransplant screening needs to be undertaken to optimize decision making prior to surgery.

Additional factors that are of particular concern when assessing patients with Sarcoidosis include the involvement of the thoracic cage. Patients with advanced disease, especially stage 4 disease associated with fibrocystic changes may present with mycetomas or pneumothoraces. Mycetomas causing haemoptysis may cause significant difficulty prior to surgery however most difficulty arises after transplantation with immunosuppression treatment (Rafferty, Biggs et al. 1983). If any fungal infection is brought through the operation there is a significant risk of anastomotic breakdown. Therefore patients with any evidence of cystic lesions on radiology investigations receive bilateral lung transplants decreasing this risk. Multiple pneumothoraces or prolonged thoracotomy tube placed as therapy may also result in pleural reaction and fibrosis that can hinder dissection at the time of transplantation. If this is extensive or if pleurodesis has been carried out the case may be too difficult with a high risk of bleeding, more often than not however, patients can be wait-listed with extra dissection time added into the protocol on the night.

In addition to pleural disease patients who have extensive mediastinal involvement need careful assessment as mediastinitis also can result in difficult dissection during surgery, in addition, if there is any evidence of impingement of the pulmonary artery with right heart failure then stenting of the pulmonary arteries may improve symptoms significantly delaying or negating the need for listing (Figure 1C). Ventilation/perfusion scans are unreliable in this instance as the significance of the obstruction may be difficult to assess and a Magnetic Resonance Angiogram gives a detailed outline of the mediastinal structures completing the workup.

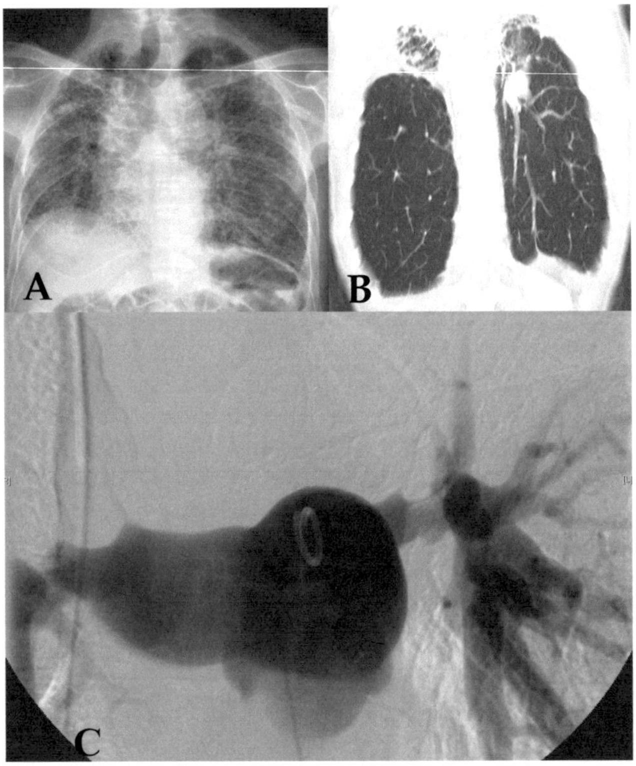

Fig. 1. Sarcoidosis Complications impacting on surgery: A) Tracheal deviation, B) pleural reaction, C) mediastinitis causing pulmonary artery outlet obstruction.

The skin, the second most common organ to be involved with up to 25% of patients affected to some degree, usually manifests itself in the form of macules, papules, plaques or indeed the classical lupus pernio involvement of the lips, cheeks and nose (Yanardag, Pamuk et al. 2003). While this type of disease is not a contraindication to lung transplantation one needs to be mindful of the potential for impaired site healing or indeed wound infection if the cutaneous region around the potential incision site is involved.

The liver and spleen may also be involved with 10 percent of patients having an elevation in their alkaline phosphatase and aminotransferases (Baughman, Teirstein et al. 2001). CT analysis of the hepatosplenic system in Sarcoidosis patients found that the liver developed granulomatous lesions in 5 percent of patients with the spleen having granulomatous involvement in 15 percent. While these figures might be higher than previously thought the nature of liver disease in Sarcoidosis is mainly of insidious onset and clinically quiescent (Scott, Berman et al. 1997). Less than 1 % of the time does significant liver disease like portal hypertension, variceal bleeding, hepatopulmonary syndrome and liver failure occur and in terms of lung transplant work up a CT scan of the abdomen in combination with laboratory parameters is usually sufficient to assess the integrity of the liver and spleen unless indicators such as haematemesis or refractory hypoxia are present.

Cardiovascular investigation represents an important area in patients with Sarcoidosis. Clinically cardiac involvement is thought to be 5 percent however cadaveric studies have shown the figure to be around 25 percent in one series (Iannuzzi, Rybicki et al. 2007). There is a low yield with cardiac biopsies and this hinders the identification of cardiac involvement. The likely reason for this is that the left free wall and septum are more commonly involved resulting in cardiomyopathy or arrhythmias. While these may be identified on routine echocardiography and electrocardiograms the use of MRI/PET with gadolinium are useful in screening for cardiac involvement (Ohira, Tsujino et al. 2008).

Immunosuppression and steroid induced diabetes post lung transplantation results in a higher risk of renal impairment. Macrophages in Sarcoidosis granulomas activate 25-hydroxy-vitamin D to 1,25-dihydroxyvitamin-D resulting in hypercalcaemia (11%), hypercalciuria (40%) and renal calculi (10%) while intrarenal calcium deposition can result in renal failure (Berliner, Haas et al. 2006). All represent a potential risk to patients post transplantation and so patients are screened with 24-hour urinary calcium excretion examination, 24-hour creatinine clearance, and CT abdomen is also performed.

Eighty percent of patients have ocular Sarcoidosis manifest by anterior and posterior uveitis. (Atmaca, Atmaca-Sonmez et al. 2009). This needs to be flagged in the pre-transplant clinic, as there is the added complication of steroid induced cataracts in the post-operative period. In addition there is an increased incidence of neurological Sarcoidosis associated with anterior uveitis, while neurosarcoid is only symptomatic 10% of the time any neurological symptoms should be investigated with an MRI with gadolinium (Menezo, Lobo et al. 2009). A positive result with significant symptoms would rule out transplantation.

3.3 Types of surgery

Sarcoidosis has been subject to most modes of lung transplantation over the decades however some are more advantageous than others. Heart lung transplantation was initially performed and can still be offered if the heart is deemed likely to be unrecoverable post transplant. This is not commonly performed now because experience has taught us that the heart can recover quite well after transplantation (Bando, Armitage et al. 1994), however, even for those in whom the heart is too impaired the paucity of donors has meant the numbers have dwindled over time.

Single lung transplantation on the other hand maximizes the donor pool and increases the chance for more patients on the list to be successfully transplanted. There is some debate as to whether single lung transplantation leaves the patient more susceptible to earlier decline in lung function due to the deficiency of the extra tissue. However we have previously published on our data showing a strong long-term survival in patients receiving a single lung transplant for interstitial lung disease of all types (Keating, Levvey et al. 2009).

Laboratory Studies	Full blood count & Coagulation testing Urea, creatinine and electrolytes Calcium, phosphorous, amylase Liver & Thyroid function tests Total protein and albumin Fasting lipids 24-hour urinary creatinine clearance Urine analysis including cotinine
Microbiology and Serology	Sputum analysis - bacterial and fungal cultures Tuberculosis – Quantiferon Testing Syphilis - RPR, VRDL Urine culture Cytomegalovirus, Epstein Barr virus, toxoplasmosis, Varicella-zoster virus, herpes simplex virus, Human immunodeficiency virus Hepatitis A, B, and C virus
Immunologic Assessment	ABO blood typing Lymphocytic cytotoxic antibody crossmatch Human leukocyte antigen typing Lymphocyte cytotoxicity screen Quantitative immunoglobulin and subclasses
Cardiac Assessment	12-lead electrocardiogram Cardiac gated blood pool scan Echocardiogram Thallium stress testing Cardiac catheterization – if > 40 yrs coronary arteries & ventriculogram, +/- right heart catheter +/- Cardiac Magnetic Resonance Imaging
Pulmonary Assessment	Spirometry, DLCO, lung volumes, arterial blood gases Computed Tomography of the chest Ventilation-perfusion scan Chest x-ray - PA and lateral, and AP supine Exercise capacity - 6-minute walk test with pulse oximetry
Vaccines	Human papilloma vaccine in females Pneumococcal Vaccine Hepatitis A (if seronegative) Hepatitis B (if seronegative)
Miscellaneous	Gynaecological exam & Mammogram > 35 years DEXA scan of spine and hips Prostate-specific antigen >55 years Nutritional assessment including BMI Dental evaluation Psychosocial Evaluation Physiotherapy consultation

Table 3. Lung Transplant work-up protocol

Others have also suggested that due to the shorter operation time single lung transplantation may be preferable for those who might benefit from a brief anesthetic exposure (Low, Trulock et al. 1992).

There are however particular situations where bilateral sequential lung transplantation is more advantageous. This particularly applies to Sarcoidosis patients who have stage IV disease. In this setting the presence of traction bronchiectasis and the presence of resistant microbes make the necessity for this procedure absolute. It is not advisable to leave a potentially infected native lung in situ if there is evidence that it harbors resistant organisms such as pseudomonas aeruginosa, scediosporum profligans or aspergillus. So while there is no research suggesting one form of surgery is superior to another in survival terms, some authors suggest bilateral transplantation should be performed on patients with severe secondary hypertension, fibrocystic Sarcoidosis, mycetomas, and bronchiectasis (Alalawi, Whelan et al. 2005).

Sarcoidosis patients most commonly have a restrictive lung disease and as a result lung size is diminished. In order to accommodate the change in size the lung function is used to compute the size a potential match should be. If there is a size discrepancy it may be necessary to perform cadaveric lobar lung transplantation. This may also be the result if there is a pediatric recipient, when the decision to perform a lobar cut down can be electively taken at the time of listing. Outcomes from this type of surgery are similar to other surgeries allowing patients previously discriminated against based on size mismatch to be transplanted successfully (Keating, Marasco et al. 2010). For similar reasons living donor lobar lung transplantation was developed in order to decrease waiting list times. While there is a theoretical 300% mortality risk, to date this has procedure has shown itself to be well tolerated (Barr, Schenkel et al. 2005). Its use has diminished recently following the introduction of the lung allocation score in the United States however it is still used in countries where culture differences with regards to brain death are still hindering donor procurement.

While the type of surgery being performed has changed, so too has the method by which it is performed. Bilateral sequential lung transplantation has superseded the en bloc approach. The use of lung transplantation over heart-lung transplantation has also developed as our experience has grown. The approach has also differed from midline approach to a clamshell horizontal incision. This now has also been modified in certain individuals to a bilateral thoracotomy incision that allows adequate access to the thoracic cavity but leaves the sternum intact. When patients such as those with Sarcoidosis have had significant exposure to corticosteroids then sternal healing may be impaired and by using this approach a more satisfactory outcome can be achieved.

3.4 Perioperative considerations

A number of issues need to be considered on the night of transplant specifically when considering the multiorgan involvement associated with Sarcoidosis. It is crucial that while on the waiting list that all personnel with a role in the transplant process are kept abreast of any new developments that might arise. This is usually achieved by regular outpatient review with follow up debriefing session with staff. It is through this attention to detail that allows coordinators, physicians and operators to organize a smooth transition through the procedure.

As part of workup patients are screened for renal impairment, if there is any suggestion that renal function may deteriorate as a result of the procedure it is possible during the perioperative period to consider alternative strategies. This might include include withholding preoperative immunosuppression and alternatively using Basiliximab a chimeric monoclonal Interleukin-2 receptor antibody with less nephrotoxicity than calcineurin inhibitors Tacrolimus and Cyclosporin. It acts as an antagonist at the interleukin-2 binding site of the p55 subunit of the high affinity Interleukin-2 receptor on the surface of the activated T lymphocytes and has been shown to decrease the incidence of acute rejection but not chronic rejection in lung transplant recipients (Borro, De la Torre et al. 2005).

3.4.1 Anesthetic considerations

As the fibrotic component of the disease advances Sarcoidosis patients develop tracheal deviation (Figure 1A). While in the majority of the cases this is not a significant issue there is a minority of patients who present on the night of transplant with a severely distorted trachea. This represents a particular problem for anesthetic staff with responsibility for inserting a double lumen endotracheal tube to allow independent lung ventilation necessary to perform a bilateral sequential lung transplant. In most cases this can be achieved, however it adds to the ischaemic time if there is a large time delay.

Routine preoperative anesthetic care involves the insertion of an epidural to adequately titre pain relief post operatively. In patients with severe end stage fibrosis this may be essential as they may have been treated preoperatively with opioid agents for excessive dyspnoea and distress thereby blunting their response to regular doses of analgesia. While in the usual setting this procedure is more routine, in the case of end stage fibrosis patients with labile oxygenation and possible vertebral fractures is requires a greater level of competence and expertise to ensure success.

3.4.2 Intraoperative considerations

Likewise for patients with stage III disease the process may extend to abut or involve the pleura. In this scenario it may be surgically challenging to remove the recipient lungs from the thoracic cavity. This can be assessed by using computed tomography of the chest and assessing the pleural involvement visually, if there is evidence of pleural thickening or adhesion it would be prudent to allow more 'dissection time' when organizing the procedure.

As stated previously the identification of pulmonary hypertension prior to listing is a useful indicator for prognosis in patients with Sarcoidosis. In addition this information is also crucial on the night of transplantation as there is a higher incidence of patients with pulmonary hypertension needing cardiac bypass. This procedure results in deoxygenated blood being removed via large bore cannula placed usually in the vena cava, being externally oxygenated, filtered, warmed and then returned to the circulation via a second large bore cannula usually placed in the ascending aorta. Some debate exists about the need for cardiac bypass in routine lung transplantation, however in the setting of pulmonary hypertension it can prevent hemodynamic collapse when the pulmonary artery is clamped. In addition is prevents any sudden increase in pulmonary pressures after clamping which might increase the after-load on the right ventricle. With underlying hypertension this could result in right heart failure and decompensation. As a result most centres will have cardiopulmonary bypass on standby in transplant cases where there is evidence of increased pulmonary pressures preoperatively (Marczin, Royston et al. 2000). In some patients with severe pulmonary hypertension and high oxygen requirements a decision to commence cardiopulmonary bypass prior to induction of anesthesia may be made. This allows the anesthetist time to correctly position the endotracheal tube without the risk of sudden and catastrophic desaturation occurring. When this is performed a different approach is used with cannulation of the femoral artery and vein.

Hyperacute rejection is one of the more devastating complications that occurs following lung transplantation surgery. On releasing the cross-clamp the flow of blood into the new lung results in an immediate reaction within minutes that can herald a terminal decline. The mechanism is thought to be pre-existing antibodies formed against ABO blood groups, endothelial cells or human leukocyte antigens (Frost, Jammal et al. 1996). This results in parenchymal damage that pathologically resembles diffuse alveolar damage characterized by mononuclear and polymorphonuclear accumulation, intravascular thrombosis and intramural vascular necrosis. Many centres now use more sensitive antibody testing such as Luminex, which allows a better assessment of the match between donor and recipient. This has decreased the incidence of hyperacute rejection and while it still represents a significant immediate complication there is some possibility that the patient can be stabilized, transferred onto extracorporeal membrane oxygenation and urgently relisted.

3.4.3 Early post-operative considerations

Most of the gains that have been achieved in lung transplantation over the last two decades have been as a result of early post-operative management. The recognition of problems that might arise not just as a result of transplantation but also in relation to the recipients underlying disease has allowed physicians to pre-empt issues rather than react to them as they arise. Some of the problems that affect Sarcoidosis patients are related to the transplant process, however some they will have a predilection to.

Immunosuppression is commenced pre-operatively and continued post operative while being closely followed using serum measurements of trough levels. Most centers use a triple immunosuppression regimen consisting of a calcineurin inhibitor (Cyclosporin or Tacrolimus), Azathioprine or mycophenylate, and corticosteroids. Basiliximab may be used in preference to the calcineurin inhibitors initially to preserve renal function. Preoperative assessment in Sarcoidosis patients usually highlights those that should be prescribed the Interleukin-2 inhibitor electively. All agents can be given intravenously initially and changed to the oral route when feasible (Snell and Westall 2007).

Ischemia reperfusion injury is used to describe non-cardiogenic edema that usually occurs approximately 24 hours after lung transplantation in up to 97% of patients. It peaks by day four, resolving usually by day seven however, it may continue for up to six months. Putative contributing factors include surgical trauma, donor lung ischemia, and interruption of bronchial circulation, lymphatic flow and donor lung innervation (Collins 2002). Features of reperfusion injury on Computed Tomography differ from those of hyperacute rejection with evidence of perihilar ground glass opacities, peribronchial and perivascular thickening and reticular interstitial or airspace opacities especially in the middle and lower lobes. In this setting it is important to rule out other causes with similar profiles such as rejection, infection, fluid overload or cardiac failure especially in Sarcoidosis patients with an increased incidence of cardiac involvement (Krishnam, Suh et al. 2007)

To avoid healing problems that may occur it is important not to induce barotrauma either to the parenchyma, which might induce an upregulation of the immune response, or direct positive pressure injury to the anastomotic area. While strategies need not necessarily be tailored for Sarcoidosis patients a strategy of low positive end expiratory pressure (5cmH_20) and tidal volumes (8-10 mL/Kg) are preferred. When patients receive single lung transplants this is especially important as the native lung will have altered compliance due to fibrosis putting the allograft at greater risk of injury using what appears to be acceptable pressures

Early weaning from mechanical ventilation is of paramount importance for a successful transplant outcome. Many patients can be weaned from the ventilator within twenty-four hours. This has significant benefits in terms of weaning of sedation, less need for airway access via suction, while the risk of infection is considerably reduced. In addition the discontinuation of positive pressure and the initiation of more natural negative ventilation helps to protect the anastomotic integrity from any barotrauma that might cause rupture. An early extubation strategy for Sarcoidosis recipients is encouraged as many patients will have been treated with prolonged courses of steroids. While this is not a contraindication for transplantation there are a number of problems that might arise if the overall burden of steroid preoperatively is excessive. Of particular concern is the patients' wound healing ability following surgery. This does not only apply to the cutaneous and underlying subcutaneous structures but also the anastomoses. The arterial and venous connections may also be compromised by significant corticosteroid doses. As a general rule most centres suggest doses of steroids to be less than 10 milligrams per day prior to transplantation, which in the majority of Sarcoidosis cases can be achieved.

Weaning from mechanical ventilation may also be affected more profoundly by the onset of critical care myopathy. While there is no indication that this affects patients with Sarcoidosis more than any other transplant recipients the long-term use of steroids in high doses certainly results in preponderance for muscle wasting (Weber-Carstens, Deja et al.). The wasting of intercostal muscles in particular may result in failure to wean from the mechanical ventilator resulting in the need to progress to tracheostomy placement and non-invasive ventilation strategies to aid recovery. A prolonged period on non-invasive ventilation through a tracheotomy leads to thicker secretions, increased frequency of infections and increased length of stay.

The diaphragm represents the main muscle of respiration and normal ventilation requires it to be healthy and functioning. Normal diaphragmatic contraction results in decreased intrapleural pressure, an expanded rib cage through its zone of apposition by generating a positive intra-abdominal pressure, and expansion of the rib cage using the abdomen as a fulcrum (Rochester 1985). The reported incidence of phrenic nerve injury in the literature varies from 3% to 30% and is dependent on the methods used to detect the defect (Maziak, Maurer et al. 1996). The putative causes of the injury include direct phrenic nerve injury during mediastinal dissection, stretch injury of the nerve as the pericardium is manipulated, and hypothermic injury during the operative period. Interruption of this phrenic nerve function leads to increased work of breathing and difficulty in weaning patients from mechanical ventilation in addition to an increased incidence of atelectasis, ventilator associated pneumonia, and hypoxemia resulting in prolongation of ICU stay in most cases (Maziak, Maurer et al. 1996; Ferdinande, Bruyninckx et al. 2004)

Physiotherapy input at this stage and indeed in the preoperative work up is essential to improve patient outcome (Kress 2009). Breathing techniques to facilitate airway secretion clearance and daily assessment of muscle function help to expedite patients' recovery and decrease infections. An earlier initiation of treatment and regular follow up exercise, in a controlled environment, has long term benefits on patients exercise capacity, lung function and quality of life (Munro, Holland et al. 2009).

3.4.4 General ICU considerations

Usually an epidural catheter placed preoperatively allows adequate analgesia to be applied at a local level and decreasing the reliance on systemic agents. If this is not possible higher doses of systemic agents may result in significant cognitive depression delaying weaning from mechanical ventilation. In addition any prolongation of mechanical ventilation should be accompanied by an attempt to awaken the patient on a daily basis to assess cognitive function, pain threshold and ability to perform even limited physiotherapy.

Although more commonly seen as a result of gastric surgery there has been a recent increase in the reported incidence of vagus nerve injury following fundoplication surgery and bariatric surgery. However, there have been reports of cases in transplantation also (Shafi and Pasricha 2007; Paul, Escareno et al. 2009)with the incidence reported to be of the order of five percent. Most cases can be managed conservatively; however there may be significant problems post lung transplantation in terms of maintaining adequate immunosuppression and nutritional absorption. Most injuries resolve over a two-year period and additional intervention is not usually required.

Malabsorption however can have additional consequences with patients often having difficulty maintaining electrolyte levels. While patients with cystic fibrosis are generally at greater risk any Sarcoidosis patients who may have occult cardiac involvement may manifest this during a period of electrolyte instability by the onset of cardiac arrhythmia. Patients are monitored daily with blood analysis while immunosuppression levels are increased to achieve adequate levels. Any evidence of renal impairment or electrolyte imbalance is treated early to avoid any cardiac arrhythmias.

Hyperammonemia has been reported to occur in up to four percent of lung transplant patients with mortality estimated to be of the order of seventy percent (Lichtenstein, Yang et al. 2000). It presents as a clinical syndrome with deteriorating neurological function despite liver function tests in the normal range within the first three months after surgery. Hyperammonemia is thought to be related to immunosuppressive agents however underlying liver and genetic abnormalities have also been suggested as alleged mechanisms of disease. Sarcoidosis patients although not shown to be at higher risk post lung transplant, may have occult disease wither due to granulomatous infiltration or to immunosuppressive agents such as azathioprine prescribed preoperatively. While the prognosis if diagnosed is poor there have been reports of patients being successfully managed, physicians however, need to maintain a high level of clinical suspicion to facilitate early intervention (Moffatt-Bruce, Pesavento et al. 2008)

3.4.5 Infections

Early infections are usually of donor origin however in the setting of severe bronchiectasis as in stage IV Sarcoidosis it is possible to have native tracheal colonization with microbes. Early antibiotic regimens are usually broad spectrum covering the commonest pathogens with the addition of cover for any microbes identified in the recipient preoperatively. Donor harvest washings are also taken to tailor the treatment if empiric treatment proves to be incomplete.

Bacterial pneumonia is frequently observed following lung transplantation; however the incidence has decreased over the last few decades. The initial six-month post operative period is when the patients are subjected to the peak level of immunosuppression and it is during this time that likelihood of bacterial infection is at its greatest. Bacterial identification has been reported in up to eighty percent of patients. In one Spanish study there was an incidence of 72 episodes of pneumonia per hundred lung transplants per year and of the established etiologies bacterial infections accounted for eighty two percent. Pseudomonas, Acinetobacter and staphylococcus accounted for the majority of the cases (Aguilar-Guisado, Givalda et al. 2007). Assessment and sampling of donor lungs during harvesting suggests that many of the early pneumonias are of donor origin; use of this information has allowed a tailoring of the post lung transplant antibiotic regime resulting in improved outcome (Dauber, Paradis et al. 1990; Weill, Dey et al. 2002). Antibiotic prophylaxis against opportunistic infections is also important and the use of sulfamethoxazole and trimethoprim three times a week has been efficacious in the prevention of Pneumocystis Jiroveci infection while it also has an effect on other microbes such as Listeria, Toxoplasma and Listeria (Fishman 2007).

Cytomegalovirus (a human herpesvirus) is probably the most important viral pathogens associated with lung transplantation due to its ability to latently infect the host allowing reactivation to occur at any stage throughout the recipients lifetime (Zamora 2004). Seronegative recipients receiving a seropositive allograft are at greatest risk of infection while previously exposed recipients have a lesser risk. CMV primary infection and reactivation is associated with a reported mortality ranging from 2- 12 percent (Fishman and Rubin 1998). While the acute effects from CMV have been identified the long term risk from latent infection or repeated activation does not have a linear relationship with the development of chronic allograft failure (Sharples, McNeil et al. 2002).

Epstein Barr Virus is a well-documented pathogen following lung transplantation with historical reports of post transplant lymphoproliferative disease in 2-5% of all lung transplant recipients and up to 30% of donor/recipient Epstein Barr virus mismatches. More recently, routine use of current antiviral prophylaxis strategies, more judicious use of immunosuppression regimens in at risk recipients, and improved treatment options have anecdotally been associated with improved outcomes (Malouf, Chhajed et al. 2002).

Other viruses such as the alphaherpesviridae (Herpes Simplex Virus 1 and 2, and Varicella Zoster Virus) were previously associated with an unacceptably high mortality however with cytomegalovirus prophylaxis the 10 percent mortality associated with these viruses has been almost eradicated (Manuel, Kumar et al. 2008)

While fungal infections post lung transplantation may include Candida, Scediosporum and Fusarium species the most problematic is Aspergillus. Aspergillus, also the commonest affecting 6.2% of all lung transplant recipients (Singh and Husain 2003), may take the form of tracheobronchitis, anastomotic infection of parenchymal invasion, although disseminated disease can also occur. Complicated surgery in addition to immunosuppressive therapy and renal impairment are recognized as risk factors for fungal infection, suggesting that extra vigilance may be warranted in Sarcoidosis patients in the weeks post procedure. Diagnosis of fungal infection is difficult but the instigation of regular surveillance bronchoscopies in most centres allows regular viewing of the anastomosis and bronchoalveolar lavage of the parenchyma, which improves the detection rate. Treatment in most centres involves fluconazole or in the case of aspergillus voriconazole or posaconazole which has been reasonably efficacious in managing the disease although eradication has proven difficult especially in the setting of single lung transplant recipients where the native lung acts as a reservoir for infection. Prophylaxis is not routinely prescribed unless isolated from the donor harvest bronchoalveolar lavage.

3.4.6 Medium and late complications

A number of conditions are associated with lung transplantation as a consequence of the long-term effects of immunosuppression. These include osteoporosis (Aris, Neuringer et al. 1996) which many Sarcoidosis patients will have a predilection to as a result of prior corticosteroid use, chronic renal failure related in part to Tacrolimus or cyclosporine (Parekh, Trulock et al. 2004) as is systemic hypertension (Morrison, Short et al. 1993). Corticosteroids and the calcineurin inhibitors can also induce diabetes mellitus (Jindal 1994), Obesity, Anaemia (End, Stift et al. 1995), hypercholesterolemia and hypertriglyceridaemia (Stephany, Alao et al. 2007). Gastroesophageal reflux disease (GORD) disease however appears to be a direct result of surgery through mechanical manipulation or impingement of the vagus nerve causing gastroparesis (Davis, Lau et al. 2003).

Lung transplantation surgery has evolved so that the recipient airway is relying on collateral and retrograde perfusion from the pulmonary artery for blood supply. Initially the bronchial arteries were re-anastomosed but this resulted in prolongation of the allograft ischaemic time; this led to the cessation of this technique. Currently evidence of diminished airway perfusion may be observed during surveillance bronchoscopies usually as variegated violet change on the endobronchial surface. These changes may subsequently develop into ischaemic injury with blackening and ulceration of the surface. Some of the sloughed endobronchial surface may result in airway obstruction with evidence of decreased FEV1 and a scalloped flow loop on lung function testing. Any sloughed areas can be debrided via the bronchoscope and closely followed to insure that secondary infection is identified and treated as early as possible.

For the majority of cases conservative management is sufficient however in 5% of patients the injury progresses to bronchial dehiscence with ulceration, perforation or stricture formation (Weder, Inci et al. 2009). It has been suggested that the technique of telescoping of the airways to adjust for size discrepancy and to add stability to the airway wall may also result in an increase in airway complications. Usually management is successful using balloon dilatations with or without the added radial cuts with argon plasma coagulation. This approach usually abrogates the need to use endobronchial stent placement. In some patients the need for stenting is unavoidable and in this scenario temporary polyflex stents can be placed which allow for their removal when the integrity of the airway wall has stiffened with scaring. Occasionally covered or uncovered stents may be placed and usually this will add architecture to the airway, however the disadvantage is that stents can fracture leading to retention of secretions around the loose wires. This may result in infection, obstruction or both and dealing with these can be problematic as the stents become embedded in the walls. On the other hand vascular anastomotic problems are not as common. Usually if present they result in pulmonary infarction on the arterial side and often occur in the early postoperative period.

Surveillance bronchoscopy is carried out regularly after transplantation at weeks 2,4,8,12,24,36, and 52. While initially this is done to assess the anastomosis and also to preempt any infection that might arise subsequently more subtle infections such as CMV and EBV can be identified earlier by using bronchoalveolar lavage thereby allowing physicians to augment therapy and avoid chronic impairment (Westall, Michaelides et al. 2004).

Bronchoscopy is also performed to monitor for acute rejection which in the early post operative period is generally diagnosed using clinical criteria. Clinically acute rejection is recognized as a constellation of symptoms including dyspnoea, fatigue, dry cough, low-grade fever, a 10mmHg decrease in PaO2, and a 10% drop in FEV1 in conjunction with radiological opacification. These clinical features are not specific and usually develop when acute rejection is more severe. Subsequently surveillance biopsies taken at bronchoscopy assist to diagnose the process. Acute rejection occurs when the host organ recipient recognizes the donor organ as foreign, based on a lack of recognition of human leukocyte antigens, and as a result attacks the organ causing it to fail. Acute rejection is classified based on the severity and extent of perivascular lymphocytic cuffing and parenchymal infiltration. No abnormality (grade A0) at one end of the scale is counterbalanced by severe rejection (grade A4) that involves the interstitium and airspaces in addition to damaged pneumocytes and vascular changes (Stewart, Fishbein et al. 2007). Most lung transplant recipients will develop at least one episode of acute rejection in the first three months and the presence of rejection grade A2 or higher is managed with a 'pulse' of methylprednisolone (500mg-1g IV x three days). Baseline immunosuppression is also augmented following this. Resistant cases may need further treatment with antilymphocyte antibody.

Chronic rejection remains the elusive 'holy grail' of transplantation. It remains the main cause of morbidity and mortality after the first year not just due to obliterative bronchiolitis but also due to increased infections (Burton, Carlsen et al. 2007). Chronic rejection is more difficult to diagnose and has a more languid onset than acute rejection. Patients usually develop a cough that may be productive and clinically produce audible squeaks on examination. Risk factors to be noted in the history include persistent or severe episodes of acute rejection, CMV infection or recurrence, organising pneumonia, ischaemic-reperfusion injury, and gastro-oesophageal reflux (Estenne, Maurer et al. 2002). Lung function may show a progressive obstruction which has been used to grade the severity of bronchiolitis obliterans syndrome while the pathological entity obliterative bronchiolitis may or may not be evident on transbronchial biopsies leaving clinicians with a diagnosis of exclusion. Treatment is generally unsatisfactory despite courses of pulsed corticosteroids, cytolytic therapy, inhaled cyclosporin, switching from Cyclosporin to Tacrolimus, total lymphoid irradiation, plasmapheresis and photopheresis, leaving retransplantation in most cases the only option provided the patient passes the assessment criteria a second time (Neuringer, Noone et al. 2009).

4. Results

Considering the numbers of transplants performed for Sarcoidosis are limited compared with other diagnosis, the specific survival data is difficult to extrapolate from the documented figures provided in international databases. Lung transplantation figures have generally improved recently, due mainly to careful choice of donors and improvements in patient management postoperatively. Recent data shows that for all deceased donor lung transplants the 1, 3, and 5 year survival is 83, 65 and 51 percent respectively (UNOS 2011). In order to address the donor shortage donor organs from patients deceased following cardiac death have been utilised, and interestingly the early outcome data suggests that the survival is improved in this cohort theoretically due to diminished neurological mediators released at the time of death although the exact reason remains to be elucidated (Snell and Levvey 2009). No direct comparison of data has been published; however one paper has shown excellent long term outcomes for all interstitial diseases following transplantation, which appears comparable to survival numbers in other organs (Keating, Levvey et al. 2009).

	Living		Deceased		Lost to Follow up		Retransplanted		Total
Year	**N**	**%**	**N**	**%**	**N**	**%**	**N**	**%**	**N**
2000	10	38.46	16	61.54	0	0	0	0	26
2001	7	22.58	22	70.97	0	0	2	6.45	31
2002	5	15.63	24	75.00	1	3.13	2	6.25	32
2003	9	42.86	11	52.38	1	4.76	0	0	21
2004	16	41.03	21	53.85	1	2.56	1	2.56	39
2005	19	39.58	27	56.25	1	2.08	1	2.08	48
2006	36	64.29	18	32.14	1	1.79	1	1.79	56
2007	25	58.14	17	39.53	1	2.33	0	0	43
2008	32	74.42	11	25.58	0	0	0	0	43
2009	37	82.22	7	15.56	0	0	1	2.22	45
2010	45	83.33	9	16.67	0	0	0	0	54
All	**241**	**55.05**	**183**	**41.78**	**6**	**1.37**	**8**	**1.83**	**438**

Table 4. Survival Data from UNOS for Sarcoidosis Recipients since 2000

Other research shows that Sarcoidosis patients, when compared to other lung transplant recipients, have a predilection for severe, acute rejection. Acute rejection is a recognised risk factor for the development of BOS or chronic rejection suggesting Sarcoidosis patients might have a worse long term outcome after transplant (Johnson, Duncan et al. 1993). On review the evidence for an increased incidence of BOS in Sarcoidosis patients is lacking and suggests that the numbers involved in this study are too small to draw definitive conclusions on long term outcomes while others have shown equivocal outcomes to other transplant diagnosis (Padilla, Schilero et al. 1997; Wille, Gaggar et al. 2008; Keating, Levvey et al. 2009).

A number of cases of Sarcoidosis have recurred post lung transplantation (Bjortuft, Foerster et al. 1994; Gisvold, Crotty et al. 2000), however only 533 patients with Sarcoidosis are registered as receiving a transplant since 1998 (OPTN/SRTR 2009). Because of the small number of recipients with a primary diagnosis of Sarcoidosis the actual prevalence of recurrence is not known definitively. To date around 21 cases are recorded with two further reports of recurrence in an undocumented number (Collins, Hartman et al. 2001). The estimated frequency is calculated as 50% but the range between reported series has been between 25 and

80% (Johnson, Duncan et al. 1993; Bjortuft, Foerster et al. 1994; Walker, Mikhail et al. 1998; Burke, Stewart et al. 2001; Milman, Burton et al. 2005). Although rates are varied Black Americans seem to have a higher recurrence rate at 66% compared to other races (Nunley, Hattler et al. 1999). Sarcoidosis, however, is not the only disease that recurs following lung transplant and a list of the other reported conditions is in Table 2.

In the majority of cases, recurrence of Sarcoidosis is not preceded by an increase in respiratory symptoms and signs (Johnson, Duncan et al. 1993; Nunley, Hattler et al. 1999). Usually cases of recurrence are identified as part of surveillance bronchoscopies carried out routinely post procedure. Recurrence is evidenced by the identification of the characteristic non-caseating granulomas present before transplantation however other causes of this such as fungal or mycobacterial infection need to be ruled out first. Radiologically the features may be of solitary or multiple nodules, or there may be no specific changes present (Collins, Hartman et al. 2001). In some cases however there may be evidence of graft dysfunction with the onset of respiratory symptoms, and in these patients there is a greater likelihood that there are coexisting infiltrates on radiological investigations (Judson 1998).

Sarcoidosis
Lymphangioleiomatosis
Diffuse Panbronchiolitis
Pulmonary alveolar proteinosis
Desquamative interstitial pneumonia
Pulmonary Langherhans Cell Histiocytosis
Bronchioloalveolar Carcinoma
Idiopathic Pulmonary Hemosiderosis
Giant Cell Interstitial Pneumonia
Alpha-1-Antitrypsin Deficiency
Pulmonary Veno-occlusive Disease

Table 5. Table of conditions known to recur after lung transplantation.

Recurrence can occur at any stage post transplantation documented from as early as 2 weeks out to 2 years (Johnson, Duncan et al. 1993; Martel, Carre et al. 1996). Some have suggested that rejection and Sarcoidosis may utilise a common pathway via the activation of T-lymphocytes however, the weight of evidence is against this. Immunosuppression used in lung transplantation to target interleukin-2, part of the CD8 cytotoxic T-lymphocyte response, has been found to be ineffective in suppressing Sarcoidosis, the granulomas of which appear to be due to a process driven by CD4 T-lymphocytes (Semenzato, Zambello et al. 1993; Wyser, van Schalkwyk et al. 1997). The recurrence of Sarcoidosis in lung transplant recipients early post operatively when immunosuppression is at its zenith would concur with a disparate immunological basis between the two pathological processes.

Notwithstanding the debate as to the frequency of recurrence of Sarcoidosis the impact of recurrence appears to be negligible. The majority of patients who have recurrence have an incidental finding with little or no effect noticeable on pulmonary function testing. Indeed while recurrence is associated with a more severe course of acute rejection, there is no evidence for increased frequency and there is no association with an increase in BOS over and above the normal LTx population.

Appropriate patients are considered for retransplantation if they are in robust enough health to allow transition through a second procedure. The evidence suggests that while the survival figures are improving retransplantation outcomes are not as good as those undergoing their first procedure. This is especially so for those who require early retransplantation within 30 days (Trulock, Edwards et al. 2003). A recent paper suggested Sarcoidosis was not a significant cause for retransplantation; of 389 patients requiring retransplantation between 1980 and 2006, only 84 patients had diffuse lung disease as the reason for initial transplantation, this number included all Sarcoidosis patients. The reason for retransplantation included BOS (52%), primary graft dysfunction (16%) and acute rejection (3%) while all other and unknown causes accounted for only 27% (59/389) (Kawut, Lederer et al. 2008). The specific Sarcoidosis numbers among these figures were not commented on, however, a previous study showed that there was no evidence to suggest a higher incidence of chronic rejection with Sarcoidosis (Padilla, Schilero et al. 1997). This taken in conjunction with the UNOS data in Table 4 shows that very few Sarcoidosis patients progress to retransplantation (n=8, 1.83%).

5. Conclusion

Sarcoidosis continues to affect significant numbers of the population and while many among this cohort spontaneously recover some progress to respiratory failure. The historical difficulty in Sarcoidosis patient receiving lung transplantation is likely to be multifactorial as the natural progression of the disease is not consistent, with no reliable markers to predict those who progress despite treatment. This meant that timing for lung transplantation was difficult to assess accurately. Recently pulmonary hypertension has been identified as a reasonable prognostic marker and all patients who develop increased pulmonary pressures on echocardiogram should be considered potential candidates. The multisystem nature of Sarcoidosis means patients still need to undergo a rigorous pre-listing assessment, but once lung transplantation has been performed outcomes are equivocal to other indications. Recurrence of Sarcoidosis is the commonest for all the indication for transplantation however it has limited impact on the long-term outcome of the recipient. The development of an LAS in score in the United States may result in Sarcoidosis receiving greater priority in the future, especially those patients with associated pulmonary hypertension. Early recognition of declining clinical and radiological status should prompt referral for lung transplant assessment with outcomes likely to improve with further improvements in transplantation.

6. Acknowledgements

UNOS data acknowledgement 'This work was supported in part by Health Resources and Services Administration contract 234-2005-370011C. The content is the responsibility of the authors alone and does not necessarily reflect the views or policies of the Department of Health and Human Services, nor does mention of trade names, commercial products, or organizations imply endorsement by the U.S. Government'.

7. References

(1999). "Statement on sarcoidosis. Joint Statement of the American Thoracic Society (ATS), the European Respiratory Society (ERS) and the World Association of Sarcoidosis and Other Granulomatous Disorders (WASOG) adopted by the ATS Board of Directors and by the ERS Executive Committee, February 1999." Am J Respir Crit Care Med 160(2): 736-55.

Aguilar-Guisado, M., J. Givalda, et al. (2007). "Pneumonia after lung transplantation in the RESITRA Cohort: a multicenter prospective study." Am J Transplant 7(8): 1989-96.

Alalawi, R., T. Whelan, et al. (2005). "Lung transplantation and interstitial lung disease." Curr Opin Pulm Med 11(5): 461-6.

Alhamad, E. H. (2009). "The six-minute walk test in patients with pulmonary sarcoidosis." Ann Thorac Med 4(2): 60-4.

Aris, R. M., I. P. Neuringer, et al. (1996). "Severe osteoporosis before and after lung transplantation." Chest 109(5): 1176-83.

Atmaca, L. S., P. Atmaca-Sonmez, et al. (2009). "Ocular involvement in sarcoidosis." Ocul Immunol Inflamm 17(2): 91-4.

Bando, K., J. M. Armitage, et al. (1994). "Indications for and results of single, bilateral, and heart-lung transplantation for pulmonary hypertension." J Thorac Cardiovasc Surg 108(6): 1056-65.

Barr, M. L., F. A. Schenkel, et al. (2005). "Living donor lobar lung transplantation: current status and future directions." Transplant Proc 37(9): 3983-6.

Baughman, R. P., U. Costabel, et al. (2008). "Treatment of sarcoidosis." Clin Chest Med 29(3): 533-48, ix-x.

Baughman, R. P., E. E. Lower, et al. (2003). "Sarcoidosis." Lancet 361(9363): 1111-8.

Baughman, R. P., A. S. Teirstein, et al. (2001). "Clinical characteristics of patients in a case control study of sarcoidosis." Am J Respir Crit Care Med 164(10 Pt 1): 1885-9.

Berliner, A. R., M. Haas, et al. (2006). "Sarcoidosis: the nephrologist's perspective." Am J Kidney Dis 48(5): 856-70.

Bjortuft, O., A. Foerster, et al. (1994). "Single lung transplantation as treatment for end-stage pulmonary sarcoidosis: recurrence of sarcoidosis in two different lung allografts in one patient." J Heart Lung Transplant 13(1 Pt 1): 24-9.

Borro, J. M., M. De la Torre, et al. (2005). "Comparative study of basiliximab treatment in lung transplantation." Transplant Proc 37(9): 3996-8.

Bresnitz, E. A. and B. L. Strom (1983). "Epidemiology of sarcoidosis." Epidemiol Rev 5: 124-56.

Burke, M., S. Stewart, et al. (2001). "Biopsy diagnosis of disease recurrence after transplantation (TX) for pulmonary sarcoidosis: a multicentre study." J Heart Lung Transplant 20(2): 154-155.

Burton, C. M., J. Carlsen, et al. (2007). "Long-term survival after lung transplantation depends on development and severity of bronchiolitis obliterans syndrome." J Heart Lung Transplant 26(7): 681-6.

Christie, J. D., L. B. Edwards, et al. (2008). "Registry of the International Society for Heart and Lung Transplantation: twenty-fifth official adult lung and heart/lung transplantation report--2008." J Heart Lung Transplant 27(9): 957-69.

Collins, J. (2002). "Imaging of the chest after lung transplantation." J Thorac Imaging 17(2): 102-12.

Collins, J., M. J. Hartman, et al. (2001). "Frequency and CT findings of recurrent disease after lung transplantation." Radiology 219(2): 503-9.

Corte, T. J., A. U. Wells, et al. (2010). "Pulmonary Hypertension in Sarcoidosis: A Review." Respirology.

Costabel, U., F. Bonella, et al. (2010). "Diagnostic modalities in sarcoidosis: BAL, EBUS, and PET." Semin Respir Crit Care Med 31(4): 404-8.

Dauber, J. H., I. L. Paradis, et al. (1990). "Infectious complications in pulmonary allograft recipients." Clin Chest Med 11(2): 291-308.

Davis, R. D., Jr., C. L. Lau, et al. (2003). "Improved lung allograft function after fundoplication in patients with gastroesophageal reflux disease undergoing lung transplantation." J Thorac Cardiovasc Surg 125(3): 533-42.

Dhote, R., O. Vignaux, et al. (2003). "[Value of MRI for the diagnosis of cardiac involvement in sarcoidosis]." Rev Med Interne 24(3): 151-7.

Egan, T. M., S. Murray, et al. (2006). "Development of the new lung allocation system in the United States." Am J Transplant 6(5 Pt 2): 1212-27.

End, A., A. Stift, et al. (1995). "Anemia and erythropoietin levels in lung transplant recipients." Transplantation 60(11): 1245-51.

Estenne, M., J. R. Maurer, et al. (2002). "Bronchiolitis obliterans syndrome 2001: an update of the diagnostic criteria." J Heart Lung Transplant 21(3): 297-310.

Fazzi, P. (2003). "Pharmacotherapeutic management of pulmonary sarcoidosis." Am J Respir Med 2(4): 311-20.

Ferdinande, P., F. Bruyninckx, et al. (2004). "Phrenic nerve dysfunction after heart-lung and lung transplantation." J Heart Lung Transplant 23(1): 105-9.

Fishman, J. A. (2007). "Infection in solid-organ transplant recipients." N Engl J Med 357(25): 2601-14.

Fishman, J. A. and R. H. Rubin (1998). "Infection in organ-transplant recipients." N Engl J Med 338(24): 1741-51.

Frost, A. E., C. T. Jammal, et al. (1996). "Hyperacute rejection following lung transplantation." Chest 110(2): 559-62.

Gilman, M. J. and K. P. Wang (1980). "Transbronchial lung biopsy in sarcoidosis. An approach to determine the optimal number of biopsies." Am Rev Respir Dis 122(5): 721-4.

Gisvold, J. J., T. B. Crotty, et al. (2000). "Sarcoidosis presenting as spiculated breast masses." Mayo Clin Proc 75(3): 293-5.

Hardy, J. D., W. R. Webb, et al. (1963). "Lung Homotransplantation in Man." JAMA 186: 1065-74.

Iannuzzi, M. C., B. A. Rybicki, et al. (2007). "Sarcoidosis." N Engl J Med 357(21): 2153-65.

Jindal, R. M. (1994). "Posttransplant diabetes mellitus--a review." Transplantation 58(12): 1289-98.

Johnson, B. A., S. R. Duncan, et al. (1993). "Recurrence of sarcoidosis in pulmonary allograft recipients." Am Rev Respir Dis 148(5): 1373-7.

Judson, M. A. (1998). "Lung transplantation for pulmonary sarcoidosis." Eur Respir J 11(3): 738-44.

Judson, M. A., R. P. Baughman, et al. (2003). "Two year prognosis of sarcoidosis: the ACCESS experience." Sarcoidosis Vasc Diffuse Lung Dis 20(3): 204-11.

Kawut, S. M., D. J. Lederer, et al. (2008). "Outcomes after lung retransplantation in the modern era." Am J Respir Crit Care Med 177(1): 114-20.

Keating, D., B. Levvey, et al. (2009). "Lung transplantation in pulmonary fibrosis: challenging early outcomes counterbalanced by surprisingly good outcomes beyond 15 years." Transplant Proc 41(1): 289-91.

Keating, D. T., S. F. Marasco, et al. (2010). "Long-term outcomes of cadaveric lobar lung transplantation: helping to maximize resources." J Heart Lung Transplant 29(4): 439-44.

Kress, J. P. (2009). "Clinical trials of early mobilization of critically ill patients." Crit Care Med 37(10 Suppl): S442-7.

Krishnam, M. S., R. D. Suh, et al. (2007). "Postoperative complications of lung transplantation: radiologic findings along a time continuum." Radiographics 27(4): 957-74.

Lichtenstein, G. R., Y. X. Yang, et al. (2000). "Fatal hyperammonemia after orthotopic lung transplantation." Ann Intern Med 132(4): 283-7.

Malouf, M. A., P. N. Chhajed, et al. (2002). "Anti-viral prophylaxis reduces the incidence of lymphoproliferative disease in lung transplant recipients." J Heart Lung Transplant 21(5): 547-54.

Manuel, O., D. Kumar, et al. (2008). "Incidence and clinical characteristics of herpes zoster after lung transplantation." J Heart Lung Transplant 27(1): 11-6.

Marczin, N., D. Royston, et al. (2000). "Pro: lung transplantation should be routinely performed with cardiopulmonary bypass." J Cardiothorac Vasc Anesth 14(6): 739-45.

Martel, S., P. C. Carre, et al. (1996). "Tumour necrosis factor-alpha gene expression by alveolar macrophages in human lung allograft recipient with recurrence of sarcoidosis. Toulouse Lung Transplantation Group." Eur Respir J 9(5): 1087-9.

Maziak, D. E., J. R. Maurer, et al. (1996). "Diaphragmatic paralysis: a complication of lung transplantation." Ann Thorac Surg 61(1): 170-3.

Mehta, D., S. A. Lubitz, et al. (2008). "Cardiac involvement in patients with sarcoidosis: diagnostic and prognostic value of outpatient testing." Chest 133(6): 1426-35.

Menezo, V., A. Lobo, et al. (2009). "Ocular features in neurosarcoidosis." Ocul Immunol Inflamm 17(3): 170-8.

Milman, N., C. Burton, et al. (2005). "Lung transplantation for end-stage pulmonary sarcoidosis: outcome in a series of seven consecutive patients." Sarcoidosis Vasc Diffuse Lung Dis 22(3): 222-8.

Moffatt-Bruce, S. D., T. Pesavento, et al. (2008). "Successful management of immunosuppression in a patient with severe hyperammonemia after lung transplantation." J Heart Lung Transplant 27(7): 801-3.

Morrison, R. J., H. D. Short, et al. (1993). "Hypertension after lung transplantation." J Heart Lung Transplant 12(6 Pt 1): 928-31.

Munro, P. E., A. E. Holland, et al. (2009). "Pulmonary rehabilitation following lung transplantation." Transplant Proc 41(1): 292-5.

Murdoch, J. and N. L. Muller (1992). "Pulmonary sarcoidosis: changes on follow-up CT examination." AJR Am J Roentgenol 159(3): 473-7.

Neuringer, I. P., P. Noone, et al. (2009). "Managing complications following lung transplantation." Expert Rev Respir Med 3(4): 403-23.

Newman, L. S., C. S. Rose, et al. (2004). "A case control etiologic study of sarcoidosis: environmental and occupational risk factors." Am J Respir Crit Care Med 170(12): 1324-30.

Newman, L. S., C. S. Rose, et al. (1997). "Sarcoidosis." N Engl J Med 336(17): 1224-34.

Niida, T., K. Isoda, et al. (2009). "Late gadolinium enhanced high resolution magnetic resonance imaging reveals pathophysiological condition of cardiac sarcoidosis." Int Heart J 50(2): 263-6.

Nunley, D. R., B. Hattler, et al. (1999). "Lung transplantation for end-stage pulmonary sarcoidosis." Sarcoidosis Vasc Diffuse Lung Dis 16(1): 93-100.

Ohira, H., I. Tsujino, et al. (2008). "Myocardial imaging with 18F-fluoro-2-deoxyglucose positron emission tomography and magnetic resonance imaging in sarcoidosis." Eur J Nucl Med Mol Imaging 35(5): 933-41.

OPTN/SRTR (2009). Chapter VII: Lung Transplantation in the United States, 1999-2008. 2009 Annual Report of the U.S. Organ Procurement and Transplantation Network and the Scientific Registry of Transplant Recipients: Transplant Data 1999-2008. U.S. Department of Health and Human Services, Health Resources and Services Administration, Healthcare Systems Bureau, Division of Transplantation, Rockville, MD., OPTN/SRTR Annual Report

Padilla, M. L., G. J. Schilero, et al. (1997). "Sarcoidosis and transplantation." Sarcoidosis Vasc Diffuse Lung Dis 14(1): 16-22.

Parekh, K., E. Trulock, et al. (2004). "Use of cyclosporine in lung transplantation." Transplant Proc 36(2 Suppl): 318S-322S.

Paul, S., C. E. Escareno, et al. (2009). "Gastrointestinal complications after lung transplantation." J Heart Lung Transplant 28(5): 475-9.

Rafferty, P., B. A. Biggs, et al. (1983). "What happens to patients with pulmonary aspergilloma? Analysis of 23 cases." Thorax 38(8): 579-83.

Rochester, D. F. (1985). "The diaphragm: contractile properties and fatigue." J Clin Invest 75(5): 1397-402.

Rybicki, B. A., K. L. Amend, et al. (2004). "Photocopier exposure and risk of sarcoidosis in African-American sibs." Sarcoidosis Vasc Diffuse Lung Dis 21(1): 49-55.

Rybicki, B. A., M. Major, et al. (1997). "Racial differences in sarcoidosis incidence: a 5-year study in a health maintenance organization." Am J Epidemiol 145(3): 234-41.

Sato, H., J. C. Grutters, et al. (2002). "HLA-DQB1*0201: a marker for good prognosis in British and Dutch patients with sarcoidosis." Am J Respir Cell Mol Biol 27(4): 406-12.

Scadding, J. G. (1961). "Prognosis of intrathoracic sarcoidosis in England. A review of 136 cases after five years' observation." Br Med J 2(5261): 1165-72.

Scott, G. C., J. M. Berman, et al. (1997). "CT patterns of nodular hepatic and splenic sarcoidosis: a review of the literature." J Comput Assist Tomogr 21(3): 369-72.

Semenzato, G., R. Zambello, et al. (1993). "Cellular immunity in sarcoidosis and hypersensitivity pneumonitis. Recent advances." Chest 103(2 Suppl): 139S-143S.

Shafi, M. A. and P. J. Pasricha (2007). "Post-surgical and obstructive gastroparesis." Curr Gastroenterol Rep 9(4): 280-5.

Sharples, L. D., K. McNeil, et al. (2002). "Risk factors for bronchiolitis obliterans: a systematic review of recent publications." J Heart Lung Transplant 21(2): 271-81.

Shorr, A. F., D. B. Davies, et al. (2002). "Outcomes for patients with sarcoidosis awaiting lung transplantation." Chest 122(1): 233-8.

Shorr, A. F., K. G. Torrington, et al. (2001). "Endobronchial involvement and airway hyperreactivity in patients with sarcoidosis." Chest 120(3): 881-6.

Shulman, J. P., P. Latkany, et al. (2009). "Whole-body 18FDG PET-CT imaging of systemic sarcoidosis: ophthalmic oncology and uveitis." Ocul Immunol Inflamm 17(2): 95-100.

Siltzbach, L. E., D. G. James, et al. (1974). "Course and prognosis of sarcoidosis around the world." Am J Med 57(6): 847-52.

Singh, N. and S. Husain (2003). "Aspergillus infections after lung transplantation: clinical differences in type of transplant and implications for management." J Heart Lung Transplant 22(3): 258-66.

Snell, G. I. and B. J. Levvey (2009). "Thoracic organ transplantation from donation-after-cardiac-death donors." Transplantation 88(2): 147-8.

Snell, G. I. and G. P. Westall (2007). "Immunosuppression for lung transplantation: evidence to date." Drugs 67(11): 1531-9.

Song, Z., L. Marzilli, et al. (2005). "Mycobacterial catalase-peroxidase is a tissue antigen and target of the adaptive immune response in systemic sarcoidosis." J Exp Med 201(5): 755-67.

Stephany, B. R., B. Alao, et al. (2007). "Hyperlipidemia is associated with accelerated chronic kidney disease progression after lung transplantation." Am J Transplant 7(11): 2553-60.

Stewart, S., M. C. Fishbein, et al. (2007). "Revision of the 1996 working formulation for the standardization of nomenclature in the diagnosis of lung rejection." J Heart Lung Transplant 26(12): 1229-42.

Studdy, P. R. and R. Bird (1989). "Serum angiotensin converting enzyme in sarcoidosis--its value in present clinical practice." Ann Clin Biochem 26 (Pt 1): 13-8.

Sulavik, S. B., R. P. Spencer, et al. (1990). "Recognition of distinctive patterns of gallium-67 distribution in sarcoidosis." J Nucl Med 31(12): 1909-14.

Trulock, E. P., L. B. Edwards, et al. (2003). "The Registry of the International Society for Heart and Lung Transplantation: Twentieth Official adult lung and heart-lung transplant report--2003." J Heart Lung Transplant 22(6): 625-35.

UNOS (2011). UNOS.

Walker, S., G. Mikhail, et al. (1998). "Medium term results of lung transplantation for end stage pulmonary sarcoidosis." Thorax 53(4): 281-4.

Wasfi, Y. S., C. S. Rose, et al. (2006). "A new tool to assess sarcoidosis severity." Chest 129(5): 1234-45.

Weber-Carstens, S., M. Deja, et al. "Risk factors in critical illness myopathy during the early course of critical illness: a prospective observational study." Crit Care 14(3): R119.

Weder, W., I. Inci, et al. (2009). "Airway complications after lung transplantation: risk factors, prevention and outcome." Eur J Cardiothorac Surg 35(2): 293-8; discussion 298.

Weill, D., G. C. Dey, et al. (2002). "A positive donor gram stain does not predict outcome following lung transplantation." J Heart Lung Transplant 21(5): 555-8.

Westall, G. P., A. Michaelides, et al. (2004). "Human cytomegalovirus load in plasma and bronchoalveolar lavage fluid: a longitudinal study of lung transplant recipients." J Infect Dis 190(6): 1076-83.

Wille, K. M., A. Gaggar, et al. (2008). "Bronchiolitis obliterans syndrome and survival following lung transplantation for patients with sarcoidosis." Sarcoidosis Vasc Diffuse Lung Dis 25(2): 117-24.

Wyser, C. P., E. M. van Schalkwyk, et al. (1997). "Treatment of progressive pulmonary sarcoidosis with cyclosporin A. A randomized controlled trial." Am J Respir Crit Care Med 156(5): 1371-6.

Yanardag, H., O. N. Pamuk, et al. (2003). "Lupus pernio in sarcoidosis: clinical features and treatment outcomes of 14 patients." J Clin Rheumatol 9(2): 72-6.

Zamora, M. R. (2004). "Cytomegalovirus and lung transplantation." Am J Transplant 4(8): 1219-26.

Part 4

Extrapulmonary Sarcoidosis

10

Clinical Features of Skin

Dilek Biyik Ozkaya
Department of Dermatology, Vakif Gureba Teaching Hospital, Istanbul, Turkey

1. Introduction

1.1 Cutaneous sarcoidosis

Sarcoidosis is a multisystem granulomatosis disease of unknown etiology, characterized pathologically by noncaseating granulomas in involved tissues[1,2]. It mainly involves the lungs but may also be associated with systemic manifestations[3]. The disease most commonly affects the lungs, lymph nodes, liver, spleen, phalangeal bones, parotid glands, eyes, and skin[4]. Skin involvement rarely causes significant morbidity or mortality. However, it can adversely affaect a patient's quality of life by causing cosmetic impairment [5].

1.2 History

Sarcoidosis is first described by Sir Jonathan Hutchinson in 1875[6]. In 1889 the dermatologist Besnier described lupus pernio (sarcoidosis of the face) as a variant of cutaneous sarcoidosis. In 1899, Boeck described benign sarcoid and miliary lupoid [4,6].

1.3 Epidemiology

Sarcoidosis occurs worldwide and affects all ages and races. Disease onset is most often in the third decade of life, although a smaller second peak occurs in people older than 50 years[7].

1.4 Etiology and pathogenesis

The cause of sarcoidosis is unknown. It has been suggested that sarcoidosis is a hypersensitivity reaction caused by prolonged exposure to a spesisic antigen[8]. Although a spesific antigen has not yet been identified for sarcoidosis , the immune response which leads to recognizable clinical lesions and functional impairment is of the type 1 variety:elevated IFN gama , IL-2, and Th1 immune regulatory monokine IL2 characterize sarkoidosis[9]. Although mycobacteria have not been identified with traditional methods, mycobacterial DNA has been found in sarcoidal lesions[10]. Infectious agents such as mycobacteria, propionibacterium acnes and Chlamydia have been associated with sarcoidosis[11]. The etiologic role of various chemicals and metals such as beryllium, aluminium, zirconium, and titanium has also been debated. Treatment with interferons can cause a variety of inflammatory conditions, including sarcoidosis[4]. Genetic susceptibility to sarcoidosis has been associated with HLA -1, HLA-B8, and HLA-DR3 alleles[6].

1.5 Cutaneous lesions

Sarcoidosis involves so many organs that it is diffucult to describe all the features. About 40-50% of patients have cutaneous involvement[10]. Lesions are divided into two: specific and nonspecific skin lesions.

Skin lesions that contain typical sarcoid granulomas histologically are classified as specific lesions. Nonspesific skin lesions are those with nondiagnostic inflamatory patterns ;the most common is erythema nodosum. Nonspecific skin lesion lack typical noncaseating granulomas[5].

1.5.1 Specific lesions

The specific lesions of sarcoidosis all contain granulomas histologically, but the clinical appearence of the lesions is inconsistent. Specific lesions of sarcoidosis can present as macules, papules, plaques, nodules, and ulcerations. The involved skin may be skin colored, hyperpigmented, hypopigmented, or violaceous in color. Epidermal changes of the lesions may include atrophy, scaling, telengiectasias, or none at all[5]. Specific sarcoidal lesions most often are found on the head and neck, and but may ocur symetrically or asymmetrically on any part of the skin and mucosa[11].

1.5.1.1 Papules and plaques

The most common presentation is papuler form[4,5,11]. Papules are eleveted skin lesions less than 5mm in size. They have a predilection for the face and especially common around the eyes and on the posterior neck. They may be skin colored, hyperpigmented, erythematous, hypopigmented, violaceous, but clasically they are described as having a yellow–brown hue with an erythematous background. When pressure is applied with a glass slide or a dermoscope the erythematous coloration is mitigated and the yellow-brown color (often described as the color of apple jelly) can be more easily appreciated[4]. The apple jelly appearence and nodules are not pathognomonic for sarcoidosis, as other granulomatous skin conditions, such as lupus vulgaris may exhibit similiar diascopic properties[11].

The plaques form of sarcoidosis is rare and involves the extremities, the face and the corpus[4]. Plaques may arise denova or from a confluence of paules.These lesions are larger than 5mm in diameter [5]. Lupus pernio describes the relatively symmetric, violaceous, indurated plaques that ocur on the nose, ear-lobes, cheeks and digits. This clinical variant of sarcoidosis is distinctive and has been associated with symmetric involvement. Lupus pernio is associated with a higher prevelance of upper respiratory tract disease[11].

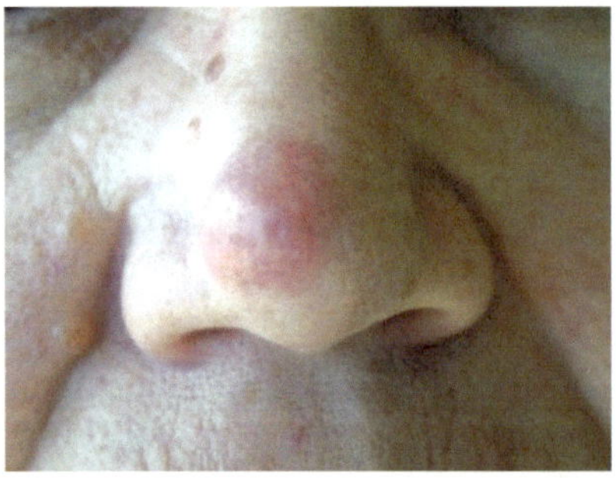

Bezmialem Vakıf University Prof. Dr. Nahide Onsun's photograph

Fig. 1. Violaceous lupus pernio lesion on the nose

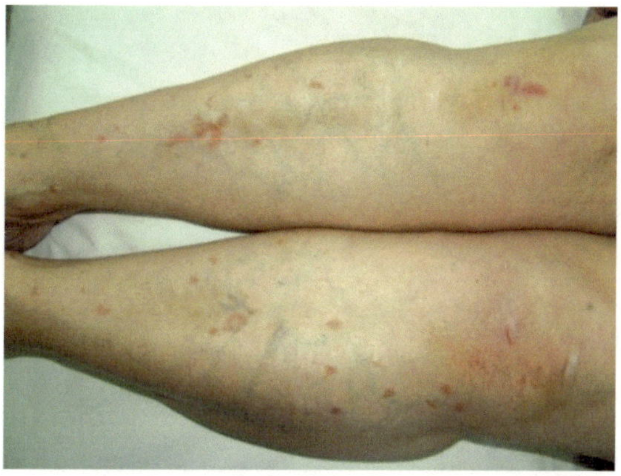

Bezmialem Vakıf University Prof. Dr. Nahide Onsun's photograph

Fig. 2. Papules and plaques at lower extremity

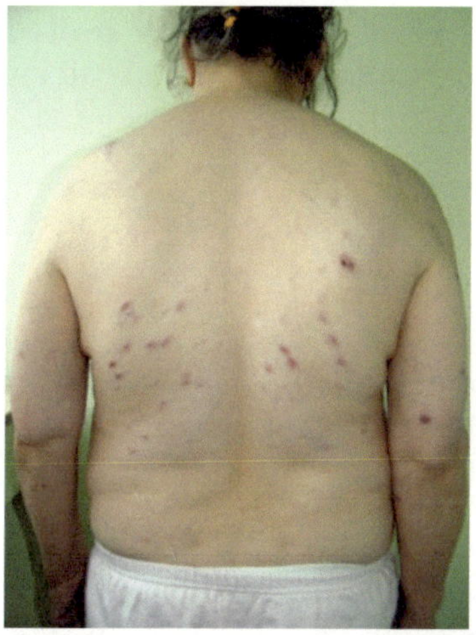

Bezmialem Vakıf University Prof. Dr. Nahide Onsun's photograph

Fig. 3. Papules and plaques

1.5.1.2 Scar sarcoidosis

Cutaneous sarcoidosis ocuuring in prior scar tisue, at traumatized areas of skin , or around foreign bodies such as tattos is common[5]. Scars become inflamed and infiltrated with sarcoidal granulomas. Inflamation of old scars may paralel or precede systemic disease activity[11]. The presence of foreign body in granuloma does not exclude sarcoidosis entirely. Many cases of scar sarcoidosis are following car accidents in which there is exposure to glass and dirt[11].

1.5.1.3 Scalp

Alopecia occurs with the involvement of the scalp. Scalp sarcoidosis may cause irrversibl cicatricial or noncicatricial sarcoidosis. Biopsy shows noncaseating granulomas. Its reversibility depends on the degree of the destruction of hair folicules [4,11].

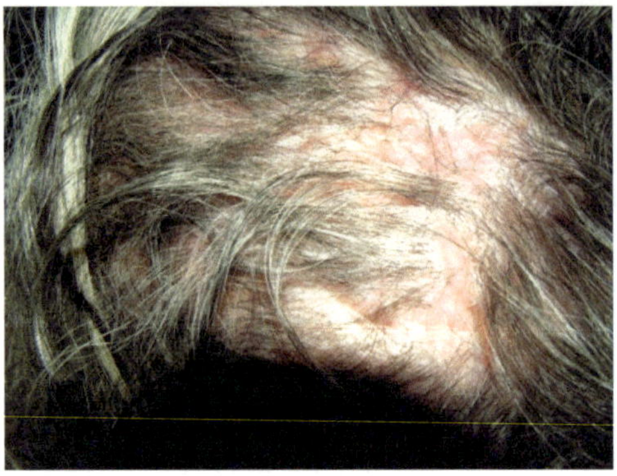

Bezmialem Vakıf University Prof. Dr. Nahide Onsun's photograph

Fig. 4. Scalp sarcoidosis

1.5.1.4 Nail

Sarcoidal inflammation around the nail matrix or within the distal bones of the digits can cause nail abnormalities[5]. Nail plate deformation and discoloration, clubbing, subungual hyperkeratosis may seen[11]. The incidence of hair and nail involvement is very low [4,11].

1.5.1.5 Mucous membranes

Sarcoidal granulomas may cause papules and plaques of the mucosal membranes and the tongue. Sarcoidosis may cause Mikulicz syndrome[11].

1.5.1.6 Ulcerations

The cutaneos lesions of sarcoidosis very rarely ulcerate. The most common site is the legs[10]. These lesions may mimic other ulcerative conditions such as venous stasis ulcerations, but they have granulomas present histologically[5]. An ulcerated necrobiosis lipoidica diabeticorum must also be considered[10].

1.5.1.7 Subcutaneous nodules

When the sarcoidal granulomas situated in the addipose tissue the skin induces clinically evident subcutaneos nodules and the classic red-brown color may not be seen. Instead the overlying skin may be normal or slightly red [5,10]. Multipl rather than solitary lesions are usually present. This granulomatous panniculitis is known as Darier -Roussy sarcoidosis [5,10].

1.5.1.8 Angiolupoid sarcoidosis (Brocq and pautrier)

This form of cronic cutaneous sarcoidosis is features red Brown papules, nodules, an plaques with prominent telengiectasies that tend to involve the mid face of the women[10]. In such cases, it is important to consider the rare granuloma eosinophlicum faciei as well as pseudolymphoma[5].

1.5.1.9 Macular

Cutaneos sarcoidosis may present as hypopigmented nonelevted areas. This variant is more common in dark skinned patients[5].

1.5.1.10 Additional presentations

Lots of additional prsentations have been reported. These includes erythroderma[12], ichtyosiform[13], rosacea like type[14], psoriasiform[15], morpheaform plaques[16], lichenoid dermatitis [17], foliкülitis like lesions, gyrate erythema, penil and vulvar lesions, palmar erythema, discoid lupus like plaques, lower extremity edema, lesions mimicking polymorphous light eruption[11].

1.5.2 Nonspecific lesions

1.5.2.1 Erythema nodosum

This is the most common nonspecific lesion. In most part of the world , it is necessary to exclude sarcoidosis when erythema nodosum is diagnosed in adults[10]. The lesions of erythema nodosum are tender and found predominantly on the lower extremities as well. The anterior surface of the lower leg is the most common location[5]. The presence of bilateral hiler adenopathy on chest radiograph with erythema nodosum is known as Löfgren syndrome[5].

Other nonspecific lesions are seen very rare. Prurigo nodules, erythema multiforme, lower extremity swelling, Sweet syndrome and pyoderma gangrenosum qualify as nonspecific cutaneous sarcoid lesions[5,11].

1.6 Treatment

The treatment of cutaneous sarcoidosis has been usually derived from agents for pulmonary sarcoidosis[18]. Standard therapeutic interventions for cutaneous sarcoidosis have traditionally included topical, intralesional and systemic corticostreoids, antimalarial drugs, methotrexate, and combinations of these agents[9].

1.6.1 Corticosteroids

Corticosteroid are the worldwide accepted standard treatment of sarcoidosis[9,18, 19]. For the patients with mild limited sarcoidosis the treatment may start with using ultrapotent topical corticosteroids[18]. Intralesional injections have been useful for some cases[18]. The concentration of the corticosteroids selected depends on the firmness and size of the lesion, but most lesions of sarcoidosis may be treated initially with intralesional triamcinolone at concentrations of 3-20 mg/mL repeated every 4 weeks until the lesions have flattened[18]. Adverse effectas are hypopigmentation and atrophy[1,7,8] Systemic corticosteroid theraphy, usually delivered orally , should be reserved for severely disfiguring or destructive lesions, widespread involvement, or lesions that have proved refractory to localized therapy [19]. The dosage of prednisone administered ranges from 40 to 80 mg/prednisone administered ranges from 40 to 80mg/day and is tapered over weeks to months depending on the clinical response [18].

1.6.2 Antimalarial agents

The effectiveness of chloroquine and hydroxychloroquine in sarcoidosis is thougt to be related to the ability of these agents to inhibit antigen processing and presentaion by APCs to CD4 T cells[8]. They have antiinflammatory properties [9,18,19]. The rate of response appears to be higher for cutaneous compared with pulmonary sarcoidosis. These drugs have been widely used for cutaneous sarcoidosis[18]. Maximum oral chloroquine dosage is 3.5 mg/kg/day and hydroxycholoroquine dosage is 6.5mg/kg/day. Lower dosages are effective and are preferred to maximal dosing [9,18]. The toxicities of antimalarials are nausea, anorexia, dizziness, headaches and blurred vision. Bleaching of the hair, agranulocytosis [9,18,19].

Agranulocytosis is rare but serious complication of theraphy. Potential ocular efffects are the most serious adverse events associated with antimalarial treatment and include the development of corneal deposits of central retinopathy[18].

1.6.3 Methotrexate

Methotrexate is a folate analogue that inhibits dihydrofolate reductase. At high doses methotrexate is antiproliferative , in low doses methotrexate has antiinflammatory properties [19].

The dose of methotrexate is varies. In adults , the average starting dosage is 10 to 15mg a week [18].Hepatotoxicity is the major long-term effect associated with methotrexate , and routine monitoring of alanine aminotransferase, aspartate aminotransferase, alkaline phosphatase and serum albumine is recomended[9,18,19]. While using methotrexate the patients must be monitored for neutropenia. Methotrexate is cleared with kidneys ; because of this serum creatinine monitoring must be done[18].

Methotrexate is associated with hematologic, gastrointestinal, pulmonary and hepatic toxicities [9,18,19]. Dose dependent toxicities are mucositis, mouth sores, and nausea. These problems can be eliminated by dividing by dividing the dose of methotrexate in half and giving oral folate [9,18,19].

1.6.4 Combination standard theraphy

Antimalarials and corticosteroids can be used in sequence. By this way complications of the long term use can be reduced. Steroids and antinalarials are steroid sparing agents. Both of them can be used in place of steroid or in combination with steroids. Combination therapies have the advantage of decreasing steroid doses[9,18,19].

1.6.5 Other therapies

Pentoxifylline[20], tetracyclines[21,22], Leflunomide[23], Thalidomide[24], Infliximab[25], Chlorambucil[26], cyclosporin-A [27], allopurinol [28], laser surgery[29] are reported for the treatment of sarcoidosis.

2. References

[1] Baughman RP,Lower EE,du Bois RM.Sarcoidosis. Lancet 2003,361(9363):1111-1118

[2] Marchell RM, Judson MA. Cutaneous Sarcoidosis. Semin Respir Crit Care Med. 2010 Aug;31(4):442-51

[3] Yamamoto M,Sharma OP,Hosodo Y,Special report-The descriptive definition of sarcoidosis. Sarcoidosis 9:33-34,1992

[4] Georgi Tchernev ;Cutaneous Sarcoidosis :The 'Great Imitator' .Am J Clin Dermatol 2006:7(6):375-82

[5] Richard M, Marchell,Marc A. Judson Cutaneous Sarcoidosis Semin Respir Crit Care Med. 2010 Aug;31(4)452-51

[6] Amy H., Clifton R.W Non infectious Granulomas.Dermatology. Jean L Bolognia, Joseph L Jorizzo,Ronald P Rapini First edition. Edinburgh, 2003, Mosby, 1455-60

[7] American Thoracic Society/ European Respiratory Society: Statement on sarcoidosis.Joint Statement of the American Thoracic Society(ATS), the European Respiratory Societ(RS) and the world Association of Sarcoidosis and Other

Granulomatous Diseases adopted by the ATS Board of directors and the ERS Executive Committee, February 1999. Am J Respir Crit Care Med 160:736,1999
[8] Kyra A Oswald-Richter, Dia C Beachboard, Xiaoyan Zhan et al. Respir Res. 2010 November 23.Doi 10.1186/1465-9921-11-161
[9] Christy B., Ted R. Cutaneous sarcoidosis therapy updated.J Am Acad Sermatol 56 (1):69-81
[10] Sergij Goert Granulomatous Diseases . Burgdorf Plewig Wolff Landthaler Third edition Springer Medizin Verlag Heidenberg Braun –Falco's Dermatology 548-555
[11] Richard M Marrchell, Bruce Thiers, Marc A. Judson Sarcoidosis. Klaus Wolff , Lowell A. Goldsmith,Stephen I .Katz et al.sevinth edition,2008 Fitzpatrick's Dermatology in General Medicine, 1484-1493
[12] Greer KE,Harman LE Jr, Kayne AL.Unusual cutaneous manifestations of sarcoidosis. South Med J 1977;70:666-668
[13] Cather JC, Cohen PR. Ichthyosiform sarcoidosis. J Am Acad Dermatol 1999;40(5 Pt 2):862-65
[14] Weber FP, Lauber HK Proc R Soc Med. 1939 Jul;32(9)1024-5
[15] Burgoyne JS, Wood MG. Psoriasiform sarcoidosis. Br. J Dermatol 1984;111:52
[16] Choi SC, Kim CR, Lee DY, Lee ES, Yang JM. Ann Dermatol. 2010 Aug;22(3):316-8.Epub 2010 Aug 5
[17] Goldberg LJ, Goldberg N, Abrahams I, Silvers DN, Szaniawski W, Halperin AJ. Giant Cell lchenoid dermatitis: a possible manifestation of sarcoidosis
[18] Robert P., Baughman , Elyse E. Lower Evidence -based therapy for cutaneous sarcoidosis. Clinics in Dermatology (2007) 25,334-340
[19] Christy B.,Ted R Evidence- Based Therapy for Cutaneous Sarcoidosis Drugs, 2008;68(10):1361-1383
[20] Park MK, Fontana Cr, Babaali H,Gilbert-Mcclain LI, Stylianou M, Joo J, Moss J, Mangansekli VC. Steroid sparing effects of pentoxifylline in pulmonary sarcoidosis. Sarcoidosis Vasc Diffuse Lung Dis. 2009 Jul;26(2):121-131
[21] Park DJ, Woog JJ,Pulido JS, Cameron JD.Minocycline for the treatment of ocular and acular adnexial sarcoidosis. Arch. Ophtalmol. 2007 May;125(5):705-9
[22] Sapadin AN,Fleischmajer R. Tetracyclines: nonantibiotic properties and their clinical implications. J Am Acad Dermatol. 2006 Feb;54(2):258-65
[23] Baughman RP, Lower EE. Leuflunomide for chronic sarcoidosis. Sarcoidosis Vasc Diffuse Lung Disease . 2004 Mar;21(1).43-8
[24] Hammond ER,Kaplin Al,Kerr DA.Spinal Cord.2007 Dec;45(12):802 Epub 2007 Aug 21
[25] Augiar M, Marcal N, Mendes AC, Bugalho de Almeida A. Infliximab for treating sarcoidosis patients. Portuguese experience. Rev port Pneumol. 2011 Apr;17(2):85-93
[26] Israel HL, McComb BL. Chlorambucil treatment of sarcoidsis. Sarcoidosis.1991 Mar;8(1):35-41
[27] Manzia TM, Bellini MI, Corona L,Frantoni S, Cillis A, Orlando G, Tisone G.Succesfull treatment of systemic de nova sarcoidosis with cyclosporine discontinuation and provision of rapamune after liver transplation. Transpl ınt 2011 Apr 19.doi:10.1111/j.1432-2277

[28] Bregnhoej A,Jemec GB. Low-dose allopurinol in the treatment of cutaneous sarcoidosis:response in four of seven patients. JDermatolog Treat.2005Apr;16(2)125-7

[29] Ross S,Raulin C,Ockenfels HM,Karsai S.Succesful treatment of cutaneous sarcoidosis lesions with the flashlamp pumped pulsed dye laser: a case report Dermatol Surg.2009 Jul;35(7):1139-40

11

Acquired Ichthyosiform Erythrodermia Sarcoidosis

Hui-Jun Ma
Department of Dermatology,
The 309 Hospital of Chinese People's liberation army,
China

1. Introduction

Sarcoidosis is a systemic disease that can involve almost any organ system. Infiltration with noncaseating granulomas is the hallmark of the disease, and it may result in various clinical manifestations [1]. Cutaneous involvement occurs in 25% of patients with systemic sarcoidosis and may occur without systemic involvement. Because lesions assume a vast array of morphologies, cutaneous sarcoidosis is known as one of the "great imitators" in dermatology [2]. The important specific lesions are lupus pernio, plaques and maculopapular eruptions. The most frequent nonspecific lesion is erythema nodosum. Other specific skin changes include subcutaneous nodules, erythema multiforme-like erythemas, alopecia, scars, verrucous outgrowths, psoriasiform lesions, ulcerative lesions, hypopigmentation, lichenoid lesions, ichthyosiform lesions and a sporadic type of erythroderma [1,2]. Ichthyosiform and erythrodermic form of cutaneous sarcodosis are all rare presentation of cutaneous sarcodosis. The association of them in one case is extremely rare. To data, there are only three cases reported in English literature [3-5].

2. Methods to use for diagnosis

Correctly diagnosing sarcoidosis may be a challenge. Unfortunately, no single test can prove the diagnosis. Patients are diagnosed with sarcoidosis when a compatible clinical or radiologic picture is present, along with histologic evidence of noncaseating granulomas, and when other potential causes, such as infections, are excluded. The following tests are needed.

Laboratory tests: Urine and blood routine examination; 24h amount of urine protein; Serum calcium and glucose, liver function and kidney function tests; Erythrocyte sedimentation rate; C-reaction protein, tuberculin test, antinuclear antibody.

Cardiologic examination: Electrocardiography; 24h Holter monitoring electrocardiogram

Ultrasonography: ultrasonography for liver, bladder, spleen, kidney, pancreas.

X-ray: computer tomography scan of chest and abdomen

Histopathologic examination: Biopsy for an eruption, a periodic acid-Schiff stain for fungi, a Ziehl-Nielsen stain for acid fast bacilli, and a Steiner stain are also needed to exclude infections.

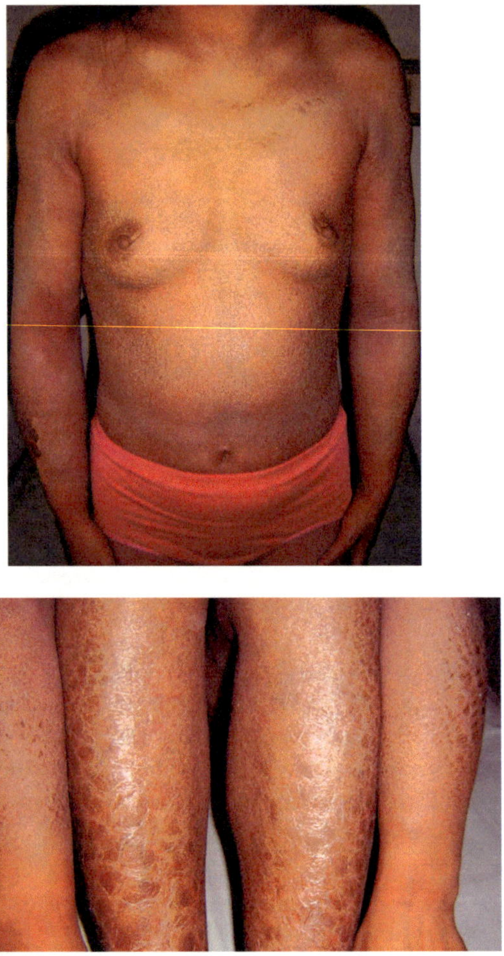

Fig. 1. The flushing, swelling and dry scaling of skin were seen throughout the whole body in a 27-year-old Chinese female patient with ichthyosiform erythrodermia Sarcoidosis. The Ichthyosiform skin lesions especially seen in upper and lower extremities.

3. Treatment protocol

The treatment of cutaneous sarcoidosis is often frustrating, because lesions may be refractory to treatment or may recur following successful treatment. Systemic glucocorticoids are the most effective agents. They are commonly used at slow, tapering dosages, starting at 20 to 40 mg of oral prednisone daily for four to six weeks. Many other medications such as hydroxychloroquine (Plaquenil), methotrexate (Rheumatrex)and thalidomide (Thalomid) may be used in refractory cases [3,6,7]

4. Different diagnoses

Acquired ichthyosis and erythrodermia in adult frequently signifies internal diseases, such as sarcoidosis, malignancy et al [8,9]. The malignant condition included lymphomas, especially

Hodgkin's disease and mycosis fungoides, multiple myeloma; carcinomas of the lung, breast, and cervix; Kaposi's sarcoma; and leiomyosarcoma [2,8,9]. Other systemic diseases that may be characterized by acquired ichthyosis include Hansen's disease, hypothyroidism, phrynoderma, and chronic malnutrition [1,10].

5. Prognosis

Sarcoidosis can affect any organ of the body but most commonly involves the lungs, lymph nodes, skin, and eyes. Less common but usually severe manifestations also occur in the central nervous system, heart, and skeletal system [2,4,8] Cutaneous manifestations are present in approximately 25 percent of patients and are classified as specific or nonspecific based upon the presence or absence of noncaseating granulomas on histopathologic examination [10]. The relationship between cutaneous and systemic sarcoidosis is being studied. Cutaneous involvement in systemic sarcoidosis may occur at any stage of the disease. However, it is most often present at the onset and may even be the presenting complaint [11]. Certain types of cutaneous lesions may have a bearing on prognosis of systemic sarcoidosis. Lesions of lupus pernio, erythrodermia, seem likely to associate with more severe systemic involvement, while erythema nodosum often indicates acute benign disease [3,4,8]. Every patient with cutaneous sarcoidosis requires an initial work-up for systemic involvement, followed by periodic screening.

6. Conclusion

Sarcoidosis is a multisystem disease that may involve almost any organ system. Therefore, it results in various clinical manifestations. Cutaneous sarcoidosis is known as one of the “great imitators” in dermatology. Ichthyosiform and erythrodermic form of cutaneous sarcodosis is extremely rare. To data, there are only three cases reported in English literature. Sarcoidosis can affect any organ of the body but most commonly involves the lungs, lymph nodes, skin, and eyes. The Correctly diagnosing sarcoidosis may be a challenge. Unfortunately, no single test can prove the diagnosis. The treatment of cutaneous sarcoidosis is often frustrating. Systemic glucocorticoids are the most effective agents.

7. References

1. Sawhney M, Sharma YK, Gera V, Jetley S. Ichthyosiform sarcoidosis following chemotherapy of Hodgkin's disease. Indian J Dermatol Venereol Leprol. 2003; 69(3):220-222.
2. Tchernev G. Cutaneous sarcoidosis: the "great imitator": etiopathogenesis, morphology, differential diagnosis, and clinical management. Am J Clin Dermatol. 2006; 7(6):375-382.
3. Feind-Koopmans AG, Lucker GP, van de Kerkhof PC. Acquired ichthyosiform erythroderma and sarcoidosis. J Am Acad Dermatol. 1996 ;35(5 Pt 2):826-828.
4. Amal S, Khadir K, Agzour K, Nejjam F, Badre L, Sqalli S, Lakhdar H. Icthyosiform erythroderma: atypical manifestation of sarcoidosis Ann Dermatol Venereol. 2000; 127(1):64-66.

5. Zhang H, Ma HJ, Liu W, Yuan XY. Sarcoidosis characterized as acquired ichthyosiform erythroderma. Eur J Dermatol. 2009; 19(5):516-517.
6. Cather JC, Cohen PR . Ichthyosiform sarcoidosis. J Am Acad Dermatol 1999; 40(5 pt2):862-865.
7. Matarasso SL, Bruce S. Ichthyosiform sarcoidosis: report of a case. Cutis. 1991; 47(6):405-408.
8. Mañá J, Marcoval J, Graells J, Salazar A, Peyrí J, Pujol R. Cutaneous involvement in sarcoidosis: relationship to systemic disease. Arch Dermatol 1997; 133(7):882- 888.
9. Yoon CH, Lee CW .Case 6. Erythrodermic form of cutaneous sarcoidosis. Clin Exp Dermatol. 2003; 28(5):575-576.
10. Rosenberg B. Ichthyosiform sarcoisis. Dermatol Online J. 2005 Dec 30; 11(4):15.
11. Katta R. Cutaneous sarcoidosis: a dermatologic masquerader. Am Fam Physician. 2002; 65(8):1581-1584.

12

Orofacial Sarcoidosis and Granulomatosis

Mohammad Hosein Kalantar Motamedi[1],
Mohammad Ghasem Shams[2] and Taghi Azizi[3]
[1]*Trauma Research Center, Oral and Maxillofacial Surgery Clinic,*
[2]*Oral and Maxillofacial Surgery Clinic,*
[3]*Pathology Department,*
[1,2,3]*Baqiyatallah Medical Center, Baqiyatallah University of Medical Sciences, Tehran, IR Iran*

1. Introduction

Sarcoidosis is a multi-systemic inflammatory disorder of unknown etiology. It is classified as an acquired systemic granulomatous disease. Because of the fact that sarcoidosis affects multiple tissues and organs it is characterized by many potential signs and symptoms, as well as by the presence of noncaseating granulomas in the organs involved. Although orofacial sarcoidosis is relatively rare, it may however, present in the oral and maxillofacial region. The respiratory system is the most commonly affected system, with approximately 90% of patients presenting pulmonary findings during the course of their disease. Cutaneous manifestations occur in around 25% of cases and are more common in chronic cases. Head and neck lesions of sarcoidosis are manifested in 10 to 15% of patients (Samtsov, 1992; Newman et al., 1997; Suresh & Radfar, 2005).

In the maxillofacial region the salivary glands may be involved, while sometimes, xerostomia and bilateral parotid swelling may be seen (Piattelli et al., 1998; Batal et al., 1999). Lesions occurring in the soft tissues of the oral cavity and/or in the jaws are rare. Orofacial granulomatosis (OFG) is a granulomatous disease. This clinicopathological entity describes patients with oral lesions characterized by persistent and/or recurrent labial enlargement, ulcers, and a variety of other orofacial features, which on biopsy have lymphedema and noncaseating granulomas. The cause is idiopathic but appears to represent an abnormal immune reaction. This may be a manifestation of Crohn's disease (CD) since some patients with oral lesions develop typical bowel symptoms of CD in ensuing months to years; tooth associated infections, viruses, food or contact allergies have been implicated in causing OFG. Sarcoidosis has also been implicated in causing OFG. Clinical features of OFG are highly variable and sometimes so insidious that signs and symptoms are frequently not severe enough to cause alarm. The lips are most commonly involved and demonstrate a nontender, persistent swelling. Because of the relatively nonspecific clinical findings associated with granulomatous diseases, a microscopic diagnosis of granulomatous inflammation per se often presents a diagnostic dilemma (Shams et al., 2007).

2. Etiology

The cause of sarcoidosis is idiopathic but appears to represent an abnormal immune reaction. OFG may be a manifestation of Crohn's disease (CD) since some patients with oral lesions develop typical bowel symptoms of CD in ensuing months to years; tooth associated infections, viruses, food or contact allergies have been implicated in causing OFG. Sarcoidosis has also been implicated in causing OFG. Although the etiology of sarcoidosis is unknown, many factors may be accused in the pathogenesis of this disease. Implicated causative factors are: infections (fungal, viral, bacterial), genetic predisposition, environmental factors and miscellaneous factors (DiAlberti et al., 1992 ; Mendelsohn et al., 1992 ; Rybicki et al., 1997 ; Armstrong et al.,2004). The specific tests for fungal (mycology tests for Candida spp-cultivation in SDA and CHROMAgar Candida), viral (Abs to HIV, EBV, CMV) and bacterial (for mycobacterium-skin test and AFB) infections may also be investigated.

3. Presentation

3.1 General findings

The respiratory system is the most commonly affected system in sarcoidosis, with approximately 90% of patients presenting pulmonary findings during the course of their disease. Cutaneous manifestations occur in around 25% of cases and are more common in chronic cases. Head and neck lesions of sarcoidosis are manifested in 10 to 15% of patients (Armstrong et al., 2004).

3.2 Oral and maxillofacial involvement

In the maxillofacial region the clinical features of OFG are highly variable and sometimes so insidious that signs and symptoms are frequently not severe enough to cause alarm. The lips are most commonly involved and demonstrate a nontender, persistent swelling (Fig. 1). Salivary glands may be involved and xerostomia and bilateral parotid swelling may be seen. Lesions occurring in the soft tissues of the oral cavity and/or in the jaws are rare. Orofacial granulomatosis (OFG) is a granulomatous disease. This clinicopathological entity describes patients with oral lesions characterized by persistent and/or recurrent labial enlargement, ulcers, and a variety of other orofacial features, which on biopsy have lymphedema and noncaseating granulomas (DiAlberti et al., 1992; Mendelsohn et al., 1992; Rybicki et al., 1997; Armstrong et al., 2004; Shams et al., 2007).

Oral involvement generally appears in patients with chronic multisystem sarcoidosis and seldom occurs in the acute stage. The oral lesions may be solitary, multiple or part of a generalized disease. In some cases, oral involvement is the first or only, manifestation of the disease and appears as a nontender well-circumscribed brownish red or violeceous swelling, as papules, or as submucosal nodules that can occasionally either show superficial ulceration or be symptomatic. Gingival involvement presents as red gingival enlargement (DiAlberti et al., 1992; Mendelsohn et al., 1992; Rybicki et al., 1997; Armstrong et al., 2004; Shams et al., 2007). In some cases the lesions are multifocal, including the lips, the gingiva and the hard palate. The clinical signs (red-violet nodular mass in the middle of the palate, and the erythematous and hyperplastic gingival in the upper incisor area) may be seen. Alternatively, oral sarcoidosis may be asymptomatic or mildly symptomatic with minimal discomfort during eating or drinking, especially if the lesions involve the tongue (Mendelsohn et al., 1992).

4. Diagnosis

In most cases of oral involvement, sarcoidosis is diagnosed before the oral manifestations become apparent. Occasionally, oral involvement is the first or only manifestation of the disease. The diagnosis of sarcoidosis is established when clinical features are supported by histopathological evidence of typical non-caseating epithelioid granulomas and other laboratory tests (Samtsov, 1992; Newman et al., 1997; Suresh & Radfar, 2005).

4.1 Differential diagnosis

The differential diagnosis of oral soft tissue lesions must consider other granulomatous conditions, such as infections (tuberculosis, leprosy, tertiary syphilis, systemic mycoses, and cat-scratch disease), Crohn's disease, Melkersson-Rosenthal syndrome (including Mieschers cheilitis or cheilitis granulomatosa), Wegener's granulomatosis, foreign body reactions and hairy cell leukaemia (Rybicki et al., 1998).

Patients with CD may present to the clinician with GI symptoms attributed to the disease or non-specific lesions in the oral cavity, nose, or larynx. Some OFG patients have both histopathological and immunopathological features that resemble those observed in CD patients. Some of these clinical manifestations have been found to be consistent with CD, but most have not (Shams et al., 2007). Often an extensive clinical, microscopic, and laboratory evaluation may be required to identify the source of the granulomatous inflammation (Piattelli et al., 1998).

4.2 Evaluation tests

As stated above, clinical microscopic, and laboratory evaluation together may be required to identify the source of the granulomatous inflammation. Negative endoscopy of the GI tract, normal ESR, normal serum albumin, Ca, folate and iron levels will rule out CD.

With regard to sarcoidosis, a normal CXR and ACE level would make sarcoidosis unlikely. Chronic granulomatous disease is ruled out by using the neutrophil nitroblue tetrazolium reduction test (DiAlberti et al., 1992; Mendelsohn et al., 1992; Rybicki et al., 1997; Armstrong et al., 2004; Shams et al., 2007).

Because of the relatively nonspecific clinical findings associated with granulomatous diseases, a microscopic diagnosis of granulomatous inflammation per se often presents a diagnostic dilemma. Clinical, microscopic, and laboratory evaluation may be required to identify the source of the granulomatous inflammation. The serum angiotensin converting enzyme (normal value: 18-55 U/L), blood calcium (normal value: 9-11 mEq/L) and 24-hrs urine calcium (normal value <180 mg) erythrocyte sedimentation rate (1-2 mm/h) should be assessed. Negative endoscopy of the GI tract, normal ESR, normal serum albumin, Ca, folate and iron levels will rule out CD. With regard to sarcoidosis, a normal CXR and ACE level would make sarcoidosis unlikely. Chronic granulomatous disease is ruled out by using the neutrophil nitroblue tetrazolium reduction test.

Another condition that may be associated with granuloma formation is cheilitis granulomatosa (CG). This is a subset of OFG, which presents clinically as persistent lip swelling. It also is a granulomatous inflammation of unknown origin. CG may be part of the triad of the Melkersson-Rosenthal syndrome (MRS). Swelling of the lips along with fissured tongue and facial paralysis constitute this syndrome. Lesions closely resemble nodules of tuberculosis (TB) and the differential diagnosis is often difficult. To make the diagnosis, other appropriate studies (special stains for acid fast bacilli,GMS and PAS stains for fungi, cultures, and so forth) to exclude tubercle bacilli, fungi, foreign bodies, or other causes of the granulomatous condition must be done. When the histopathological findings are compatible with sarcoidosis, in order to confirm the diagnosis, we must proceed with laboratory tests that support the diagnosis for sarcoidosis (DiAlberti et al., 1992 ; Mendelsohn et al., 1992 ; Rybicki et al., 1997 ; Armstrong et al.,2004; Shams et al.,2007).

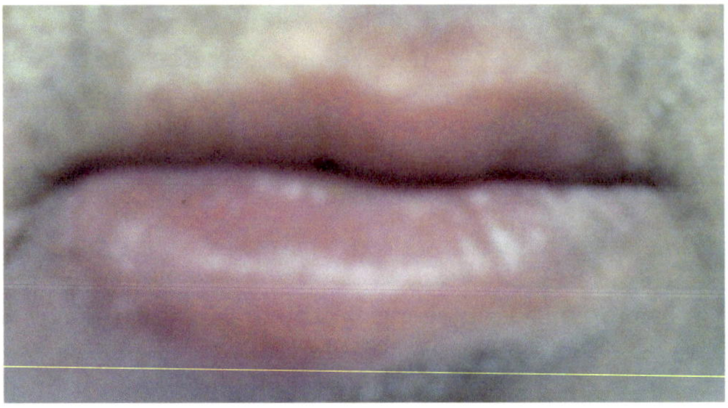

Fig. 1. Typical swelling of the lips.

5. Histopathology

Histopathologically, OFG lesions closely resemble nodules of tuberculosis (TB) and the differential diagnosis is often difficult. To make the diagnosis other appropriate studies (special stains for acid fast bacilli, GMS and PAS stains for fungi, cultures, etc.) to exclude tubercle bacilli, fungi, foreign bodies, or other causes of the granulomatous condition must be done. Photomicrographs of OFG lesions (Figs.2-8) show edema, scattered and clustered lymphocytes in the connective tissue as well as several well-defined, granulomas consisting of collections of epithelioid histiocytes and multinucleated giant cells (Shams et al.,2007).

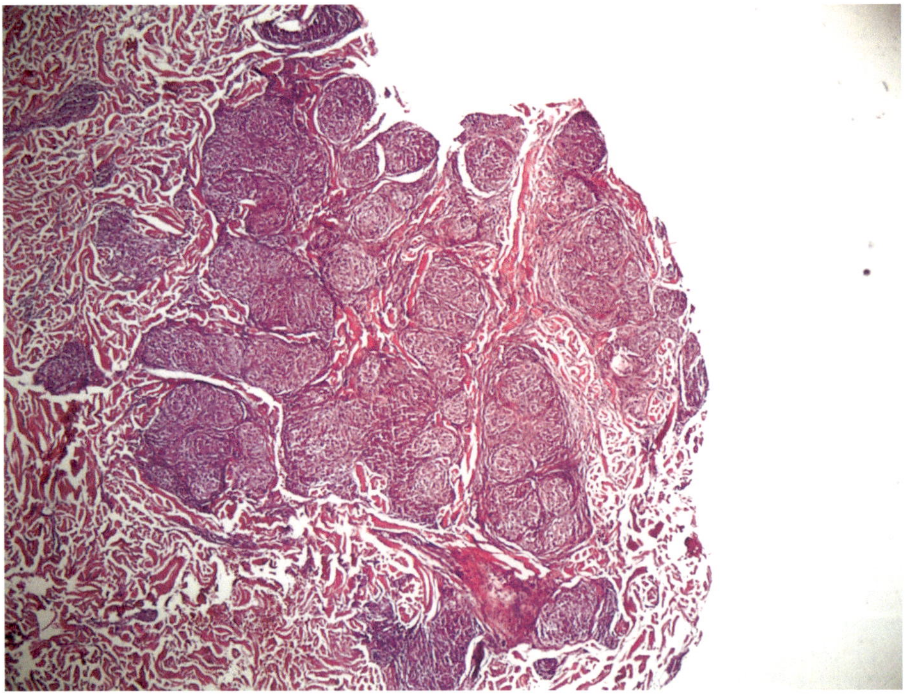

Fig. 2. Confluent noncaseating granulomatous inflammation (H&E low power view).

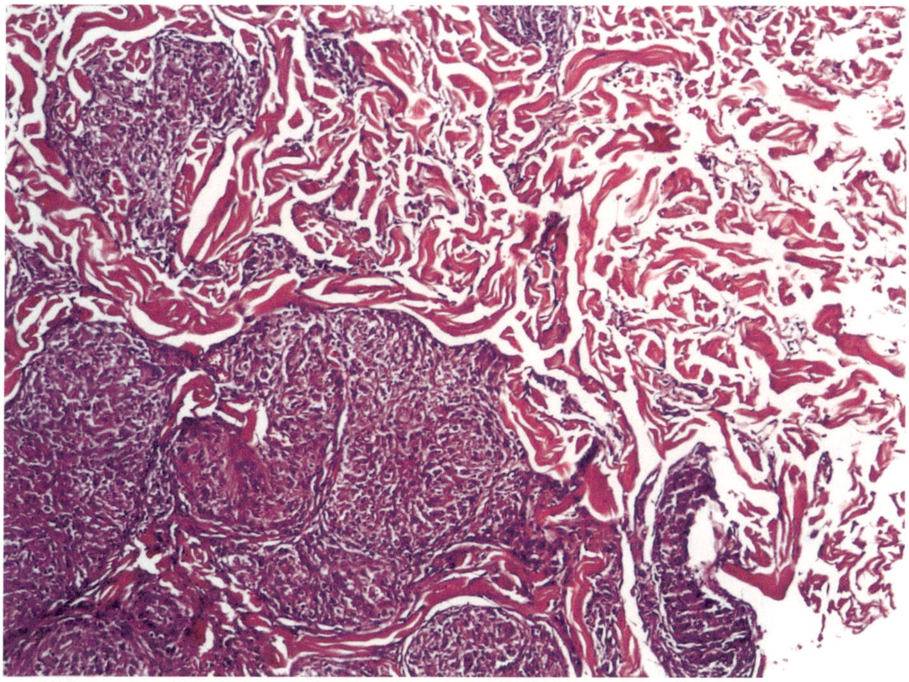

Fig. 3. Confluent noncaseating granulomatous inflammation (H&E medium power view).

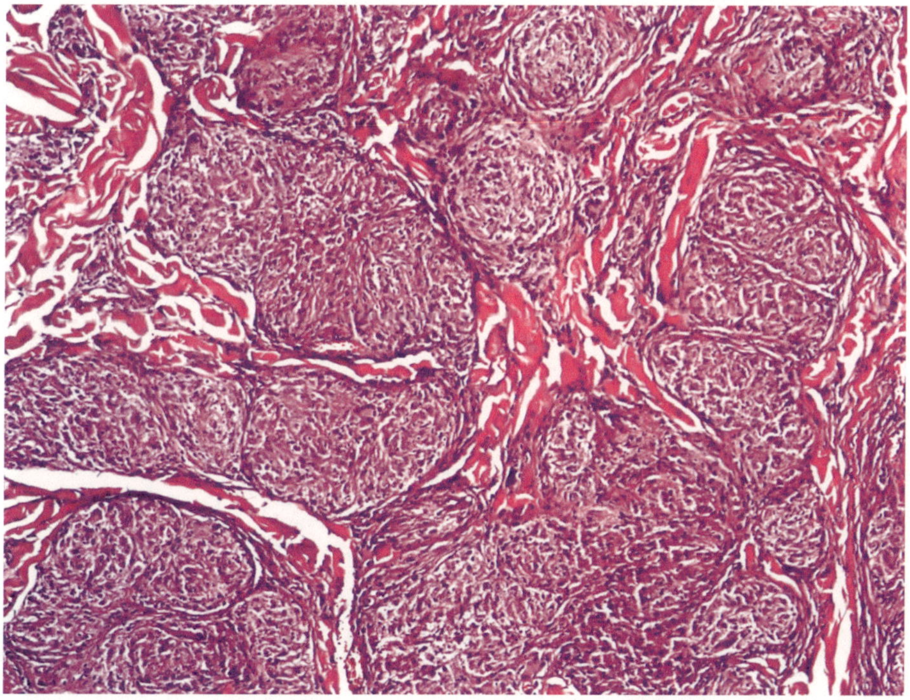

Fig. 4. Confluent noncaseating granulomatous inflammation (H&E high power view).

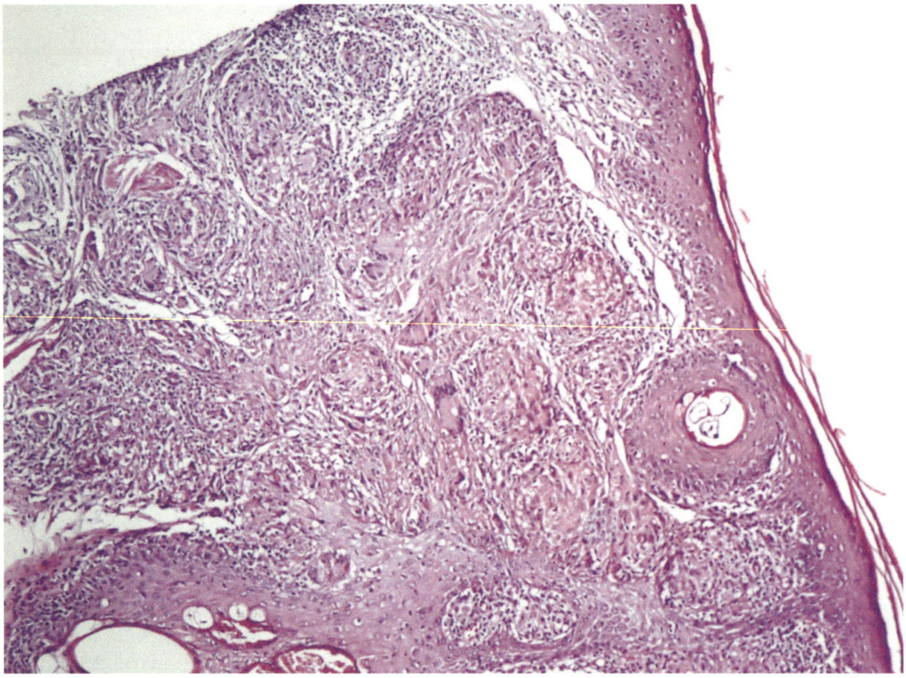

Fig. 5. Sarcoidosis of skin, noncaseating granulomatous inflammation (H&E low power).

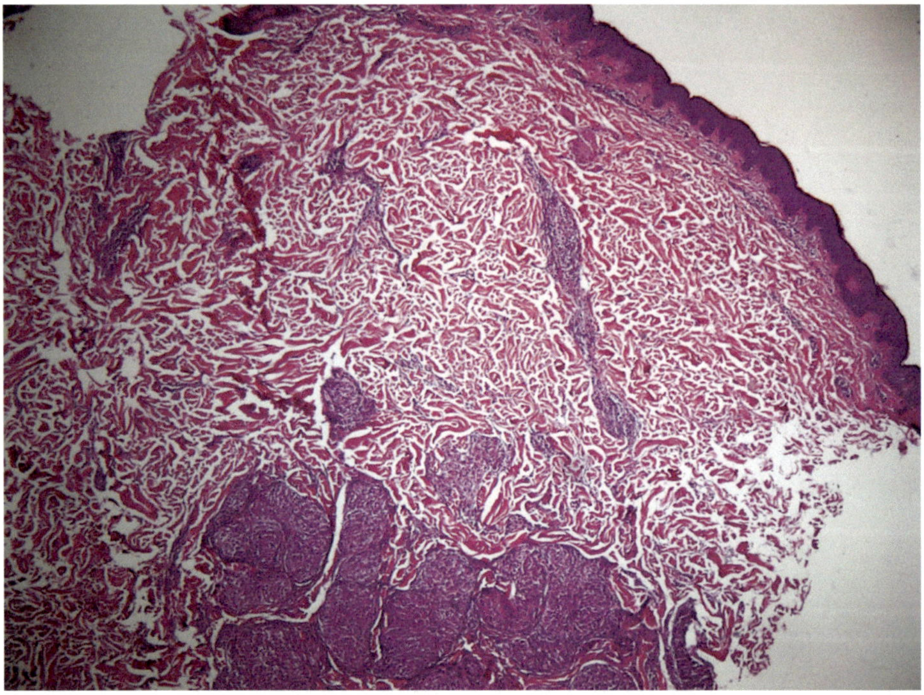

Fig. 6. Sarcoidosis of skin, noncaseating granulomatous inflammation (H&E low power view).

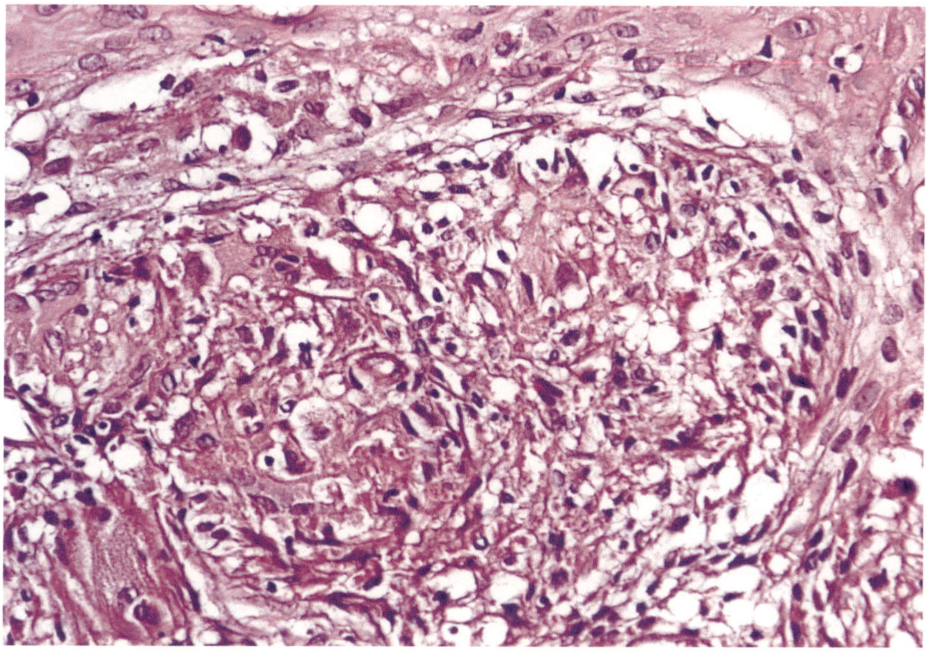

Fig. 7. Sarcoidosis asteroid bodies and multinucleated giant cells (H&E high power view).

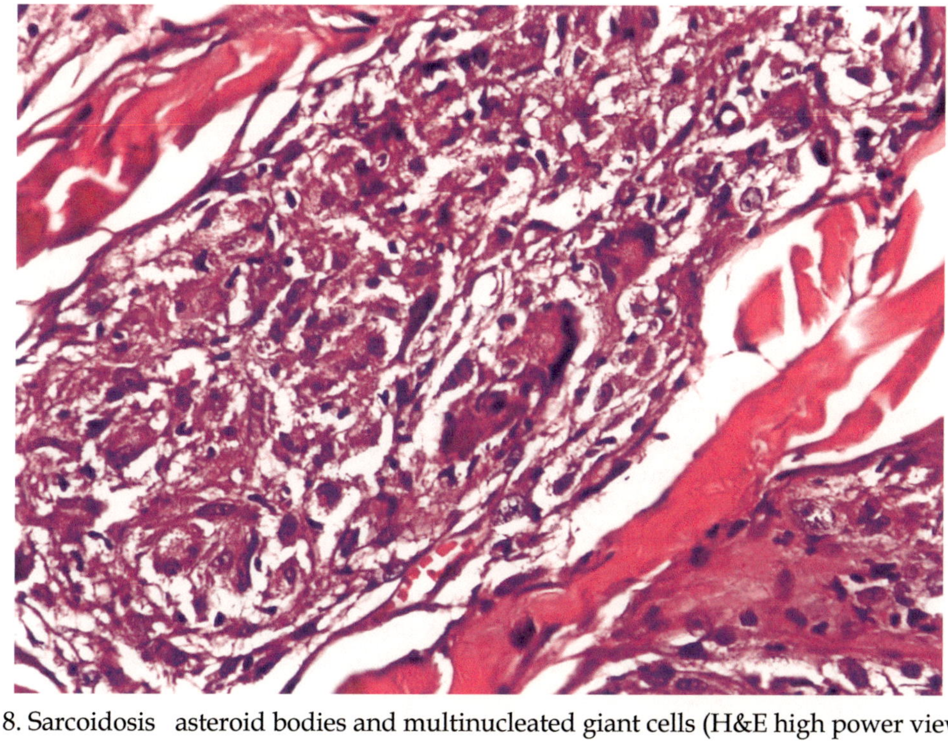

Fig. 8. Sarcoidosis asteroid bodies and multinucleated giant cells (H&E high power view).

6. Treatment

Oral glucocorticoids are the first-line treatment. Other medications include cytotoxic drugs such as methotrexate, azathioprine, chlorambucil, cyclosporine and cyclophosphamide. Some authors suggest the surgical excision for treatment of oral soft tissue or jaw lesions. A variety of drugs have been tried in treatment of OFG including corticosteroids. Surgery in these patients is usually unnecessary as treatment is primarily pharmacological. Systemic corticosteroids are considered the best treatment. Glucocorticoids effectively suppress the activated T-helper-induced cell processes occurring at the site of disease in 50 percent of the patients. The usual therapy is prednisolone 1 mg/kg for 4 to 6 weeks followed by a slow tapering over 2 to 3 months. This is repeated if the disease again becomes active. Intralesional steroid injections are also an alternative treatment method that one might also consider. The prognosis is generally favourable (Shams et al., 2007).

7. Prognosis

Oral lesions may be the first or the only sign of sarcoidosis in an otherwise healthy patient. Although, oral involvement of the disease is very rare and often localized, however, the prognosis of orofacial sarcoidosis correlates with mode of onset, initial clinical course, characteristics of the host and extent of the disease. However, this multisystem disorder may never be completely cured. Moreover, it is important to endorse a periodic follow- up of patients in order to evaluate the status of the patient and course of the disease. Many of those affected remain asymptomatic and remission sometimes occurs spontaneously (Shams et al., 2007).

8. Discussion

The nomenclature of OFG lacks specificity. Recently, a question has been posed to determine whether OFG is a manifestation of a separate and specific inflammatory bowel disease. Other authors also suggested that OFG is a descriptive term and the specific cause of these lesions is unknown (Shams et al., 2007).
Some authors (Edmondstone & Wilson, 1985 ; Hills et al., 1987 ; Edmondstone, 1988;Bardinas et al., 1989 ;Panayeas et al., 1991 ; Rybicki et al.,1997) have reported a familial, (i.e. among people in the same household), seasonal and occupational clustering of sarcoidosis, suggesting a multifactorial origin that includes genetic predisposition, infectious organisms and environmental exposures as probable underlying mechanisms.

8.1 Organ involvement

Sarcoidosis is known to affect a wide array of organs and tissues, including the lung, heart, liver, spleen, bones, skin, eyes, lymph nodes, parotid glands and, on occasion, the oral cavity(Cahn et al., 1964 ; Tilman, 1964). The extent of the disease and its complications vary, ranging from mild symptoms in some patients to major incapacitation in others (Tilman, 1964 ; Steinberg & Mueller,1994). Many patients experience no symptoms and are identified incidentally. The most prominent manifestations of the disease involve the lungs, as evidenced clinically by the presence of dyspnea in patients. Lung volumes and diffusing capacity often are reduced, and chest radiographs reveal bilateral hilar lymphadenopathy, diffuse parenchymal infiltrates or both (Reed, 1988; Steinberg & Mueller, 1994; Quernheim, 1998; Hong & Farish, 2000).

8.2 Disease course

The pattern of onset in sarcoidosis, the site involved determines the course and prognosis of the disease. Skin, eyes and lymph nodes are the most frequent sites of extrapulmonary involvement. Cutaneous sarcoidosis has been reported to occur in 25 percent of patients, and it may suggest chronicity and poor prognosis (Hong & Farish, 2000). Similarly, one of four patients is affected with ocular sarcoidosis with the potential for progression to blindness (Steinberg & Mueller, 1994). Cardiac sarcoidosis and neurosarcoidosis are uncommon, but they may lead to fatal complications such as dysrhythmias and conduction block, as well as seizures and encephalopathy. Other possible systemic effects include liver and spleen enlargement, thrombocytopenia, abnormal calcium metabolism, renal dysfunction, arthropathy and skeletal deformities (Hillerup, 1976; Johns, 1988 ; Reed, 1988 ; Steinberg & Mueller, 1994).

8.3 Diagnosis of exclusion

Owing to the absence of a diagnostic gold standard, sarcoidosis is a diagnosis of exclusion (Quernheim, 1998 ; Hong & Farish, 2000). First, the clinician establishes a compatible clinical picture based on symptomatology and physical and radiographic findings. Next, the clinician performs a biopsy of the most accessible organ, such as skin or lymph nodes, to obtain histologic evidence of noncaseating granulomas. These structures are composed of focal aggregates of lymphocytes, macrophages and multinucleated giant cells, but they are not unique to this disease. Therefore, it is necessary to exclude other sources of granulomatous inflammation, such as foreign-body implantation, tuberculosis, Crohn's disease and deep fungal infections (Israel & Sones, 1964; Reed, 1988 ; Steinberg & , Mueller, 1994).

8.4 Comprehensive assessment

Clinicians confronting patients with oral granulomatosis must perform a comprehensive assessment of potential target organs in patients suspected of having sarcoidosis, with special attention paid to the lungs, heart, central nervous system (CNS), eyes, skin and lymph nodes. A chest radiograph and a thorough ophthalmic evaluation are required, even for patients without specific pulmonary or ocular complaints. Baseline laboratory tests include complete blood cell counts, erythrocyte sedimentation rate, liver and renal function tests, serum calcium and SACE levels, pulmonary function tests, electrocardiography and tuberculin testing. Periodic follow-up is essential for the clinician to evaluate the progression of the disease and to detect new organ involvement (Reed, 1988; Steinberg & , Mueller, 1994 ; Rybicki et al.,1996; DiAlberti et al.,1997 ; Rybicki et al.,1998).

8.5 Laboratory markers

The SACE level has been studied extensively as a laboratory marker in sarcoidosis. Secretion of ACE by granuloma-forming epithelioid cells results in high serum levels in 80 to 90 percent of patients with sarcoidosis. However, because of the lack of specificity, an elevated SACE level is only suggestive of, rather than diagnostic for, sarcoidosis. The reported false-positive and false-negative rates for the SACE level as a laboratory marker of sarcoidosis are 10 and 40 percent, respectively. (Schultz et al., 1979 ; Chesnutt & Enigmas, 1995 ; Shah et al., 1997 ; Rybicki et al.,1998)

8.6 Pattern of onset

The pattern of onset in sarcoidosis determines the course and prognosis of the disease, as well as the patient's therapeutic response. Although spontaneous resolution is common in cases of acute sarcoidosis, chronic disease often is associated with a gradual onset, a progressive course and many potential complications. Poor prognostic indicators include older age at onset, black race, hypersplenism and advanced pulmonary involvement. It is uncommon for patients to die of sarcoidosis and death often is attributed to terminal fibrosis of critical organs such as the lungs, heart or CNS (Steinberg & , Mueller, 1994;Mana et al., 1994; Newman et al., 1997; Quernheim, 1998).

8.7 Head and neck involvement

Sarcoidosis typically is diagnosed before orofacial sequelae appear. Sarcoidosis may affect the head and neck lymph nodes, osseous and soft oral tissues, as well as the major and minor salivary glands. Parotid glands are affected in 4 to 6 percent of cases of sarcoidosis, with a self-limiting or permanent enlargement as the outward presentation. Enlargements often are bilateral, asymptomatic, firm and smooth on palpation, with no changes in size when eating. Associated xerostomia may or may not be present. Although these clinical features are characteristic of Sjögren's syndrome, occasionally they may be associated with sarcoidosis. A labial gland biopsy is a highly sensitive and specific diagnostic test in the histologic assessment of Sjögren's syndrome, but it also can assist in the differentiation of Sjögren's syndrome from sarcoidosis when clinical presentations are similar (Greenberg et al., 1964; Gold &, Sager, 1976; James et al., 1976; Giotaki et al., 1986;, Melsom et al., 1988; Drosos et al., 1999; Levy et al., 2001).

Sarcoid lesions of the jaw bones may appear as diffuse, poorly defined radiolucencies on dental radiographs, and they can result in tooth mobility on clinical examination.

Several studies have shown sarcoid infiltration of the minor salivary glands with or without clinical involvement of the major salivary glands. Therefore, when accessible and clinically involved tissues are not available, the clinician can perform a biopsy of normal-appearing tissue to confirm the histologic diagnosis in a patient with compatible clinical findings (Hughes & Gross, 1972; Tarpley et al,1972; Rasmussen & Neukirch, 1976; Nessan & Jacoway, 1979).

8.8 Labial minor salivary gland biopsy

Several cases of sarcoidosis-induced parotid enlargement confirmed via biopsy of the labial minor salivary gland have been reported in the literature. This technique has a lower diagnostic yield in sarcoidosis compared with biopsies of the liver, lung, lymph node or parotid gland, perhaps because of the uncommon, delayed (after other clinical signs develop) and less intense histologic involvement of the minor salivary glands. On the other hand, this procedure is simple, minimally invasive and associated with significantly less morbidity than is a parotid gland biopsy. In addition, the tissue is readily accessible from the lower labial mucosa, and the clinician can perform the procedure under local anesthesia at chairside (Chisholm et al., 1971 ;Tannenbaum et al.,1974 ; Siltzbach,1980 ; Marx et al., 1988).

Owing to the complexity of disease manifestation, clinicians tailor therapy to each patient. Many patients experience temporary or long-term remission without medical therapy. Therefore, treatment often is deferred for three to 12 months to assess the overall disease progression. Immediate medical treatment is reserved for patients with neurological, cardiac, severe ocular, advanced pulmonary and disfiguring cutaneous disease, as well as persistent hypercalcemia (Turiaf et al., 1976 ; van Maarsseveen et al.,1982; Nagata et al., 1999). Clinicians focus treatment on the suppression of the immune system, and corticosteroids are the mainstay of therapy. Topical, inhalational, intralesional or systemic steroids may be used to control the disease, depending on its severity. Physicians closely monitor patients receiving long-term systemic steroid therapy for potential adverse effects of these medications. They also can consider steroid-sparing immunosuppressive agents for patients with critical organ involvement that is poorly controlled with systemic steroid therapy. Implanted cardiac defibrillators or heart and lung transplantation may be indicated for patients with cardiac and pulmonary sarcoidosis in which the organs are not salvageable. Splenectomy may be necessary to treat sarcoidosis-induced splenomegaly associated with a risk of rupture (Russo & Millikan,1994; Baughman,1997 ; Judson, 1998 ; Crystal, 1998 ; Pietinalho et al.,1999).

8.9 Dental considerations

Dentists need to consider a number of issues regarding the dental care of patients with sarcoidosis. Sarcoid lesions of the jaw bones may appear as diffuse, poorly defined radiolucencies on dental radiographs, and they can result in tooth mobility on clinical examination. Approximately 1 to 6 percent of patients with sarcoidosis may have an obstruction of the nasal passages or chronic sinusitis. Steroid supplementation before major oral surgery may be indicated for patients with adrenal suppression secondary to long-term steroid therapy. These patients also may be susceptible to infection and require prophylactic antibiotics before undergoing invasive dental procedures (Clayman, 1998).

In addition, platelet retention associated with hypersplenism may lead to occasional thrombocytopenia, necessitating preoperative blood count studies. Anemia and other hematologic changes also may result from granulomatous infiltration of bone marrow (Yanardag et al.,2002). Practitioners also need to evaluate patients for leukopenia, anemia, thrombocytopenia and oral mucositis secondary to the administration of drugs that are toxic to bone marrow. Clinicians should defer dental procedures performed in hospitals under general anesthesia until a patient's medical status and degree of vital organ dysfunction have been evaluated. Sarcoid infiltration of major salivary glands and subsequent xerostomia predispose patients to caries, periodontal disease and candidiasis, highlighting the need for frequent recall appointments and aggressive preventive measures with salivary stimulants, topical fluoride and anti-fungal medications (Yanardag et al.,2002).

9. Conclusion

Orofacial granulomatosis is a generic term applied to manifestations of several diseases including sarcoidosis, Crohn's disease, Melkersson-Rosenthal syndrome, cheilitis granulomatosa of Miescher and foreign-body reactions. What bonds these diseases together is the presence of noncaseating granulomas. A typical clinical manifestation of orofacial granulomatosis is recurrent labial swellings that eventually persist (Kim & Lee, 2010; Martini, 2010).

Orofacial granulomatosis (OFG) is the presence of persistent enlargement of the soft tissues of the oral and maxillofacial region, characterized by non-caseating granulomatous inflammation in the absence of diagnosable systemic Crohn's disease (CD) or sarcoidosis. Over 20 years have passed since OFG was first described and an extensive review of the literature reveals that there is no consensus whether OFG is a distinct clinical disorder or an initial presentation of CD or sarcoidosis. Furthermore, the precise cause of OFG is still unknown although several theories have been suggested including infection, genetic predisposition and allergy. OFG is a rare granulomatous disorder, characterized by persistent enlargement of the soft tissues of the oral and maxillofacial region . Recurrent facial swelling, with/without intraoral manifestations, is the single most common presentation at onset.

Several prior studies have suggested different treatment modalities for oral CD, ranging from the use of mouthwash with corticosteroids to intravenous infusions of an infliximab. Consistent with the findings of previous reports, a favourable outcome in our patient, using intralesional triamcinolone, is suggestive that this can be used as a treatment option for patients with CD that have oral lesions. The symptoms associated with CD usually show a clinical course that waxes and wanes. If patients with CD complain of symptoms associated with these oral lesions during the course of their disease, treatment of the oral lesions with intralesional triamcinolone can improve the quality of life of the patients by ameliorating associated disease symptoms.

In conclusion, patients presenting with an OFG should be carefully evaluated for gastrointestinal signs and symptoms such as diarrhea, hematochezia and abdominal pain. Even in cases with no presenting gastrointestinal symptoms, intestinal disease might exist on closer examination, thus investigation of the GI tract is highly suggested. Intralesional triamcinolone injections can be successful in relieving symptoms associated with oral lesions in a CD patient. (Kim & Lee, 2010; Martini, 2010).

The clinical outcome of OFG patients continues to be unpredictable. Current therapies remain unpredictable. Regular clinical review is indicated to identify the development of gastrointestinal or systemic involvement. The aim of this review was to analyze the developments in our understanding of the aetiology, pathogenesis and treatment protocols, with particular emphasis on management and outcomes of this disease.

10. Acknowledgments

The authors are professors at the Baqiyatallah University of Medical Sciences and would like to thank the faculty and staff of the Trauma Research, Maxillofacial and Pathology departments of the Baqiyatallah Medical Center.

11. References

Armstrong C, Napier S, Linden GJ. Sarcoidosis with gingival involvement: A case report. J Periodontol. 2004;75:608–612.

Bardinas F, Morera J, Fite E, Plasencia A. Seasonal clustering of sarcoidosis. Lancet 1989;2:455–6.

Batal H, Chou LL, Cottrel DA. Sarcoidosis: Medical and dental implications. Oral Surg Oral Med Oral Pathol Oral Radiol Endod. 1999;88:386–390.

Baughman RP, Lower E. Steroid-sparing alternative treatments for sarcoidosis. Clin Chest Med 1997;18:853–64.

Cahn LR, Eisenbud L, Blake MN, Stern D. Biopsies of normal-appearing palates of patients with known sarcoidosis: a preliminary report. Oral Surg Oral Med Oral Pathol 1964;18:342–5.

Chesnutt AN. Enigmas in sarcoidosis. West J Med 1995;162:519–26.

Chisholm DM, Lyell A, Haroon TS, Mason DK, Beeley JA. Salivary gland function in sarcoidosis: report of a case. Oral Surg 1971;31:766–71.

Clayman L, MacLennan M, Dolan R. Nonpainful swelling of the palate and loosening of the maxillary incisors. J Oral Maxillofac Surg 1998;56:1327–35.

Crystal RG. Sarcoidosis. In: Harrison TR, Fauci AS, eds. Harrison's principles of internal medicine. 14th ed. New York: McGraw-Hill, Health Professions Division;1998:1922–8.

DiAlberti L, Piatteli A, Artese L, et al. Human herpesvirus 8 variants in sarcoid tissues. Lancet. 1997;350:1655–1661.

Drosos AA, Voulgari PV, Psychos DN, Tsifetaki N, Bai M. Sicca syndrome in patients with sarcoidosis. Rheumatol Int 1999;18:177–80.
Edmondstone WM, Wilson AG. Sarcoidosis in Caucasians, Blacks and Asians in London. Br J Dis Chest 1985;79:27–36.
Edmondstone WM. Sarcoidosis in nurses: is there an association? Thorax 1988;43:342–3.
Giotaki H, Constantopoulos SH, Papadimitriou CS, Moutsopoulos HM. Labial minor salivary gland biopsy: a highly discriminatory diagnostic method between sarcoidosis and Sjögren's syndrome. Respiration 1986;50:102–7.
Greenberg G, Anderson R, Sharpstone P, James DG. Enlargement of parotid gland due to sarcoidosis. Br Med J 1964;5413:861–2.
Gold RS, Sager E. Oral sarcoidosis: review of the literature. J Oral Surg 1976;34:237–44.
Hillerup S. Diagnosis of sarcoidosis from oral manifestation. Int J Oral Surg 1976;5:95–9.
Hills SE, Parkes SA, Baker SB. Epidemiology of sarcoidosis in the Isle of Man, part 2: evidence for space-time clustering. Thorax 1987;42:427–30.
Hong J, Farish SE. Intraosseous sarcoidosis of the maxilla: case report. J Oral Maxillofac Surg 2000;58:435–9.
Hughes RV, Gross NJ. Diagnosis of sarcoidosis by labial gland biopsy. Br Med J 1972;3:215.
Israel HL, Sones M. Selection of biopsy procedures for diagnosis of sarcoidosis. Acta Med Scand Suppl 1964;425:222–4.
James D, Neville E, Siltzbach L. A worldwide review of sarcoidosis. Ann N Y Acad Sci 1976;278:321–34.
Johns CS. Sarcoidosis. In: Fishman AP, ed. Pulmonary diseases and disorders. 2nd ed. New York: McGraw-Hill; 1988:619–46.
Judson MA. Lung transplantation for pulmonary sarcoidosis. Eur Respir J 1998;11:738–44.
Kim SK, Lee ES. Orofacial granulomatosis associated with Crohn's disease. Ann Dermatol. 2010 May;22(2):203-5. Epub 2010 May 18.
Levy O, Topilski M, Brazowski E, Yaron M, Tishler M. Sarcoidosis presenting as primary Sjögren's syndrome. Isr Med Assoc J 2001;3:63–4.
Mana J, Salazar A, Manresa F. Clinical factors predicting persistence of activity in sarcoidosis: a multivariate analysis of 193 cases. Respiration 1994;61:219–25.
Martini MZ, Galletta VC, Pereira EM, De Sousa SC, Lemos CA, Migliari DA. Orofacial granulomatosis of the lip: a report of 2 cases with histological and immunohistochemical analyses and intralesional corticotherapy. Minerva Stomatol. 2010 Oct;59(10):579-81.
Marx RE, Hartman KS, Rethman KV. A prospective study comparing incisional labial to incisional parotid biopsies in the detection and confirmation of sarcoidosis, Sjögren's disease, sialosis and lymphoma. J Rheumatol 1988;15:621–9.
Melsom RD, Speight PM, Ryan J, Perry JD. Sarcoidosis in a patient presenting with clinical and histological features of primary Sjögren's syndrome. Ann Rheum Dis 1988;47:166–8.
Mendelsohn SS, Field EA, Woolgar J. Sarcoidosis of the tongue. Clin Exp Dermatol. 1992;17:47–48.
Nagata Y, Kanekura T, Kawabata H, et al. A case of sarcoidosis involving tongue. J Dermatol 1999;26:666–70.
Nessan VJ, Jacoway JR. Biopsy of minor salivary glands in the diagnosis of sarcoidosis. New Engl J Med 1979;301:922–4.
Newman LS, Rose CS, Maier LA. Sarcoidosis. N Engl J Med 1997;336:1224–35.
Panayeas S, Theodorakopoulos P, Bouras A, Constantopoulos S. Seasonal occurrence of sarcoidosis in Greece. Lancet 1991;338:510–1.

Piattelli A, Favia GF, DiAlberti L. Oral ulceration as a presenting sign of unknown sarcoidosis mimicking a tumour: report of 2 cases. Oral Oncol. 1998;34:427–430.

Pietinalho A, Tukiainen P, Haahtela T, Persson T, Selroos O. Oral prednisolone followed by inhaled budesonide in newly diagnosed pulmonary sarcoidosis: a double-blind, placebo-controlled multicenter study. Finnish Pulmonary Sarcoidosis Study Group. Chest 1999;116:424–31.

Quernheim JM. Sarcoidosis: clinical manifestations, staging and therapy (part II). Respir Med 1998;92:140–9.

Rasmussen SM, Neukirch F. Sarcoidosis: a clinical study with special reference to the choice biopsy procedure. Acta Med Scand 1976;199:209–16.

Reed TM. Sarcoidosis: a review and case report. J Am Podiatr Med Assoc 1988;78:279–86.

Russo G, Millikan LE. Cutaneous sarcoidosis: diagnosis and treatment. Compr Ther 1994;20:418–21.

Rybicki BA, Harrington D, Major M, et al. Heterogeneity of familial risk in sarcoidosis. Genet Epidemiol 1996;13:23–33.

Rybicki BA, Major M, Popovich J Jr, Maliarik MJ, Iannuzzi MC. Racial differences in sarcoidosis incidence: a 5-year study in a health maintenance organization. Am J Epidemiol 1997;145:234–41.

Rybicki BA, Mallarik M, Major M, et al. Epidemiology, demographics and genetics of sarcoidosis. Semin Respir Infect. 1998;13:166–173.

Samtsov AV. Cutaneous sarcoidosis. Int J Dermatol. 1992;117:203–207.

Schultz T, Miller WC, Bedrossian CW. Clinical application of measurement of angiotensin-converting enzyme level. JAMA 1979;242:439–41.

Shah UK, White JA, Gooey JE, Hybels RL. Otolaryngologic manifestations of sarcoidosis: presentation and diagnosis. Laryngoscope 1997;107:67–75.

Shams MG, Motamedi MH, Azizi T. Orofacial granulomatosis of the lower lip and cheek: report of a case. Oral Surg Oral Med Oral Pathol Oral Radiol Endod. 2007 Oct;104(4):e42-4. Epub 2007 Aug 20.

Siltzbach LE. Sarcoidosis. In: Fishman AP, ed. Pulmonary diseases and disorders. New York: McGraw-Hill; 1980:885–915.

Steinberg MJ, Mueller DP. Treating oral sarcoidosis. JADA 1994;125:76–9.

Suresh L, Radfar L. Oral Sarcoidosis: a review of literature. Oral Diseases. 2005;11:138–145.

Tannenbaum H, Anderson LG, Rosenberg EH, Sheffer AL. Diagnosis of sarcoidosis by lip biopsy of minor salivary glands. Can Med Assoc J 1974;111:1323–4.

Tarpley TM, Anderson L, Lightbody P, Sheagren JN. Minor salivary gland involvement in sarcoidosis: report of 3 cases with positive lip biopsies. Oral Surg Oral Med Oral Pathol 1972;33:755–62.

Tilman HH. Sarcoidosis with unsuspected oral manifestations: report of a case. Oral Surg Oral Med Oral Pathol 1964;18:130–5.

Turiaf J, Johns CJ, Terstein AS, Tsuji S, Wurm K. The problem of the treatment of sarcoidosis: report of the subcommittee on therapy. Ann N Y Acad Sci 1976;278:743–51.

van Maarsseveen AC, van der Waal I, Stam J, Veldhuizen RW, van der Kwast WA. Oral involvement in sarcoidosis. Int J Oral Surg 1982;11:21–9.

Yanardag H, Pamuk GE, Karayel T, Demirci S. Bone marrow involvement in sarcoidosis: an analysis of 50 bone marrow samples. Hematologica 2002;32:419–25.

13

Diagnostic and Therapeutic Management of Cardiac Sarcoidosis -Application of High Resolution Electrocardiography

Kenji Yodogawa
Division of Cardiology, Department of Internal Medicine, Nippon Medical School Chiba Hokusoh Hospital, Japan

1. Introduction

Sarcoidosis is a common multisystem granulomatous disease of unknown etiology. Overall the prognosis is not necessarily deleterious because organ involvement is usually asymptomatic except for ocular or cutaneous involvements and the disease is often self-limiting. Cardiac Sarcoidosis is rare (5%) but once the heart is involved, the patient's prognosis is poor because of the development of fatal arrhythmias, atrioventricular conduction disturbance or refractory congestive heart failure (Newman et al., 1997). Despite advanced research, a clear cause and pathogenesis for sarcoidosis remains unknown. Sarcoidosis is thought to be caused by an abnormal, exaggerated response of the immune system. Infectious agents such as *Propionibacterium acnes, Mycobacteria* suspected of causing sarcoidosis (Nishiwaki et al., 2004; Hance, 1998) , but The American Thoracic Society's wide-ranging *Statement on Sarcoidosis* suggested that there is no clear evidence of an infectious agent causing sarcoidosis. Genetic factors such as the human leucocyte antigens (specifically HLA-DRB1) may be a predisposition for sarcoidosis (Maliark et al., 1998), but not the only cause. Currently, sarcoidosis is considered to be caused by multiple factors.

2. Diagnostics

There are no specific symptoms or signs of CS. Clinical manifestations such as dyspnea, palpitations, syncope are often associated with arrhythmias or heart failure. There is no golden standard for diagnosis of CS. Since 1993, the Japanese Ministry of Health and Welfare (JMHW) guidelines (Hiraga et al., 1993) have been widely used as the reference standard (table 1).
Endomyocardial biopsy is specific but it shows noncaseating granulomas no more than 25% of CS (Uemura et al., 1999; Ardehali et al., 2005). Diagnosis of CS is often made by combination of cardiac abnormality and pathology of other organs.

1 Histologic diagnosis group: endomyocardial biopsy demonstrates epithelioid granulomata without caseating granulomata.

2 Clinical diagnosis group: in patients with histologic diagnosis of extracardiac sarcoidosis, cardiac sarcoidosis is suspected when "a" and at least one of criteria "b" to "d" is present, and other etiologies such as hypertension and coronary artery disea have been excluded:

a. Complete RBBB, left-axis deviation, AV block, VT, PVC, or pathological Q or ST-T change on resting or ambulatory electrocardiogram.

b. Abnormal wall motion, regional wall thinning, or dilation of the left ventricle.

c. Perfusion defect by 201thallium-myocardial scintigraphy or abnormal accumulation by 67Ga-citrate or 99mTc-PYP myocardial scintigraphy.

d. Abnormal intracardiac pressure, low cardiac output, or abnormal wall motion or depressed ejection fraction of the left ventricle.

AV atrioventricular; LBBB left bundle branch block; PVC premature ventricular contraction; RBBB right bundle branch block; VT ventricular tachycardia.

Table 1. Modified Guidelines for the Diagnosis of Cardiac Sarcoidosis Based on the Study Reporton Diffuse Pulmonary Diseases From the Japanese Ministry of Health and Welfare, 1993.

2.1 Electrocardiography

Electrocardiographic conduction abnormalities, atorioventricular block (AVB) or bundle branch block (BBB) are well known as the characteristic manifestation of CS. These manifestations have been detected in less than 5% of patients with sarcoidosis (Silverman et al., 1978). Nevertheless, in autopsy studies, cardiac involvements have been found in 20% to 58% of the cases, indicating latent CS does exist in a larger part of the sarcoidosis patients, even if routine electrocardiogram (ECG) shows no abnormal findings (Loncope et al., 1952; Iwai et al., 1994; Bargout et al. 2004). Previously, we reported the results of signal averaged electrocardiography (SAECG) in 10 cardiac sarcoidosis patients, 52 pulmonary sarcoidosis patients with normal ECG, and 52 normal controls (Yodogawa et al., 2007). We found that late potentials (LP) were positive in 80% of cardiac sarcoidosis patients, 46.2% in pulmonary sarcoidosis patients, and 5.8% in normal control ($P < 0.0001$). These results suggested that latent cardiac abnormality may exist in sarcoidosis patients even if ECG is normal. In a similar point of view, there is increasing concern about "subclinical" cardiac sarcoidosis. Soejima et al stated that many patients who have cardiac sarcoidosis are asymptomatic, and Positron Emission Tomography (PET) and Magnetic Resonance Imaging (MRI) are useful for early detection of cardiac abnormality (Soejima & Yada, 2009).

2.2 Echocardiography

In the early stage, regional wall thickness caused by granulomatous infiltration may be noted (Yazaki et al., 1998; Matsumori et al., 2000). Later, myocardial scar occurred as the result of healed sarcoid granulomas. In the progressed stage, thinning of myocardium, wall motion abnormality, and sometimes aneurysms (Sato et al., 2010) are seen. Valantine et al. reported that thinning at the base of the intra-ventricular septum is pathognomonic for CS (Valantine et al., 1987). However, the sensitivity is reported to be relatively low (20%) (Uemura et al., 2005).

2.3 Gallium-67 scintigraphy

Gallium-67 scintigraphy has been widely used in diagnosis and management of CS. Gallium uptake in the heart indicates active inflammation, which is a useful finding in predicting the response to corticosteroid therapy (Okayama et al. 1995). Futamatsu et al. recently reported that gallium-67 scintigraphy is useful for evaluation of CS with ventricular tachycardia (VT) (Futamatsu et al., 2006). According to the study, accumulation of gallium-67 in the heart at the time of diagnosis was detected more frequently in the VT group than in the non-VT group (14.3 vs 71.4%, $P < 0.05$). Thus, Gallium-67 uptake is highly specific to inflammatory disease and a useful for detection of disease activity of cardiac sarcoidosis. Meanwhile, the main disadvantage is lack of sensitivity (20%, 36%) (Okayama et al., 1995; Kiuchi et al., 2007).

2.4 Positron Emission Tomography (PET)

PET is noninvasive imaging technique using small amounts of radioactive positrons for measuring the metabolic activity of cells in the human body. Fluorine-18 fluorodeoxyglucose-(18F-FDG) is accumulated by inflammatory cells, and widely used radiotracer for PET imaging studies. Yamagishi *et al.* reported a significantly higher sensitivity of 18F-FDG uptake for detection of CS compared with that of Gallium-67 uptake (Yamagishi et al., 2003). They also showed improvement of 18F-FDG uptake after corticosteroid therapy. Hence, FDG-PFT is considered to be useful not only for detection but therapeutic monitoring of cardiac involvement. The biggest advantage of PET is its high sensitivity (87.5%, 100%, and 100%), but the specificity is obscure (38.5%, 81.5%, and 90.9%) (Ohira et al., 2008; Ishimaru et al., 2005; Okumura et al., 2004). This may be due to the possibility of detecting subclinical CS or natural accumulation with interindividual variability.

2.5 Magnetic Resonance Imaging (MRI)

Cardiac MRI is a noninvasive diagnostic testing to detect structural abnormalities. Increased signal intensity of T2-weighted images is considered to indicate active inflammation area, and Gadolinium-DTPA enhanced the detection of the region. Cardiac MRI has been reported to be useful for detecting areas of inflammation associated with sarcoid granulomas (Shimada et al., 2001). Several reports have shown high sensitivity (100%) and specificity (78% and 100%) for diagnosis of CS (Smedema et al., 2005; Tadamura et al., 2005). However, one of the main disadvantages is that MRI is not recommended for patients with implantable cardiac devices, such as pacemaker, or implantable cardioverter-defibrillator (ICD).

3. Treatment

In patients with definite diagnosis of CS, corticosteroid therapy should be considered. In general, the initial dosage is 30 mg/day of prednisone or its equivalent on alternate days, which was tapered over a period of 6 months to a maintenance dosage of 5-10 mg/day. Initiation of corticosteroid therapy is reported to preserve LV function and improve outcomes (Yazaki et al., 2001; Chiu et al., 2005). Concerning arrhythmias, Kato et al. described that AVB resolved in 4 of the 7 CS patients by corticosteroid therapy, but did not resolve or improve in any of the patients without corticosteroid therapy (Kato et al., 2003). Recently, Banba et al evaluated the effect of corticosteroids in CS patients presenting VT or CAVB. In their cohort, atrioventricular conduction improved in 5 of 9 CAVB patients after corticosteroid therapy albeit the fact that ventricular arrhythmias were not improved after corticosteroid therapy (Banba et al., 2007). In regard to ventricular arrhythmias, we evaluated the effect of corticosteroids in CS patients presenting VT (Yodogawa et al., 2008). After corticosteroid therapy, VT was suppressed in 6 of 15 patients (Responder group). Accumulation of gallium-

67 was detected more frequently in the responder group than in the non-responder group (66.7% vs. 11.1%, $p<0.05$). All patients underwent SAECG in which the filtered QRS duration (f-QRS), the root mean square voltage of the terminal 40 ms (RMS_{40}) in the filtered QRS complex and the duration of low-amplitude signals < 40μV (LAS_{40}) in the terminal filtered QRS complex were measured. In the responder group, f-QRS and LAS_{40} were significantly decreased and RMS_{40} was significantly increased compared with those before corticosteroid therapy (f-QRS: 136.3+/-30.6msec vs 116.8+/-25.4msec, $p<0.05$ LAS_{40}: 68.2+/-24.0msec vs 47.8+/-22.9msec, $p<0.05$ RMS_{40}: 7.2+/-3.3 msec vs 13.3+/-7.6msec, $p<0.05$). However, SAECG parameters did not change significantly in non-responder group. In addition, we recently reported the effect of corticosteroid therapy in CS patients presenting ventricular arrhythmias (Yodogawa et al., 2010). The less advanced LV dysfunction patients (EF ≥ 35%) showed improvement of ventricular arrhythmias after corticosteroid therapy, and had a significantly higher prevalence of Gallium-67 uptake compared with the advanced LV dysfunction patients (EF < 35 %). Remission of Gallium-67 uptake was observed in 5 of 6 CS patients after corticosteroid therapy. These results suggested that active and reversible inflammation might play an important role for the occurrence of ventricular arrhythmias in CS. Thus, CS patients with gallium-67 uptake and relatively preserved LV function are thought to be good candidates for treatment of the steroid therapy. On the contrary, CS patients with advanced LV dysfunction and no gallium-67 uptake are considered to be non-responders to corticosteroid therapy, and require earlier initiation of additional therapy such as catheter ablation, permanent pacemaker or ICD implantation. In patients with no response to corticosteroid therapy or intolerant to steroid side effects, alternative therapy such as methotrexate, cyclosporine is the treatment of choice. Although rare, cardiac transplantation may be needed for severe CS patients unresponsive to these therapies.

4. Prognosis

The prognosis of symptomatic CS is not well elucidated. Although it has been considered poor, recent studies have shown better prognosis in patients treated with corticosteroids. Yazaki et al. showed 5-year survival rates of 75% in the steroid-treated patients and of 89% in patients with a left ventricular ejection fraction > or = 50% (Yazaki et al., 2001). According to a report by Chiu et al., survival rate of CS patients was relatively good, at 98% after 1 year, 93% after 3 years, 90% after 5 years, and 84% after 10 years. Especially, there were no cardiac deaths in preserved EF patients (initial LV ejection fractions >55%), during the follow-up period of 10 years (Chiu et al., 2005). Therefore earlier initiation of corticosteroid therapy is mandatory for CS patients before the deterioration of cardiac function.

5. Conclusion

The early detection of CS is critical for successful treatment and improved prognosis. Although MRI and PET scan have renewed the awareness of CS, the early detection still remains difficult. Currently, no single test has proven consistently reliable in detecting CS. A combination of multiple testing methodologies is considered to be the most reliable approach for the early identification. Refinements in noninvasive electrocardiographic studies may help in the early detection and management for CS.

6. References

Lima Newman LE, Rose CS, Maier LA. Sarcoidosis. N Engl J Med 1997;336:1224– 1234.

Nishiwaki T, Yoneyama H, Eishi Y, Matsuo N, Tatsumi K, Kimura H, Kuriyama T, Matsushima K: Indigenous pulmonary *Propionibacterium acnes* primes the host in the development of sarcoid-like pulmonary granulomatosis in mice. Am J Pathol 2004;165:631-639.

Hance AJ. The role of Mycobacteria in the pathogenesis of sarcoidosis. Seminars in Respiratory Infections 1998;13:197-205.

American Thoracic Society. Medical Section of the American Lung Association: Statement on sarcoidosis. Am J Respir Cri Care Med 1999;160:736-55.

Maliark MJ, Chen KM, Major ML, Sheffer RG, Popovich J, Rybicki BA, Iannuzzi MC. Analysis of HLA-DPB1 polymorphism in African-Americans with sarcoidosis. Am J Respir Crit Care 1998;158:111-4.

Hiraga H, Yuwai K, Hiroe M. Guideline for diagnosis of cardiac sarcoidosis: study report on diffuse pulmonary disease from the Japanese Ministry of Health and Welfare (in Japanese). 1993;6:23–24.

Uemura A, Morimoto S, Hiramitsu S, et al. Histologic diagnostic rate of cardiac sarcoidosis: evaluation of endomyocardial biopsies. Am Heart J 1999;138:299-302.

Ardehali H, Howard DL, Hariri, A, et al. A positive endomyocardial biopsy result for sarcoid is associated with poor prognosis in patients with initially unexplained cardiomyopathy. Am heart J 2005;150:459-463.

Silverman KJ, Hutchins JM, Bulkley BH. Cardiac sarcoid: A clinicopathologic study of 84 unselected patients with systemic sarcoidosis. *Circulation* 1978; 58: 1204– 1211.

Loncope WT, Freiman DGH. A study of sarcoidosis: Based on a combined investigation of 160 cases including 30 autopsies from the Johns Hopkins Hospital and Massachusetts General Hospital. *Medicine* 1952; 31: 1–132.

Iwai K, Sekiguchi M, Hosoda Y, DeRemee RA, Tazelaar HD, Sharma OP, et al. Racial difference in cardiac sarcoidosis incidence observed at autopsy. *Sarcoidosis* 1994;11:26-31

Bargout R, Kelly RF. Sarcoid heart disease: Clinical course and treatment. *Int J Cardiol* 2004; 97: 173 - 182.

Yodogawa K, Seino Y, Ohara T, et al. Non-invasive detection of latent cardiac conduction abnormalities in patients with pulmonary sarcoidosis. Circ J. 2007;71:540-545.

Soejima K, Yada H. The work-up and management of patients with apparent or subclinical cardiac sarcoidosis: with emphasis on the associated heart rhythm abnormalities. J Cardiovasc Electrophysiol. 2009;20(5):578-83.

Yazaki Y, Isobe M, Hayasaka M, Tanaka M, Fujii T, Sekiguchi M. Cardiac sarcoidosis mimicking hypertrophic cardiomyopathy: clinical utility of radionuclide imaging for differential diagnosis. Jpn Circ J. 1998 ;62(6):465-8.

Matsumori A, Hara M, Nagai S, Izumi T, Ohashi N, Ono K, Sasayama S. Hypertrophic cardiomyopathy as a manifestation of cardiac sarcoidosis. Jpn Circ J. 2000 ;64(9):679-83.

Sato T, Kanzaki H, Ishida Y, et al. Second left ventricular aneurysm newly developed in a patient with untreated cardiac sarcoidosis. Circ J. 2010 ;74(11):2477-8.

Valantine HA, Tazelaar HD, Macoviak J, et al. Cardiac sarcoidosis: response to steroids and transplantation. J Heart Transplant 1987;6: 244– 50.

Uemura A, Morimoto S, Kato Y, Hiramitsu S, Ohtsuki M, Kato S, Sugiura A, Miyagishima K, Iwase M, Hishida H. Relationship between basal thinning of the interventricular septum and atrioventricular block in patients with cardiac sarcoidosis. Sarcoidosis Vasc Diffuse Lung Dis. 2005 ;22(1):63-5.

Okayama K, Kurata C, Tawarahara K, et al. Diagnostic and prognostic value of myocardial scintigraphy with thallium-201 and gallium-67 in cardiac sarcoidosis. Chest 1995;107:330-334.

Futamatsu H, Suzuki J, Adachi S, et al. Utility of gallium-67 scintigraphy for evaluation of cardiac sarcoidosis with ventricular tachycardia. Int J Cardiovasc Imaging 2006;22:443–448.

Kiuchi S, Teraoka K, Koizumi K, et al. Usefulness of late gadolinium enhancement combined with MRI and 67-Ga scintigraphy in the diagnosis of cardiac sarcoidosis and disease activity evaluation. Int J Cardiovasc Imaging 2007;23:237-41

Yamagishi H, Shirai N, Takagi M, Yoshiyama M, Akioka K, Takeuchi K, Yoshikawa J: Identification of cardiac sarcoidosis with (13)N-NH(3)/(18)F-FDG PET. J Nucl Med 2003;44:1030-1036.

Ohira H, Tsujino I, Ishimaru S, Oyama N, Takei T, Tsukamoto E, Miura M, Sakaue S, Tamaki N, Nishimura M. Myocardial imaging with 18F-fluoro-2-deoxyglucose positron emission tomography and magnetic resonance imaging in sarcoidosis. Eur J Nucl Med Mol Imaging. 2008 ;35(5):933-41.

Ishimaru S, Tsujino I, Takei T, et al. Focal uptake on 18F-fluoro-2-deoxyglucose positron emission tomography images indicates cardiac involvement of sarcoidosis. Eur Heart J 2005;26: 1538-43.

Okumura W, Iwasaki T, Toyama T, et al. Usefulness of fasting 18FFDGPET in identification of cardiac sarcoidosis. J Nucl Med 2004;45:1989-98.

Shimada T, Shimada K, Sakane T, et al.: Diagnosis of cardiac sarcoidosis and evaluation of the effects of steroid therapy by gadolinium-DTPA-enhanced magnetic resonance imaging. Am J Med 2001,110:520-527.

Smedema JP, Snoep G, Van Kroonenburgh MP, et al. Evaluation of the accuracy of gadolinium-enhanced cardiovascular magnetic resonance in the diagnosis of cardiac sarcoidosis. J Am Coll Cardiol 2005;45:1683-90.

Tadamura E, Yamamuro M, Kubo S, et al. Effectiveness of delayed enhanced MRI for identification of cardiac sarcoidosis: comparison with radionuclide imaging. Am J Roentgenol 2005; 185: 110–115.

Yazaki Y, Isobe M, Hiroe M, et al. Central Japan Heart Study Group. Prognostic determinants of long-term survival in Japanese patients with cardiac sarcoidosis treated with prednisolone. Am J Cardiol 2001;88:1006 –1010.

Chiu CZ, Nakatani S, Zhang G, et al. Prevention of left ventricular remodeling by long-term corticosteroid therapy in patients with cardiac sarcoidosis. Am J Cardiol 2005;95:143-146.

Kato Y, Morimoto S, Uemura A, et al. Efficacy of corticosteroids in sarcoidosis presenting with atrioventricular block. Sarcoidosis Vasc Diffuse Lung Dis 2003 ; 20:133-137.

Banba K, Kusano KF, Nakamura K, et al. Relationship between arrhythmogenesis and disease activity in cardiac sarcoidosis. Heart Rhythm 2007;4:1292-1299.

Yodogawa K, Seino Y, Ono N, et al. Therapeutic Evaluation of Corticosteroid Therapy for Ventricular Tachycardia Associated with Cardiac Sarcoidosis -Application of High Resolution Electrocardiography- (abstr). Circulation 2008;118:S_671.

Yodogawa K, Seino Y, Ohara T, et al. Effect of corticosteroid therapy on ventricular arrhythmias in patients with cardiac sarcoidosis. Ann Noninvasive Electrocardiol 2011;16(2):140-147.

Yazaki Y, Isobe M, Hiroe M, et al. Prognostic determinants of longterm survival in Japanese patients with cardiac sarcoidosis treated with prednisone. Am J Cardiol 2001;88:1006-10.

Chiu CZ, Nakatani S, Zhang G, Tachibana T, Ohmori F, Yamagishi M, Kitakaze M, Tomoike H, Miyatake K. Prevention of left ventricular remodeling by long-term corticosteroid therapy in patients with cardiac sarcoidosis. Am J Cardiol. 2005 ;95(1):143-6.

14

Neurological Sarcoidosis

J. Chad Hoyle and Herbert B. Newton
Departments of Neurology and Neurosurgery,
The Ohio State University Medical Center and James Cancer Hospital,
USA

1. Introduction

Sarcoidosis is a granulomatous, inflammatory disease that can affect multiple systems of the body. Most commonly this involves the lungs, skin, and eyes, but also can affect the nervous system in about 5% of cases (Delaney1977, Stern et al 1985). Neurological sarcoidosis may be associated with virtually any aspect of the nervous system, but just like the predilection for certain organ systems in systemic disease, neurological involvement also may demonstrate characteristic clinical patterns to aid in the recognition of the disorder. This is especially important because the presenting manifestations may be neurological in nearly 50% of these patients (Stern et al 1985). The first large review of the trends of clinical involvement of the nervous system in sarcoidosis was outlined over 60 years ago (Colover 1948). Subsequent reviews and case reports have built on that foundation. This chapter will outline the clinical manifestations, diagnostic considerations, and management options, including new trends in therapy of neurological sarcoidosis.

2. Clinical manifestations

The most classic clinical patterns of nervous system involvement in sarcoidosis include cranial neuropathy, meningeal based disease, and hypothalamic-pituitary axis symptomatology. Cranial neuropathy is the most common neurological deficit with an incidence of 50 to 75% of patients (Delaney 1977, Stern et al 1985). In general, meningeal based disease is a common hallmark of neurosarcoidosis and can manifest in a variety of ways as outlined below. Hypothalamic-pituitary axis involvement may yield only relatively nonspecific symptomatology, but can be a frequent and important manifestation, as well.

The most common cranial neuropathy is a facial palsy. In hindsight, the first historically described cases occurred early in the 20th century, when unusual presentations of parotid enlargement, uveitis, and facial palsies were described (Heerfordt 1909). Years later facial palsy was documented in half of neurosarcoidosis patients (Colover 1948, Stern et al 1985), making it the most predominant clinical association. A third of these cases are bilateral (Colover 1948, Stern et al 1985), and those presentations or recurrent facial palsy in general should trigger a suspicion for a secondary cause of facial palsy, such as Lyme disease or neurosarcoidosis.

The second most common cranial neuropathy is of the optic nerve. The incidence of this presenting complaint is rather high, and actually in more recent papers, some have described this as being even more common than facial palsy (Pawate et al 2009, Joseph and Scolding 2009). Referral bias was considered as a cause of this as Pawate's data came from a multiple sclerosis center, whereas Stern's prior data noted above came from a sarcoidosis clinic. Regardless, sarcoidosis needs to be in the differential of secondary causes of optic neuritis within the appropriate clinical context, and bilateral optic neuritis, in particular, may herald an even stronger neurological suspicion for sarcoidosis, along with other conditions that may classically present that way, such as neuromyelitis optica. Unfortunately, bilateral optic neuritis tends to have a markedly worse prognosis for recovery compared to unilateral optic neuritis (Pawate et al 2009). Of note, it is important to keep in mind that the most common ocular symptoms in sarcoidosis are still primary ophthalmological manifestations, such as uveitis.

The eighth cranial nerve is affected in up to one fifth of patients. This involvement tends to be bilateral, and appears to be related to granulomatous meningitis in most cases. Patients may experience hearing loss or have vestibular dysfunction. This may present suddenly or with a fluctuating course. Recovery of function is less common than with facial palsies. (Stern et al 1985) The most common extraocular muscle palsy is of the sixth nerve (Joseph and Scolding 2009). Trigeminal neuropathies have also been well described in association with sarcoidosis (Armin A and Balderacchi JL 2010). Cranial nerve nine and ten palsies may result in dysphagia, hoarseness, or vocal cord paralysis (Delaney 1977). Though an ENT study documented neurosarcoidosis of the vagus nerve to be rare in their general patient population, they noted it should still be considered in the differential diagnosis of vocal cord paresis or paralysis (Alon and Ekbom 2010). Although felt to be uncommon, decreased smell might be an underreported complication given that the 1st cranial nerve is not commonly tested on examination. Significant, symptomatic anosmia from sarcoidosis is more commonly encountered in patients with significant generalized disease and it can be refractory to treatment (Aubart et al 2006). Essentially, any cranial nerve may be affected by the granulomatous infiltration of sarcoidosis, though the rest of the cranial nerves not outlined above would only very rarely be involved.

Meningeal based disease is another classic finding of neurosarcoidosis. In fact this meningeal based disease is also not only responsible for many of the cranial neuropathic complications, but presents in a variety of other ways, as well. Significant basilar disease can be associated with a polycranial neuropathy from meningeal infiltration. Meningeal disease may cause headache related to acute aseptic or chronic meningitis. In one large review series at the Mayo Clinic, chronic meningitis was actually the most common initial manifestation of neurosarcoidosis (Aksamit and Norona 1999). If cerebrospinal fluid flow becomes obstructed, then headache might also be a manifestation of hydrocephalus. Weakness, pain, and sensory dysfunction can be seen in some cases with polyradicular involvement from spinal meningeal infiltration. All together, some form of meningeal involvement is a very common and suggestive feature of neurological sarcoidosis.

Hypothalamic-pituitary axis symptomatology can be rather nonspecific, but taken into context with other features of neurosarcoidosis, it might help tip the balance of clinical evidence to proceed further with testing for sarcoidosis. Diabetes insipidus is considered the most common manifestation, accounting for half of all neuroendocrine abnormalities (Chapelon et al 1990). Of note, an organic primary polydipsia may also be the cause of polyuria and polydipsia, and hypercalcemia from sarcoidosis can cause nephrogenic diabetes insipidus (Stuart et al 1980). Other relatively common neuroendocrine manifestations of sarcoidosis include amenorrhea or galactorrhea. Serum prolactin levels have been high in up to a third of patients in general with sarcoidosis (Turkington and Macindoe JH 1972), and that unexpected high percentage could reflect that some degree of subclinical neurological involvement is associated with many more systemic sarcoidosis patients than previously thought. A more complete list of possible endocrine manifestations of sarcoidosis includes morbid obesity, dysregulation of body temperature, insomnia, personality change, SIADH, diabetes insipidus, hyperprolactinemia, hypothyroidism, hypoadrenalism, growth hormone deficiency, and impaired counter-regulatory response to hypoglycemia (Porter et al 2003).

In addition to the above classical neurological manifestations of sarcoidosis, there are several other neurological entities that are seen with intermediate frequency and less specificity. This may include seizures, which have been reported in 10% to 17% of patients (Delaney 1977, Pawate et al 2009, Joseph and Scolding 2009). Seizures correlate with a worse prognosis overall, likely as a reflection of more significant underlying parenchymal disease. In addition to seizures, central nervous system granulomatous mass lesions can cause headache, lethargy, or other localization related symptomatology. (Stern et al 1985) Spinal cord disease also can present with intermediate frequency. Leptomeningeal infiltration in the region of the spinal cord is associated with sarcoidosis, but intraparenchymal infiltration can occur, too, causing fusiform spinal cord enlargement, focal or diffuse intramedullary disease, or spinal cord atrophy (Junger et al 1993). Based on recent reports, greater than 15% of initial clinical presentations of neurosarcoidosis can be related to myelopathy or spinal cord disease in general (Pawate et al 2009, Joseph and Scolding 2009). A longitudinal myelitis can be the presenting symptom of neurosarcoidosis, making this a consideration with other longitudinally extensive cord inflammatory syndromes (Sierra-Hidalgo et al 2010), such as neuromyelitis optica or connective tissue disorders such as Sjogren's disease or Lupus. Neuropsychiatric disorders also have an intermediate incidence. The symptomatology related to this can include encephalopathy, psychosis, depression, bipolar disorder, apathy, irritability, and lethargy (Joseph and Scolding 2007, De Mulder and Vandenberghe 2008, Spiegel et al 2010, Friedman and Gould 2002, Bona et al 1998, O'Brien et al 1994, Sabaawi et al 1992). One should consider these neuropsychiatric symptoms to potentially be organic and possibly responsive to immunomodulatory therapy rather than just primary psychological causes. Interestingly, a patient has been described as having abnormal cerebrospinal fluid with isolated psychiatric symptoms (Gilmore et al 1980). Peripheral nervous system involvement occurs in about 15% of neurosarcoidosis cases and typically has a better prognosis than central nervous system involvement (Delaney 1977). A subacute generalized axonal sensorimotor polyneuropathy is the typical subtype of polyneuropathy seen in sarcoidosis (Zuniga et al 1991), but one must take into account that asymmetrical peripheral neuropathic limb symptomatology can be seen with polyradiculoneuropathy, which is a very well documented presentation in this disorder (Burns et al 2006). Sarcoidosis can also cause mononeuropathy with a notable increased incidence of carpal tunnel syndrome (Niemer et al 2001) among other mononeuropathy presentations. A more diffuse mononeuritis multiplex picture may occur (Zuniga et al 1999, Garg et al 2005), purely sensory neuropathy may be seen, and even rare associations of lumbosacral plexopathy have been encountered (Zuniga et al 1991). Small fiber neuropathy needs to be considered in sarcoidosis, as well (Tavee and Culver 2011, Hoitsma et al 2002). Finally, there have even been reports of Guillain-Barre like illnesses associated with neurosarcoidosis (Fahoum et al 2009).

Muscle involvement symptomatically ranges from less than 1% to potentially up to 26% of patients (Oksanen 1986, Chapelon et al 1990). Symmetrical myopathic weakness or myalgias can be experienced. There may be isolated palpable nodules within the muscle. More often, though, muscle involvement is asymptomatic. This asymptomatic involvement can be seen in up to 50% of muscle biopsies (Delaney 1977). Vascular infiltration is remarkably rare, with a very low incidence of hemorrhage or stroke. Movement disorders other than cerebellar ataxia are very rare, with only isolated reports of extrapyramidal symptoms from basal ganglia involvement, such as chorea, hemiballism, and Parkinsonism (Delaney 1977).

To summarize, the classical clinical findings include cranial neuropathy, meningeal based disease, and hypothalamic-pituitary axis symptomatology. Intermediate frequency symptomatology, such as seizures, spinal cord disease, peripheral neuropathy, muscle disease, or neuropsychiatric manifestations can be rather non-specific. Early recognition of systemic signs and symptoms of ocular disease, lung disease, and skin disease increases the yield of recognizing the disorder. In addition, 30% of patients present with more than one neurological manifestation (Stern et al 1985), which may increase the clinical context for suspecting the diagnosis, even in cases without systemic disease. As there is no gold standard test, except for biopsy, clinical acumen is necessary to combine clinical suspicion with optimal understanding of non-invasive test strategies to select appropriate patients without a known diagnosis of sarcoidosis for pathological tissue studies to confirm the diagnosis. The next section will expand upon diagnostic considerations.

Classical features
Cranial neuropathy
Meningeal based disease
Hypothalamic-pituitary axis dysfunction
Intermediate frequency features
Seizures
Encephalopathy/psychiatric symptomatology
Spinal cord disease
Peripheral neuropathy

Table 1. Major clinical features of neurosarcoidosis

Most common cranial neuropathies in sarcoidosis in order of frequency
Bell's palsy (Cranial Nerve 7)
Optic neuropathy/neuritis (Cranial Nerve 2)
Vestibulocochlear neuropathy (Cranial Nerve 8)
Other cranial nerves with intermediate frequency
Cranial Nerves 5, 6, 9, or 10

Table 2. Cranial nerve involvement in sarcoidosis

3. Diagnostic considerations

Once neurosarcoidosis is considered in the differential diagnosis, the next step is to further evaluate this with non-invasive supportive diagnostic testing. MRI with contrast, lumbar puncture, and ACE levels should all be considered in the initial work-up, though these tests lack specificity. In cases without systemic involvement, routine chest imaging should be undertaken at a minimum, and further supportive testing such as gallium scanning or bronchoalveolar lavage should also be considered. Nevertheless, pathological confirmation of tissue, demonstrating non-caseating granulomas, is necessary to justify treatment for this disorder. The proposed criteria for the diagnosis of neurosarcoidosis has been partitioned into definite, probable, or possible disease (Zajicek et al 1999). Definite disease consists of a clinical presentation compatible with neurosarcoidosis, exclusion of other possible causes, and confirmation with biopsy of nervous system tissue, such as the meninges or another source. Probable disease is defined as a clinical presentation compatible with neurosarcoidosis, non-invasive neurodiagnostic support of the diagnosis, exclusion of other possible causes, and evidence of systemic sarcoidosis by biopsy. Possible neurosarcoidosis is defined as a clinical presentation compatible with neurosarcoidosis clinically and with noninvasive neurodiagnostic studies, along with exclusion of other possible causes.

Developing a focused differential diagnosis based on the site of neurological involvement is critical to effectively excluding other disorders that may mimic neurosarcoidosis. Classical disease that involves a meningeal process would require the exclusion of infectious and malignant etiologies. Examples of this would range from chronic infectious processes, such as fungal infections and tuberculosis to malignant processes such as carcinomatous or lymphomatous meningitis. These would all be highly pertinent considerations in patients with basilar infiltration causing polycranial neuropathies. Restricted cranial nerve lesions, such as unilateral Bell's palsy may be clinically indistinguishable from idiopathic cases, though recurrent or bilateral disease should invoke consideration of secondary causes such as sarcoidosis, Lyme disease, or a rare disorder, Melkersson-Rosenthal syndrome. Similarly, unilateral optic neuritis might suggest multiple sclerosis in the differential, whereas bilateral disease increases the suspicion of sarcoidosis or other disorders, such as neuromyelitis optica. Transverse myelitis might be difficult to distinguish from idiopathic demyelination or multiple sclerosis, but longitudinally extensive lesions, which can be seen in neurosarcoidosis, bring several diagnostic considerations to the forefront, such as neuromyelitis optica, connective tissue disorders such as Sjogren's or Lupus, or vascular disorders, such as dural A-V fistula. White matter disease on MRI would necessitate differentiation from multiple sclerosis, nonspecific vascular disease, inflammatory/vasculitic etiologies, or infectious considerations like Lyme disease. HIV can masquerade as having many of the features of neurosarcoidosis, in general. Multi-systemic disease may suggest other uncommon syndromes, such as amyloidosis. Mass lesions in the brain from sarcoid granulomas need differentiation from other lesions such as tumor or abscess. Dural lesions can mimic meningioma. A vasculopathy appearance with encephalopathy must be differentiated from CNS vasculitis or neurosyphilis. Finally, peripheral nervous system involvement is much more nonspecific. With peripheral neuropathic processes, the differential diagnosis depends on the location, neurophysiology, and timing of the neuropathy. For instance, the most common polyneuropathy of an axonal sensorimotor polyneuropathy might be difficult to distinguish from the common causes of metabolic polyneuropathy, such as diabetes, thyroid disease, vitamin deficiency, connective tissue disease, toxins, or monoclonal gammopathies associated with or without significant underlying hematological disease. A subacute onset might help lean more towards an acquired, inflammatory cause in the differential, though. With a mononeuritis multiplex picture, one would need to differentiate between vasculitis, diabetes, or less common infectious etiologies such as hepatitis, Lyme, or HIV. Isolated mononeuropathy would be difficult to distinguish from common entrapment neuropathies. As mentioned above, an acute polyneuropathy with a Guillain-Barre phenotype can be seen. A Guillain-Barre like illness with unexpected cerebrospinal fluid pleocytosis (Fahoum et al 2009) in addition to the expected high protein level might signal other considerations like HIV or sarcoidosis as underlying etiologies.

Compatible epidemiological features such as younger patients and an African American predominance can be clues, though very non-specific given the differential diagnosis above. In cases of known systemic sarcoidosis, the diagnosis mainly entails ruling out other etiologies of neurological involvement, especially infectious causes given these patients may already be immunosuppressed. In cases without systemic involvement, the diagnosis can be challenging and further experience with the details of the diagnostic workup is necessary. We will discuss the noninvasive diagnostic strategies first. This will include MRI studies with contrast, cerebral spinal fluid studies, ACE levels, chest imaging, and gallium studies. Analyzing five large case reviews (Zajicek et al 1999, Christoforidis et al 1999, Aksamit and Norona 1999, Pawate et al 2009, Joseph and Scolding 2009), the following trends and details regarding specific diagnostic tests emerge.

MRI of the brain with contrast, as well as the spinal cord, if symptomatology and exam findings suggest localization there, is a key to the diagnostic workup. The sensitivity rate for an abnormal brain MRI with contrast in patients with symptoms referable to the central nervous system may be as high as 80 to 90% (Christoforidis et al 1999, Pawate et al 2009). Overall, spinal cord abnormalities are seen in 10-20% of cases (Zajicek et al 1999, Pawate et al 2009). However, when spinal cord symptomatology is present, imaging is abnormal in roughly 60-70% of cases (Aksamit and Norona 1999, Pawate et al 2009).

On MRI of the brain, nonspecific white matter lesions are common, with roughly 40% of cases showing these findings (Zajicek et al 1999). Patients with isolated white matter disease tend to have a good prognosis. Nevertheless, this is a very nonspecific finding and a contrast enhanced study with gadolinium will demonstrate much more of the classical features of sarcoidosis. Meningeal enhancement is quite common and can be seen in nearly 40% of cases (Zajicek et al 1999). There are multiple other enhancing abnormalities that can be encountered, too. Strictly dural enhancement may be seen, as well as isolated cranial nerve enhancement, focal parenchymal enhancement associated with a white matter lesion or with a focal mass (in general parenchymal enhancement has a relative predilection for the hypothalamic-pituitary axis), or periventricular radial vascular enhancement. In 10-15% of neurosarcoidosis patients, hydrocephalus can be present (Zajicek et al 1999). Vasculitic infarcts are very rare, but do occur (Pawate et al 2009). Interestingly, 40% of cranial nerve deficits were not associated with their respective cranial nerves having enhancement on MRI, though conversely 44% of patients had MRI evidence of cranial nerve involvement with no symptoms related to that radiologically affected site (Christoforidis et al 1999). The findings of Christoforidis also noted that even though hypothalamic-pituitary axis enhancement is not a rare finding on imaging, 50% of patients with symptoms related to the hypothalamic-pituitary axis had no abnormal findings on imaging in that region. Spinal cord lesions most typically consist of meningeal enhancement, spinal cord swelling, or enhancing myelitis of the cord (Pawate 2009).

Common MRI Brain features of neurosarcoidosis
Non specific white matter changes
Meningeal thickening/enhancement
Cranial nerve enhancement
Parenchymal enhancement of white matter lesion or a focal mass
Parenchymal enhancement has a relatively greater predilection for the hypothalamic-pituitary axis
Hydrocephalus
MRI Spine features of neurosarcoidosis
Meningeal or radicular enhancement/thickening
Cord swelling
Myelitis (often enhancing)

Table 3. Imaging findings in neurological sarcoidosis

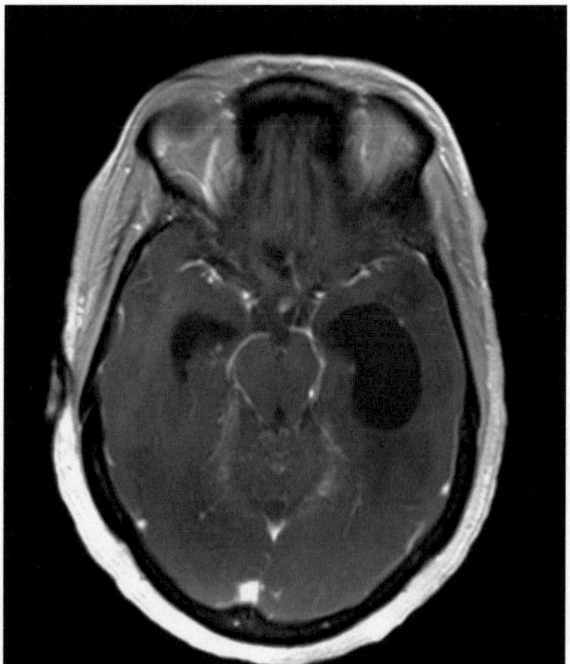

Fig. 1. Gadolinium enhanced MRI of the brain demonstrating basilar leptomeningeal enhancement and hydrocephalus

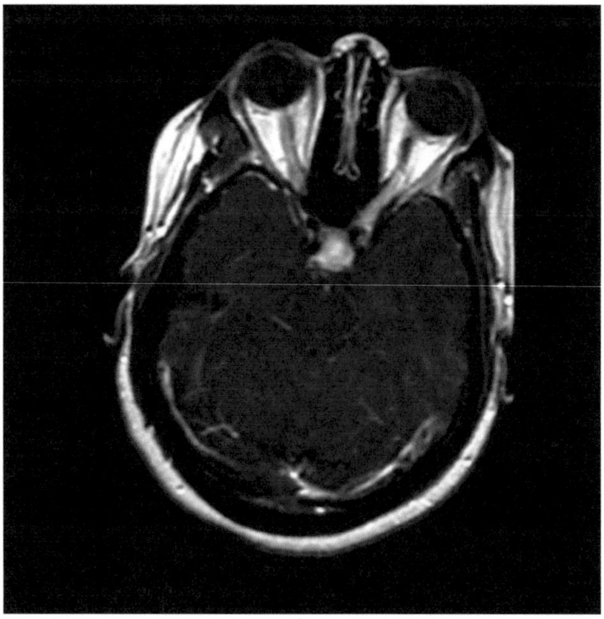

Fig. 2. Gadolinium enhanced MRI of the brain demonstrating bilateral optic nerve and pituitary axis enhancement

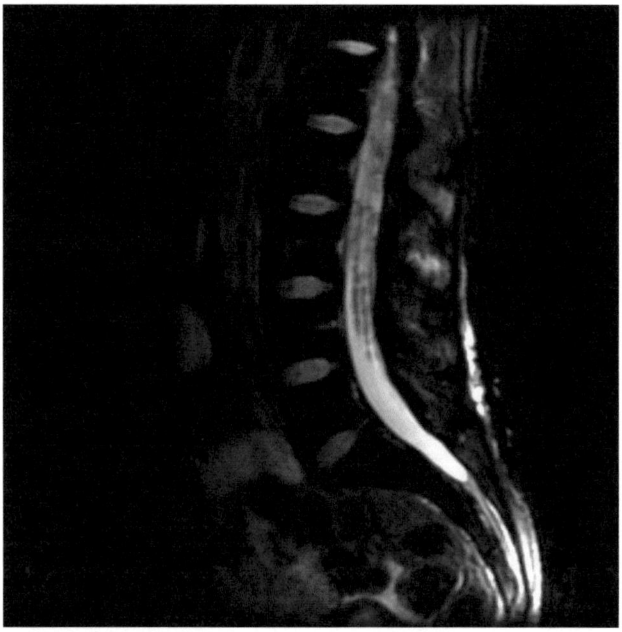

Fig. 3. MRI of the lumbosacral spine demonstrating diffuse radicular nodularity

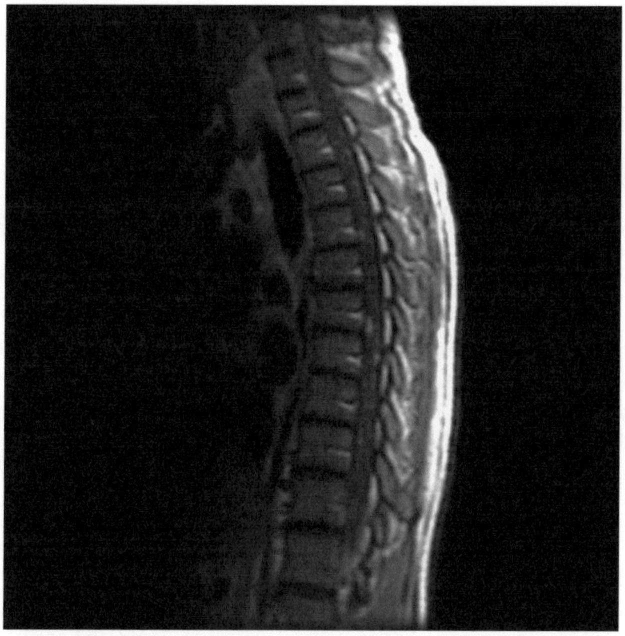

Fig. 4. Gadolinium enhanced MRI of the thoracic spine demonstrating scattered nodular enhancement.

Spinal fluid evaluation is indicated for all patients suspected of having neurosarcoidosis, assuming that there is not a risk for herniation based on CNS imaging. Cerebrospinal fluid evaluation serves two purposes. First, it has a high sensitivity for demonstrating abnormalities in patients with neurosarcoidosis, even if they are relatively nonspecific. In addition, spinal fluid studies may be sent to help rule out other mimicking conditions of this disorder, such as infectious and malignant causes.

Neurosarcoidosis reviews (Aksamit and Norona 1999, Zajicek et al 1999) offer insight into the details of cerebrospinal fluid findings. The cerebrospinal fluid protein is typically elevated in roughly 70 to 80% of patients. The value may be very highly elevated and an average case would be above 100. Spinal fluid pleocytosis is seen in 55-72% of patients with a mean value of around 50, but values of several hundred can be seen. This is typically a lymphocytosis. Oligoclonal bands are positive in around 20% of patients. An elevated protein typically accompanies this, which might lead one to consideration of sarcoidosis, rather than a more typical multiple sclerosis case. Cerebrospinal fluid ACE levels are positive in only about 1/4 to 1/3 of patients. This low sensitivity is also coupled with concerns of specificity. Five of nine elevated cerebrospinal fluid ACE levels in the Mayo Clinic review were related to infectious or carcinomatous meningitis (Aksamit and Norona 1999).

Serum ACE levels have a relatively high sensitivity for undiagnosed sarcoidosis patients in general, and may approach 75% (Studdy and Bird 1989). Observations for patients presenting with neurosarcoidosis demonstrate potentially lower sensitivities overall with Joseph and Scolding (2009) having data of only a 29% positivity rate. This is likely due to many patients having a more localized expression of sarcoidosis in the nervous system. In addition, this test also suffers from specificity limitations with false positives in 2-4% of normals and high false positive rates in patients with infection, liver disease, renal disease, hyperthyroidism, Gaucher's, and some cases of other disorders (Wallach 2000).

Around 90% of sarcoidosis patients have pulmonary involvement (Baughman 2004); nevertheless, due to the potentially more isolated disease of neurosarcoidosis, those numbers are not as high in series of patients presenting with neurological complications. Regardless, 50-60% of patients still had abnormalities and so this is still a very useful screening method in patients with a possible diagnosis of neurosarcoidosis (Pawate et al 2009, Joseph and Scolding 2009). Chest CT can enhance the sensitivity of pertinent findings, though in Pawate's series, only two patients with a normal chest x-ray had chest CT findings. This demonstrated that even a routine chest x-ray is a very useful initial screening measure (Pawate et al 2009). Gallium scanning can demonstrate characteristic uptake patterns in sarcoidosis, including the lung and parotid regions, for example, and informative abnormalities appear to be present in roughly half of patients presenting with neurosarcoidosis (Zajicek et al 1999, Joseph and Scolding 2009).

Taking into account all of the diagnostic information noted above, the main purpose is to guide the decision of whether to obtain a biopsy for suspicion of neurosarcoidosis, as well as to rule out other mimicking conditions. This confirmatory strategy is necessary in order to proceed with aggressive immunomodulatory medication. If there is evidence of systemic disease, then biopsy of the appropriate lung (transbronchial), skin, or lymph node tissue would be an appropriate strategy (Aksamit and Norana 1999, Aksamit 2008, Pawate et al 2009). In patients without this possibility, biopsy of a clinically relevant nervous system lesion, such as an enhancing area of the meninges or accessible significant parenchymal lesion could be considered for a definitive diagnosis (Aksamit 2008). Peripheral nervous system involvement could be biopsied, as well, with symptomatology and exam findings helping to guide that decision. A muscle biopsy could be considered even in patients without muscle related symptoms as 50% of patients have abnormalities on a muscle biopsy, which is well above the clinical incidence of muscle involvement (Delaney 1977). Other biopsy approaches of "clinically silent" areas would include a bone marrow biopsy or a conjunctival biopsy, which have a 30-40% chance of a positive result (Aksamit and Norona 1999). A conjunctival biopsy was recommended as an initial strategy by Aksamit due to its relatively non-invasive nature and question of whether the yield of muscle biopsy is as high as mentioned above (Aksamit 2008).

4. Treatment

Neurological involvement of sarcoidosis is, by definition, an indication for the initiation of medical treatment (Hunninghake et al 1999). The first line therapy is oral corticosteroids (Selroos 1994). For neurological disease, prednisone is to be started at around 1 mg per kilogram per day and continued for 6-8 weeks of high-dose therapy before beginning a very slow taper (Hoitsma et al 2004). Overall, treatment is suggested for last at least 6-12 months to help avoid progression or relapse of the disease (Aksamit 2008). Exceptions to this could include more benign or monophasic expressions of neurosarcoidosis, such as isolated Bell's palsy or aseptic meningitis, potentially being treated on the order of weeks rather than more chronically, given the favorable prognosis (Luke et al 1987). Along those lines the general rule is central nervous system disease, especially with significant parenchymal involvement or seizure activity, is more likely to have a poor prognosis and require more aggressive treatment than peripheral nervous system disease (Ferriby et al

2001, Stern et al 1985, Luke et al 1987, Scott 1993, Zajicek et al 1999). With more significant disease, not only is at least 6-12 months of corticosteroid treatment indicated, but steroid sparing agents may be necessary in cases that appear more likely to run a refractory course during the steroid taper or if the patient is not tolerating steroid treatment. Some options include methotrexate, cyclosporin, azathioprine, cellcept, or cytoxan (Androdias et al 2011, Agbogu et al 1995, Stern et al 1992, Soriano et al 1990, Elkin and Willcox 1985). These medications will likely need to be continued for 6-12 months or longer with significant disease. With severe disease onset, a pulse of IV methylprednisolone for 5 days before starting oral corticosteroids might be necessary, and, in addition, a steroid sparing agent might need to be started early in the course of therapy (Scott et al 2007). Management of corticosteroids and the immunosuppressants outlined above should be undertaken by a clinician who is familiar with these medications and their practice. Further details of the dosing and possible toxicity are similar to the general treatment principles with systemic disease. Finally, hydroxychloroquine is a medication that inhibits antigen presentation to MHC peptide complexes and their transport to the cell surface (Moller 2003). This medication theoretically could be considered as an add-on medication with an additional mechanism of action to treat sarcoidosis, but does not have much efficacy in the primary treatment of neurosarcoidosis. It may be beneficial in helping to maintain longer remissions in patients who have difficulty maintaining steroid remission without a relapse (Aksamit 2008). It is a well tolerated medication, though monitoring for retinal toxicity is necessary (Baughman and Lynch 2003). Finally, radiation therapy has been utilized in patients refractory to all medication therapy as a last resort (Bruns et al 2004, Menninger et al 2003).

Unfortunately, despite the treatment approach outlined above, patients with neurosarcoidosis can be steroid resistant and another 20-40% of those further resistant to the use of conventional immunosuppressive agents (Hoitsma et al 2004). The rationale for utilizing these treatments is to generically suppress the inflammatory response generated by a TH 1 mediated reaction to the antigen stimulus of sarcoidosis. The TH 1 mediated response to MHC-II complexes formed from antigen stimuli in sarcoidosis heavily involves interleukin-2, interleukin-12, interferon-γ, and tumor necrosis factor-α (Moller 2003). Tumor necrosis factor-α is the main cytokine of interest, and there have been several clinical trials of direct therapy to block it with encouraging results. The predominant examples of this include infliximab and thalidomide. Infliximab is a monoclonal antibody that blocks tumor necrosis factor-α. Concerns of infection related to immunosuppression, cytopenias, a paradoxical provocation of multiple sclerosis, allergic reactions, and significant cost of the medication are all factors that could limit its use. Nevertheless, there is a large and growing support for its efficacy, though lacking any confirmatory prospective study. Its use may be considered in patients refractory to other medical treatment (Pereira et al 2011, Santos et al 2010, Aksamit 2008). Likewise, thalidomide also has properties that involve tumor necrosis factor-α blockade. This medication is most known for its concerns for teratogenic effects, such as phocomelia, and it now has to be prescribed through the system for thalidomide education and prescribed safety (STEPS), only available to be prescribed through select physicians. In addition, toxicity such as an axonal sensory polyneuropathy develops in about 20% of patients. Sedation is the main limitation of the medication otherwise, which is very slowly titrated as tolerated from 100 mg to a max of 800 mg as needed (though typically 400 mg or less for maintenance). Other side effects could include rash, thromboembolism, dizziness, and constipation. (Wu et al 2005) In contrast to other immunosuppressive therapies, there is not a significantly increased risk of infection with patients on thalidomide (Baughman and Lower 2004). Our experience is consistent with other authors, and demonstrates the efficacy of thalidomide in patients with steroid and immunosuppressant-refractory neurosarcoidosis (Hoyle, Newton, Katz 2008, Hammond et al 2007, Nguyen et al 2004).

The future trends in therapy will likely involve the use of drugs targeted to the underlying pathophysiology of sarcoidosis, such as the new tumor necrosis factor-α inhibitors currently under investigation. Also, future prevention or possible treatment of neurosarcoidosis could be enhanced by a better understanding of the antigen responsible for initiating sarcoidosis, and why such a small percentage of patients develop neurological involvement. Proprionibacterium and mycobacterium have been two antigenic candidates that have not resulted in any significant disease modification with attempts at treatment. Other environmental antigens have been proposed, as well. Further exploration of the antigenic source of initiation of sarcoidosis, the conditions that allow the host response to become susceptible to the development of non-caseating granulomas and, more specifically, how this can selectively occur in the nervous system will hopefully yield progress in the field.

5. Conclusion

Neurosarcoidosis is a complex disorder that may involve virtually any aspect of the nervous system. Nevertheless, it may present with certain classical features, such as cranial nerve involvement, meningeal based disease, or hypothalamic-pituitary axis symptomatology to alert one to the possibility of this diagnosis. Seizures, spinal cord involvement, encephalopathy/psychiatric symptomatology, and peripheral neuropathy occur with intermediate frequencies and less specificity for suspecting this condition, but need to be understood in the context of other clues systemically or otherwise to the disorder.

Diagnosis in cases of known systemic sarcoidosis is more straightforward, but in the absence of systemic features on presentation, diagnosis may be complicated. MRI of the brain with contrast (and potentially spinal cord) and cerebrospinal fluid studies are mandatory in the initial evaluation to not only demonstrate features suggesting a need to pursue a pathological tissue diagnosis, but also important in evaluating for other mimickers of the disease, chief among those being infection or malignancy. ACE levels have relatively poor sensitivity and specificity, but can increase suspicion of the disorder in cases without other apparent clues. A detailed clinical understanding of the features of systemic disease is important background knowledge for evaluating patients with potential neurosarcoidosis. Routine chest imaging and potentially gallium studies if needed can be helpful noninvasive adjuncts. Nevertheless, tissue diagnosis remains the gold standard and is necessary before committing to significant immunomodulatory therapy.

Corticosteroids remain the first-line therapy of neurosarcoidosis with steroid sparing agents reserved for more severe or refractory disease, or for patients who are intolerant to corticosteroids. Selective therapy of downstream inflammatory features of sarcoidosis, such as with tumor necrosis factor-α antagonists, are becoming more recognized as options in refractory disease. Further exploration of targeted immunomodulatory therapy, better understanding of the antigenic initiation of the disease, and discovery of host factors that make one susceptible not only to sarcoidosis, but specifically nervous system involvement, are important areas for future progress in treating this disorder.

6. References

Agbogu BN, Stern BJ, Sewell C, Yang G. Arch Neurol. Therapeutic considerations in patients with refractory neurosarcoidosis. 1995 Sep;52(9):875-9.

Aksamit AJ, Norona F. Neurosarcoidosis without systemic sarcoid. Ann Neurol 1999;46:471.

Aksamit. Neurosarcoidosis. Continuum. 2008;14(1):181-196.

Alon EE, Ekbom DC. Neurosarcoidosis affecting the vagus nerve. Ann Otol Rhinol Laryngol. 2010 Sep;119(9):641-5.

Androdias G, Maillet D, Marignier R, Pinède L, Confavreux C, Broussolle C, Vukusic S, Sève P. Mycophenolate mofetil may be effective in CNS sarcoidosis but not in sarcoid myopathy.Neurology. 2011 Mar 29;76(13):1168-72.

Armin A, Balderacchi JL. Trigeminal neurosarcoidosis: case report and literature review. Ear Nose Throat J. 2010 Jul;89(7):320-2.

Aubart FC, Quayoun M, Brauner M, Attali P, Kambouchner M, Valeyre D, Nunes H. Sinonasal involvement in sarcoidosis: a case-control study of 20 patients. 2006 Nov;85(6):365-71.

Baughman RP. Pulmonary sarcoidosis. Clin Chest Med. 2004;25(3):521.

Baughman RP, Lower EE: Newer therapies for cutaneous sarcoidosis - the role of thalidomide and other agents. Am J Clin Derm 2004, 5(6):385-94.

Baughman RP, Lynch JP. Difficult treatment issues in sarcoidosis. Journal of Internal Medicine. 2003;253;41-45.

Bona JR, Fackler SM, Fendley MJ, Nemeroff CB. Neurosarcoidosis as a cause of refractory psychosis: a complicated case report. Am J Psychiatry. 1998 Aug; 155 (8): 1106 -8.

Bruns F, Pruemer B, Haverkamp U, Fischedick AR. Neurosarcoidosis: an unusual indication for radiotherapy. Br J Radiol 2004 Sep; 77(921):777-9.

Burns TM, Dyck PJ, Aksamit AJ, Dyck PJ. The natural history and long-term outcome of 57 limb sarcoidosis neuropathy cases. J Neurol Sci. 2006 May 15; 244 (1-2):77-87.

Chapelon C, Ziza JM, Piette JC, et al. Neurosarcoidosis: signs course and treatment in 35 confirmed cases. Medicine 1990;69:261-76

Christoforidis GA, Spickler EM, Reccio MV, Mehta BM. MR of CNS sarcoidosis: correlation of imaging features to clinical symptoms and response to treatment. AJNR1999; 20:655 -669

Colover J. Sarcoidosis with involvement of the nervous system. Brain 1948; 71:451-75.

De Mulder D, Vandenberghe J. Neurosarcoidosis as a cause of manic psychosis.Tijdschr Psychiatr. 2008;50(11):741-5. Dutch.

Delaney P. Neurologic manifestations in sarcoidosis: review of literature, with a report of 23 cases. Ann Intern Med 1977;87(3):336-45.

Elkin R, Willcox PA. Neurosarcoidosis. A report of 5 cases. S Afr Med J. 1985 Jun 8;67(23):943-6.

Fahoum F, Drory VE, Issakov J, Neufeld MY. Neurosarcoidosis presenting as Guillain-Barre like syndrome. A case report and review of the literature. J Clin Neuromuscul Dis. 2009 Sep;11(1):35-43.

Ferriby D, de Seze J, Stojkovic, T, Hachulla E, Wallaert B, Destee A, Hatron PY, Vermersch P. Long-term follow-up of neurosarcoidosis. Neurology 2001;57;927-929.

Friedman SH, Gould DJ. Neurosarcoidosis presenting as psychosis and dementia: a case report.Int J Psychiatry Med. 2002;32(4):401-3.

Garg S, Wright A, Reichwein R, Boyer P, Towfighi J, Kothari MJ. Mononeuritis multiplex secondary to sarcoidosis.Clin Neurol Neurosurg. 2005 Feb;107(2):140-3.

Gilmore K, Rudden M, Kalman TP. Psychiatric manifestations of sarcoidosis. Can J Psychiatry 1980;25:329-31.

Hammond ER, Kaplin AI, Kerr DA. Thalidomide for acute treatment of neurosarcoidosis. Spinal Cord 2007;45(12):802-3.

Heerfordt CF. Uber eine "Febris uveo-parotidea subchronica" an der glandula parotis und der uvea des anges lokalisiert und haufig mit paresen cerebrospinaler nerven kompliaiert. V Graef Arch Klin Exp Ophthalmol 1909;70:254.

Hoitsma E, Faber CG, Drent M, Sharma OP: Neurosarcoidosis: a clinical dilemma. Lancet Neurol 2004, 3(7):397-407.

Hoitsma E, Marziniak M, Faber GC, Reulen JP, Sommer C, De Baets M, Drent M. Small fibre neuropathy in sarcoidosis. Lancet 359 (2002), pp 2085-2086.

Hoyle JC, Newton HB, Katz S. Prognosis of refractory neurosarcoidosis altered by thalidomide: a case report. Journal of Medical Case Reports 2008, 2:27

Hunninghake GW, Costabel U, Ando M, Baughman R, Cordier JF, du Bois R, Eklund A, Kitaichi M, Lynch J, Rizzato G, Rose C, Selroos O, Semenzato G, Sharma OP: ATS/ERS/WASOG Statement Sarcoidosis. Sarcoidosis Vasc Diffuse Lung Dis 1999, 16:149-173.

Joseph FG, Scolding NJ. Neurosarcoidosis: A study of 30 new cases. Neurol Neurosurg Psychiatry 2009 Mar;80(3):297-304.

Joseph FG, Scolding NJ. Sarcoidosis of the nervous system. Pract Neurol 2007;7:234-244.

Junger SS, Stern BJ, Levine SR, Sipos E, Marti-Masso JF. Intramedullary spinal sarcoidosis: Clinical and magnetic resonance imaging characteristics. Neurology 1993; 43: 333-337.

Luke RA, Stern BJ, Krumholz A, Johns CJ. Neurosarcoidosis: the long-term clinical course. Neurology 1987 Mar;37(3):461-3.

Menninger MD, Amdur RJ, Marcus RB Jr. Am J Clin Oncol 2003 Aug;26(4):e115-8.

Moller DR: Treatment of sarcoidosis – from a basic science point of view. Journal of Internal Medicine 2003, 253:31-40.

Nguyen YT, Dupuy A, Cordoliani F, Vignon-Pennamen MD, Lebbe C, Morel, P, Rybojad M. Treatment of cutaneous sarcoidosis with thalidomide. J Am Acad Dermatol 2004;50:235-241.

Niemer GW, Bolster MB, Buxbaum L, Judson MA. Carpal tunnel syndrome in sarcoidosis. Sarcoidosis Vasc Diffuse Lung Dis. 2001;18(3):296.

O'Brien GM, Baughman RP, Broderick JP, Arnold L, Lower EE. Paranoid psychosis due to neurosarcoidosis. Sarcoidosis. 1994 Mar;11(1):34-6.

Oksanen V. Neurosarcoidosis: clinical presentations and course in 50 patients. Acta Med Scand 1986;73:283-90.

Pawate S, Moses H, Sriram S. Presentations and outcomes of neurosarcoidosis: a study of 54 cases.QJM. 2009 Jul;102(7):449-60.

Pereira J, Anderson NE, McAuley D, Bergin P, Kilfoyle D, Fink J. Medically refractory neurosarcoidosis treated with infliximab. Intern Med J 2011 Apr;41(4):354-7.

Porter N, Beynon HL, Randeva HS. Endocrine and reproductive manifestations of sarcoidosis. QJM. 2003 Aug;96(8):553-61.

Sabaawi M, Gutierrez-Nunez J, Fragala MR. Neurosarcoidosis presenting as schizophreniform disorder. Int J Psychiatry Med. 1992;22(3):269-74.

Santos E, Shaunak S, Renowden S, Scolding NJ. Treatment of refractory neurosarcoidosis with infliximab. J Neurol Neurosurg Psychiatry. 2010 Mar;81(3):241-6.

Scott, TF. Neurosarcoidosis: Progress and clinical aspects. Neurology 1993;43:8-12.

Scott TF, Yandora K, Valeri A, Chieffe C, Schramke C. Aggressive therapy for neurosarcoidosis: long-term follow-up of 48 treated patients. Arch Neurol. 2007;64(5):691.

Selroos O. Treatment of sarcoidosis. Sarcoidosis 1994;11:80-83.

Sierra-Hidalgo F, Moreno-Ramos T, Martinez de Aragon A, Correas-Callero E, Erana I, de Pablo-Fernandez E. Longitudinal myelitis as the presenting symptom of neurosarcoidosis. Rev Neurol 2010 Sep 1;51(5):302.

Soriano FG, Caramelli P, Nitrini R, Rocha AS. Neurosarcoidosis: therapeutic success with methotrexate. Postgrad Med J. 1990 Feb;66(772):142-3.

Spiegel DR, Thomas CS, Shah P, Kent KD. A possible case of mixed mania due to neurosarcoidosis treated successfully with methylprednisolone and ziprasidone: another example of frontal-subcortical disinhibition?Gen Hosp Psychiatry. 2010 May-Jun;32(3):342.

Stern BJ, Krumholz A, Johns C, Scott P, Nissim J. Sarcoidosis and its neurological manifestations. Arch Neurol. 1985 Sep;42(9):909-17. Review.

Stern BJ, Schonfeld SA, Sewell C, Krumholz A, Scott P, Belendiuk G. The treatment of neurosarcoidosis with cyclosporine. Arch Neurol. 1992 Oct;49(10):1065-72.

Stuart C, Neelon F, Lebovitz H. Disordered control of thirst in hypothalamic-pituitary sarcoidosis. N Engl J Med 1980; 303:1078–82.

Studdy PR, Bird R. Serum angiotensin converting enzyme in sarcoidosis--its value in present clinical practice. Ann Clin Biochem. 1989;26 (Pt 1):13.

Tavee J, Culver D. Sarcoidosis and small fiber neuropathy. Curr Pain Headache Rep 2011 June;15(3):201-6.

Turkington RW, MacIndoe JH. Hyperprolactinemia in sarcoidosis. Ann Intern Med 1972;76(4):545-9.

Wallach J. Interpretation of Diagnostic Tests, 7th Ed., 2000.

Wu JJ, Huang DB, Pang KR, Hsu S, Tyring SK: Thalidomide: dermatological indications, mechanisms of action and side-effects. British Journal of Dermatology 2005, 153:254-73.

Zajicek JP, Scolding NJ, Foster O, et al. Central nervous system sarcoidosis-diagnosis and management. QJM 1999;92(2):103-117.
Zuniga G, Ropper AH, Frank J. Sarcoid peripheral neuropathy. Neurology. 1991;41(10):1558.

15

Spinal Cord Sarcoidosis Accompanied with Compressive Cervical Myelopathy

Yoshihito Sakai[1], Yukihiro Matsuyama[2] and Shiro Imagama[3]
[1]*Department of Orthopaedic Surgery, National Center for Geriatrics and Gerontology,*
[2]*Department of Orthopaedic Surgery, Hamamatsu University School of Medicine,*
[3]*Department of Orthopaedic Surgery, Nagoya University School of Medicine,*
Japan

1. Introduction

Spinal cord Sarcoidosis was first described by Longcope in 1941 (Longcope, 1941), and since then, spinal cord involvement has been reported in less than 10% of patients with neurosarcoidosis (Bogousslavsky et al., 1982, Fried et al., 1993) Spinal cord sarcoidosis is a chronic, granulomatous, systemic inflammatory disease, although precise understanding of the pathogenesis remains unclear, and most commonly occurs at the cervical level, presenting with subacute or chronic myelopathy frequently progressing to paraplegia (Sauter et al., 1991, Morita et al., 1992). The mainstay of treatment of spinal cord sarcoidosis is high-dose corticosteroid therapy, and surgery is undertaken when suggested by biopsy results and histopathological diagnosis (Jallo et al., 1997). However, since the lower middle cervical segments are more frequently affected (Nagai et al., 1985), it is difficult to differentiate cervical spinal cord sarcoidosis from cervical spondylotic myelopathy when gradually occurring in elderly patients. Magnetic resonance imaging (MRI) findings with high signal intensity on T2 weighted images and vagueness of diffuse enlargement of the spinal cord due to spinal canal stenosis often leads to the surgeons to diagnose spinal cord sarcoidosis only after decompressive surgery has been performed for compressive cervical myelopathy.

More than 80 cases of spinal cord sarcoidosis have been reported, most of which were studied using MRI (Kanzaki et al., 2004). There are no papers on the coexistence of compressive cervical myelopathy and cervical spinal cord sarcoidosis, and it is uncertain not only whether compressive cervical myelopathy triggers the development of inflammatory granuloma in spinal cord sarcoidosis but also the effect of decompressive surgery. In this chapter, the outcome of decompressive surgery performed for cervical spinal cord sarcoidosis accompanied with compressive cervical myelopathy and the effect of steroid therapy provided after decompressive surgery is expressed, comparing the outcome of the treatment of spinal cord sarcoidosis with no compressive cervical myelopathy shown by MRI.

2. Diagnosis

Nagoya Spine Group (NSG) was established since April 2006 by the spine surgeons of Nagoya University Hospital and 15 referral hospitals to evaluate the outcome of surgical treatment of spinal disorders in a prospective and/or retrospective multicenter clinical series. The NSG database included 6,187 cases of patients who underwent spinal surgery, of which 1,560 cases were of compressive cervical myelopathy treated with cervical laminectomy or laminoplasty from January 2001 to December 2005. Of the 1,560 patients, a total of 12 (0.08%) patients were identified with spinal cord sarcoidosis, which was treated with decompressive surgery during the study period. The medical records of these 12 patients were retrieved, and the demographic data collected included age, sex, duration of disease, surgical outcome, and effectiveness of steroid therapy. The study was independently reviewed and approved by the institutional review boards at all participating institutions.

The medical records of the patients were reviewed. The patients comprised 5 men and 7 women, in the age range of 47 to 74 years (median, 57.8 years). Postoperative follow-up period ranged from 1 to 5 years (median, 2.0 years). Preoperative MRI was performed in all the cases and all lesions were observed to be present in the cervical region. Surgical outcome was evaluated using the Japanese Orthopaedic Association (JOA) scoring system, the JOA score was established prospectively at the time of treatment. This score comprises a total of 17 points; 4 points each for motor dysfunction of the upper and lower extremities, respectively; 2 points each for sensory dysfunction of the upper and lower extremities and the trunk, respectively; and 3 points for bladder dysfunction. The recovery rate was calculated using Hirabayashi's method.

Zajicek's diagnostic criteria (Zajicek et al., 1999), those of "definite", "probable", and "possible" were adopted for neurosarcoidosis. In brief, neurosarcoidosis was defined as "definite" when histopathological findings showed sterile, noncaseating granuloma in the spinal cord tissue. Neurosarcoidosis was defined as "probable" in the case of presence of spinal cord inflammation (elevated cerebrospinal fluid (CSF) protein level and/or increased cell number or spinal cord MRI findings comparable with those indicating neurosarcoidosis). Neurosarcoidosis was defined as "possible" when suggested by clinical presentation. After surgery, the diagnosis of neurosarcoidosis was confirmed, and the duration between the diagnosis and surgery ranged from 0 to 6 months (median, 3.9 weeks).

3. Treatment

3.1 Surgical treatment

All the 12 patients underwent decompressive surgery, including laminectomy (2 patients) and laminoplasty (10 patients). Preoperative diagnosis was intramedullary spinal cord tumor with compressive cervical myelopathy in 8 cases and cervical spondylotic myelopathy in 4 cases. That is all patients had compressive cervical myelopathy and spinal canal stenosis, with intramedullary T2 hyperintensity extending to the cervical level on MRI. The duration between the onset of initial symptoms and the operation ranged from 3 weeks to 1.5 years (median 7.3 months). Spinal cord biopsy was performed with the intraoperative motor-evoked potential (MEP) monitoring in 8 cases because intramedullary lesion was suspected on preoperative MRI or intraoperative ultrasonography; in the other 4 cases, only decompressive surgery was performed owing to the preoperative diagnosis of cervical spondylotic myelopathy. Radical surgical removal of the intramedullary sarcoid granuloma was possible only in 1 case.

3.2 Steroid therapy

All the 12 patients were provided high-dose corticosteroid therapy postoperatively. The duration between the operation and initiation of steroid administration ranged from 1 week to 3 months (median, 31.3 days). The effect of the steroid administred was evaluated on the basis of the JOA score. As control subjects, 8 patients with spinal cord sarcoidosis but showing no compressive lesion on MRI and who received high-dose steroid therapy from a neurologist without surgery were recruited to compare the effectiveness of the steroid and the outcome of spinal cord sarcoidosis. Their demographic data are presented in Table 1. The JOA score assigned of the non-surgery group was calculated on the basis of the retrospective review of the charts of the patients. There were no significant differences in the initial dose of the corticosteroid between the surgery and the non-surgery groups.

	Surgery group (N=12)	Non-surgery group (N=8)
Age (years)	57.8±9.8	62.4±8.2
Gender (M/F)	5/7	2/6
Follow-up period (month)	24.0±15.2	30.2±15.0
Period from onset to surgery (week)	17.6±5.7	—
Period from onset to steroid (day)	44.9±15.9	43.5±12.8
Initial dose of steroid (mg/day)	54.0±7.0	51.3±4.2
JOA score before treatment (point)	8.2±2.4	8.9±2.4

Table 1. Demographics of surgery and non-surgery group

Non-surgery group indicates the patients with spinal cord sarcoidosis without compressive cervical myelopathy on MRI finding who underwent steroid therapy without operation.

3.3 Statistical analysis

StatView 5.0 software (ABACUS, Berkeley, CA) was used to calculate the statistical difference. Equality of means for continuous variables was assessed by using the Mann-Whitney test. A P value of 0.05 or less was considered to be statistically significant.

4. Results

In the surgery group, 8 and 4 patients were identified with definite and probable neurosarcoidosis, respectively after decompressive surgery. The diagnosis in all the 8 cases of definite neurosarcoidosis was confirmed by biopsy results. The other 4 cases of probable neurosarcoidosis were diagnosed by a neurologist on the basis of laboratory data for inflammation of the spinal cord and biopsy of the lung, skin or eye. Spinal cord sarcoidosis was preoperatively suspected in 4 patients; however, they all showed negative results on clinical examination and other tissue biopsies. In the non-surgery group, all the 8 patients were diagnosed by a neurologist as having probable neurosarcoidosis without performing spinal cord biopsy.

4.1 Clinical presentation

There were no acute spinal cord symptoms that progressed within 1 month in both the surgery and the non-surgery groups. The characteristic spinal cord symptoms included chronic symptoms, which progressed over 3 months in 7 (58.3%) and 6 patients (75.0%) in the surgery and non-surgery groups, respectively, and subacute symptoms, which progressed within 3 months in 5 (41.7%) and 2 patients (25%) in the surgery and non-surgery groups, respectively. All the patients in both the groups presented with insidious paresthesias in the extremities. In the surgery group, a discrepancy was observed between the narrowest portion and the neurological findings in the case of 7 (58.3%) patients. Other presentations such as hand clumsiness, gait disturbance, and bladder dysfunction in both the groups are shown in Fig. 1. The surgery group exhibited a slight tendency to show serious neurological findings; however, there were no significant differences between the 2 groups.

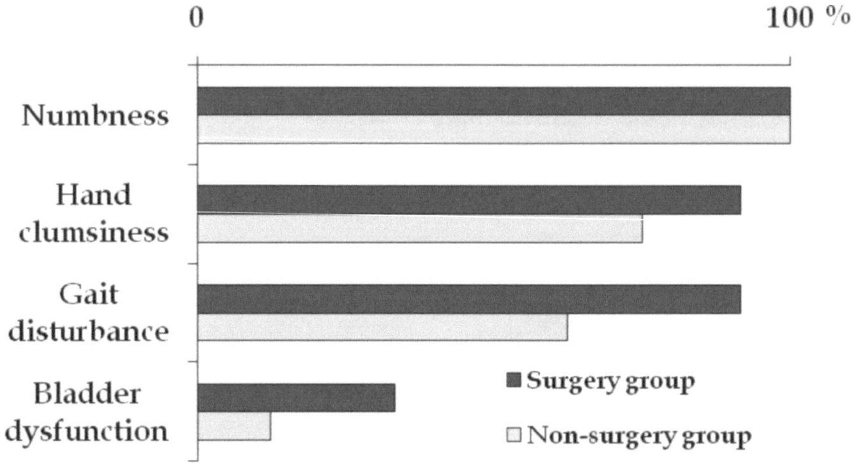

Fig. 1. Neurological symptoms

4.2 MRI findings

All the patients had fusiform enlargement of the spinal cord with high signal intensity on T2-weighted images and enhancing lesions in the spinal cord. Meningeal patchy enhancement occurred in 4 cases (33.3%) and 3 cases (37.5%) in the surgery and non-surgery groups, respectively. In the surgery group, high signal intensity on T2-weighted images extended from C2 to Th1, and the maximum compression levels were present in the high signal intensity area. Enhancing lesions were observed at C5-6 in 7 cases, C6-7 in 2 cases, C4/5 in 1 case, C2/3-Th1 in 1 case and C3/4-C6 in1 case, which coincided with the maximum compression levels observed in all the cases. (Fig.2)

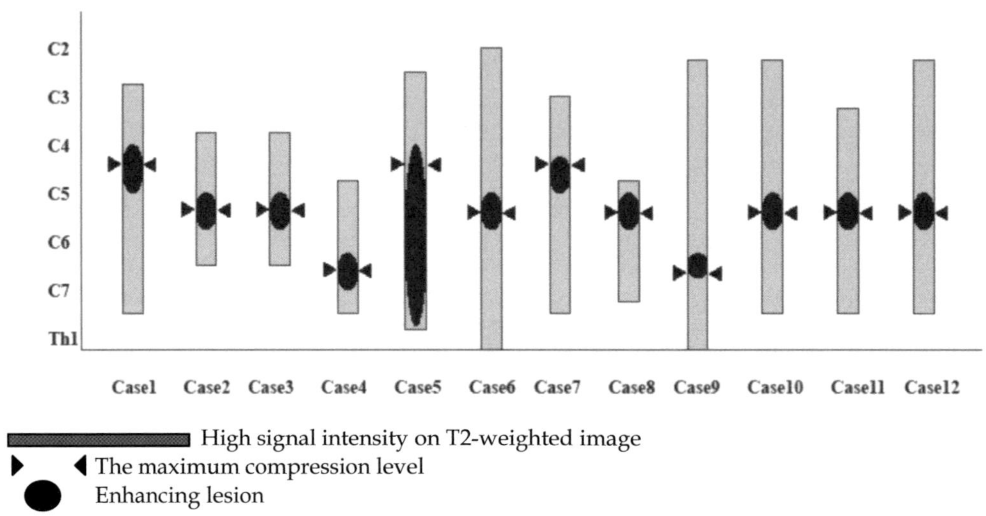

Fig. 2. The distribution of the affected spinal segments.

4.3 Surgical outcome

Preoperative JOA score in the surgery group was 8.2 points (2.0-11.0 points), and that in the non-surgery group was 9.0 points (5.0-13.0 points), with no significant differences. ($p=0.52$) Postoperative JOA score in the surgery group slightly decreased at 1 week and 4 weeks, and postoperative recovery rates in the surgery group at 1 week and 4 weeks were -7.4% (from -52.9% to 25.0%) and -1.1% (from -41.2% to 25.0%), respectively (Fig.3). Only 5 of the 12 patients showed clinical improvement after decompressive surgery, but their condition worsened again at an average of 7.4 weeks (2-12 weeks) after surgery. The average postoperative recovery rate of these 5 patients at 4 weeks was in 17.4% (9.5%-25.0%). After surgery, these 5 patients showed reduction in high signal intensity on T2-weighted images and enhancing lesions in the spinal cord; however, the improvement in MRI findings was not always consistent with neurological improvement. Only 2 of the 5 patients who showed temporary neurological improvement showed regression of the intramedullary sarcoid lesions. There was no correlation between the MRI findings after decompressive surgery and the clinical results.

As postoperative complications, C5 palsy and infection were seen in 1 patient each. Sensory deterioration was seen in 4 of the 8 patients who underwent spinal cord biopsy. No motor deterioration was seen immediately after surgery except in 1 case of C5 palsy. No abnormal wave patterns on MEP monitoring were observed during biopsy as well as the whole procedure in any patient who underwent spinal cord biopsy.

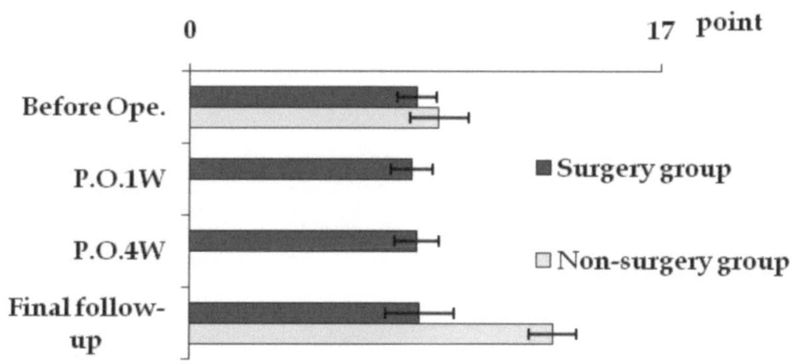

Fig. 3. JOA scores before and after each treatment

4.4 Effect of steroid therapy

Postoperative diagnosis of spinal cord sarcoidosis was made on the basis of pathological findings of the spinal cord in 8 patients, lung biopsy results in 2 patients, skin biopsy findings in 1 patient, and eye biopsy results in 1 patient at an average of 3.9 weeks (1-24 weeks). Postoperative oral steroid therapy was initiated at an average of 6.4 weeks (2-25 weeks), and the average initial dose was 54.0 mg (40-60 mg) in the surgery group and 51.3 mg (30-60 mg) in the non-surgery group. There was no statistical significance in the initiated dose between the 2 groups. No patients were provided steroid therapy before decompressive surgery in the surgery group. Two patients in the surgery group died of another disease irrelevant to spinal cord sarcoidosis at 1 year and 22 months. The JOA score before steroid therapy, at 4 weeks and 1 year after steroid therapy and the recovery rate at the final follow-up are shown in Fig. 4 and Fig.5. Significant differences were observed in the JOA scores at 4 weeks and 1 year after steroid therapy. ($p<0.05$) At the final follow-up, the recovery rate of the JOA score, which increased after steroid therapy, was significantly higher in the non-surgery group (62.5%) than in the surgery group (18.6%) (p<0.01).

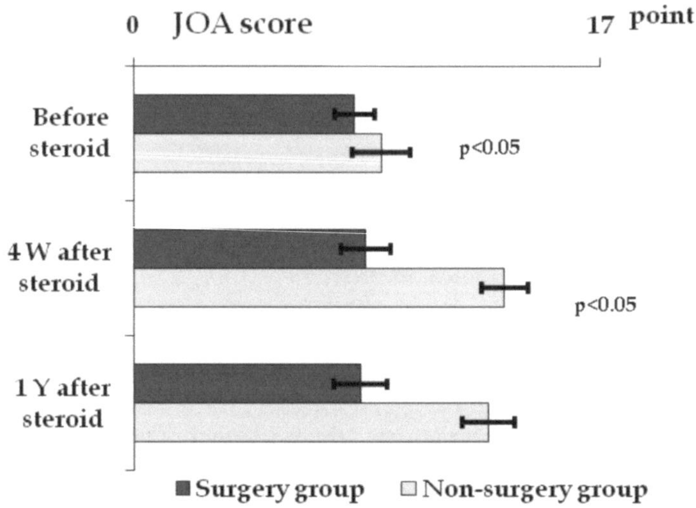

Fig. 4. JOA score before and after steroid administration.

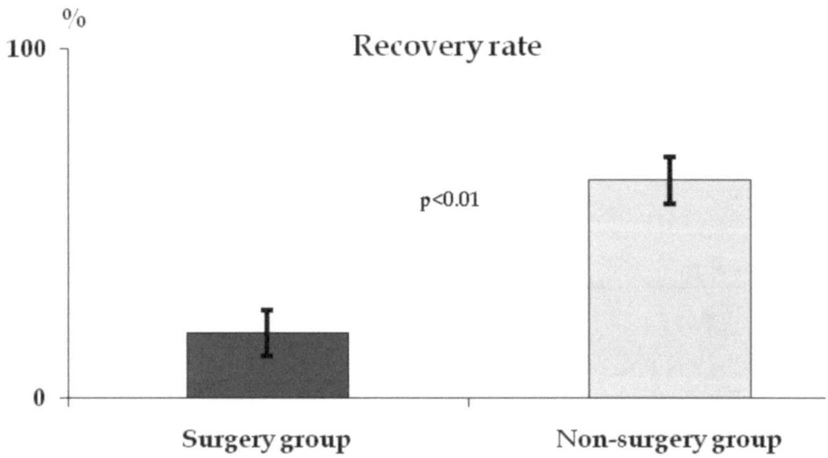

Fig. 5. Recovery rate in JOA score after steroid administration.

4.5 Representative case (Fig.6)

A 63-year-old woman presented with an 8 year history of gradual progression of numbness in the upper and lower extremities, bilateral hand clumsiness, gait disturbance and bladder dysfunction. MRI showed spinal cord compression and T2 hyperintensity extending from C4/5 to C5/6. Gadolinium enhancement was seen at the same levels as those of compression in sagittal slice and of multiple white-matter lesions in axial slice. Spinal cord sarcoidosis was suspected but other investigations including lymph node biopsy and bronchoalveolar lavage fluid analysis showed no abnormality. Anterior decompression/corpectomy should be reasonable for anterior compression and slight kyphosis at C4/5 observed on MRI; however, posterior approach was adopted. After laminoplasty from C3 to C7 and spinal cord biopsy, the patient's numbness and motor dysfunction were slightly reduced for 2 weeks, but T2 hyperintensity and gadolinium enhancement increased. After diagnosis of spinal cord sarcoidosis on the basis of pathological findings of the spinal cord, high-dose corticosteroid therapy (60mg) was initiated. Improvement was observed in the symptoms and MRI findings, but motor dysfunction persisted in the hands.

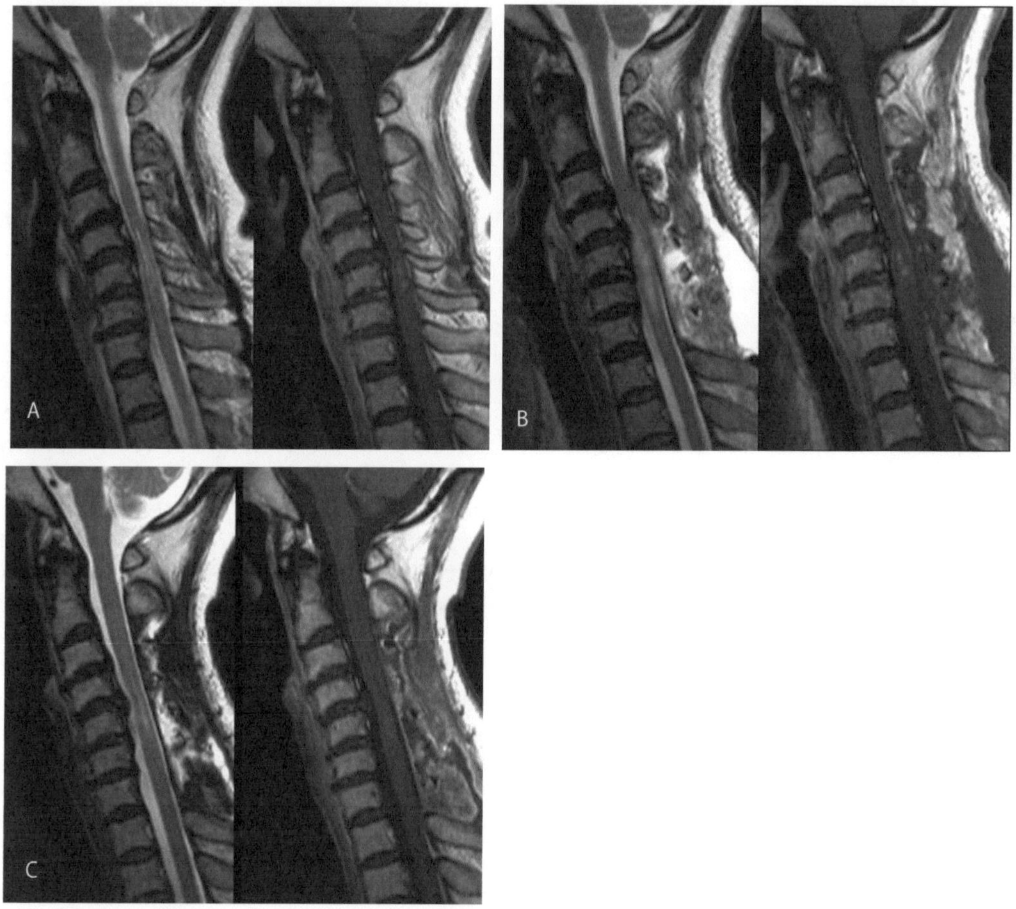

Fig. 6. Representative case (63 years, female). A. Preoperative MRI showing spinal cord compression at C4/5 and T2 hyperintensity and gadolinium enhancement at C5. B. Postoperative MRI showing extended T2 hyperintensity and gadolinium enhancement. C. After administration of corticosteroid, T2 hyperintensity and gadolinium enhancement remarkably improved.

5. Discussion

Histopathogenesis of sarcoidosis of the central nervous system is considered as the flow of primary leptomeningeal inflammatory exudate from the subarachnoid space along the Virchow-Robin spaces into the brain parenchyma (Mirfakhraee et al., 1986). It remains unknown if this hypothesis applies to spinal cord sarcoidosis; however, inflammatory granuloma formation and progressive fibrosis caused by immunological reaction play an important role (Newman et al., 1997). Clinical diagnosis of spinal cord sarcoidosis is often difficult since the nervous system is a relatively uncommon site for the occurrence of the disease. Biopsy of the nervous system tissue is required for definite diagnosis of neurosarcoidosis, and Zajicek et al. proposed definite diagnosis of the disease on the basis of positive histological findings of the nervous system (Zajicek et al., 1999). Unfortunately, biopsy is not possible or desirable in many cases because of the site of involvement. A presumptive diagnosis of sarcoidosis can be made on the basis of clinical or imaging evidence such as MRI findings, CSF angiotensin-converting enzyme (ACE) level, increased lysosome count and raised beta 2-microglobulin level, an increased helper-suppresor T-lymphocyte ratio, or a CD4/CD8 ratio of >5 (Joseph et al., 2007). A comprehensive search for any systematic feature is required for the diagnosis of sarcoidosis after clinical confirmation of neurological involvement.

On the other hand, it is well known that while increased pressure within the spinal cord and sequential hypoxia and ischemic changes play important roles in the progression of lesions in cervical spondylotic myelopathy (Ito et al., 1996), involvement of inflammatory processes has also been indicated (Frank et al., 1995, Demircan et al., 2007). It is uncertain whether compressive cervical myelopathy triggers the development of inflammatory granuloma in spinal cord sarcoidosis. In the present study, MRI findings showed that area of enhancing sarcoid lesions coincided with the maximum compression levels. However, further study should be conducted to identify the relation between compressive myelopathy and lesions in sarcoidosis.

Diagnosis of sarcoidosis is expected to be difficult when the disease id accompanied with spinal cord compression due to cervical spondylosis; however, in this regard, a few reports are available. Ando et al. mentioned that spinal cord swelling without serious compression and disagreement between the level of compression and the extent of T2 hiperintensity challenge the presence of sarcoidosis (Ando et al., 2006). The present study demonstrated that the maximum compression levels in cervical spondylotic myelopathy coincided with the area of enhancing lesions, resulting in the inability to identify as sarcoidosis on the basis of MRI findings. Another study reported that inconsistency between the area with sensory disturbance and the affected level in cervical spondylotic myelopathy responsible for the main functional disorder enables differentiation (Oe et al., 2006). The fact that a discrepancy was observed between the narrowest portion and neurological findings in 58.3% patients indicates the difficulty in discriminating the affected levels in spinal cord sarcoidosis, especially in cases with multilevel stenosis. In addition, MRI findings concerning clinically silent compression of the spinal cord in elderly patients and the difficulties encountered in determining the exact responsible level in multisegmental compression (Boden et al., 1990) prompt many surgeons to perform multisegmental decompression by laminoplasty (Yonenobu et al., 1992, Satomi et al., 1994, Seichi et al., 2001). Neurological findings would not be reliable for diagnosis when spinal cord sarcoidosis develops at the level of stenosis.

Decompressive surgery produced temporary improvement in the condition of one-third of the patients with spinal cord sarcoidosis accompanied with compressive cervical myelopathy. However, the neurological symptoms relapsed postoperatively after a few months, and all the patients were provided steroid therapy. Spinal cord biopsy would have affected sensory deterioration immediately after surgery. In the previous study, neurological changes secondary to spinal cord biopsy occurred in 6 of 38 patients who underwent biopsy; further, all postoperative complications were all mild and completely resolved in most cases at 3 months after surgery (Cohen-Gadol et al., 2003). Gradual neurological deterioration after decompressive surgery indicates insufficient decompression for lesions in sarcoidosis. In general surgical results of laminoplasty for cervical spondylotic myelopathy have been shown to be good, helping to prevent neurological deterioration and resulting in 50%-70% recovery rates (Sakai et al., 2005, Yukawa et al., 2007). The present study demonstrated that the average recovery rate of the patients who showed neurological improvement after surgery was 17.4%, which was extremely lower than that observed in cervical spondylotic myelopathy; further, the improvement was only transitory.

While steroid administration after decompressive surgery was shown to be effective for spinal cord sarcoidosis accompanied with compressive cervical myelopathy, the outcome was poorer than that of the treatment of spinal cord sarcoidosis without compressive cervical myelopathy. This may be ascribed to the irreversible change produced in the spinal cord due to mechanical compression. In spinal cord sarcoidosis accompanied with compressive cervical myelopathy, decompressive surgery including laminoplasty should not be the first choice of treatment except for cases with appropriate differentiation of intramedullary spinal cord tumor and early diagnosis of sarcoidosis. Although there are no distinct signal characteristics for spinal cord sarcoidosis, diffuse increase in intramedullary T2 hyperintensity, presence of enhancing nodules, and leptomeningeal involvement suggest the disease. The mainstay of medical treatment of spinal cord sarcoidosis is steroid therapy, thus, it should be preferred after early diagnosis rather than decompressive surgery. Postoperative neurological deterioration after resection of sarcoid granulomas has been reported (Day et al., 1977, Baruah et al., 1978). Mathieson et al demonstrated that among 31 cases of histologically proven intramedullary sarcoidosis, postoperative deterioration in neurological function occurred in 50% cases (Mathieson et al., 2004). Thus, several reports suggest that the first surgery should be limited to decompression of the spinal cord and biopsy without complete extirpation in cases of suspected spinal cord sarcoidosis (Rubinstein et al., 1984, Vighetto et al., 1985, Kayama et al., 1993Jallo et al., 1997, Yukawa et al., 1999). However, there has been no report describing the effects of spinal cord decompression on lesions in sarcoidosis. In spinal cord sarcoidosis accompanied with compressive cervical myelopathy such as in our series, it is difficult to determine which lesion is responsible for the neurological symptoms. Early treatment with a suitable steroid decreases inflammation in sarcoidosis (Soucek et al., 1993) and MRI findings are dramatically improved by corticosteroid therapy (Koike et al., 2000). A long interval between the onset of the disease and the initiation of steroid therapy contributes to poor functional recovery (Stern et al., 1985). Decompressive surgery should be undertaken when steroid therapy proves to be insufficient for the treatment of spinal cord sarcoidosis accompanied with cervical compressive myelopathy. In addition in cases with unsatisfactory results of decompressive surgery for compressive cervical myelopathy, presence of spinal cord sarcoidosis should be considered, if spinal cord swelling and/or increase in intramedullary T2 hyperintensity are observed after decompression. In some cases, enlarged spinal cord appears unclear with coexisting compressive cervical lesions. Spinal cord enlargement is occasionally underestimated when cervical spondylotic compression coexists. Spinal cord biopsy is indispensable if the diagnosis of sarcoidosis is not proved; however, the risks involved in performing biopsies for nonspecific spinal cord lesions may lead to the preference for generalized screening and diagnosis of sarcoidosis on the basis of less invasive procedures before subjecting the patient to surgery. The patients should be informed that the prognosis of surgery is guarded in any case of spinal cord sarcoidosis.

6. Conclusions

The effectiveness of decompressive surgery for spinal cord sarcoidosis accompanied with compressive cervical myelopathy is transitory and not adequate. Steroid therapy after decompressive surgery is also less effective for spinal cord sarcoidosis accompanied with compressive cervical myelopathy, compared with the treatment of spinal cord sarcoidosis without compressive cervical myelopathy. Early diagnosis of sarcoidosis and steroid therapy is preferred.

7. References

Ando, T.; Kameyama, T.; Suzuki, K.; Yoshida, A. & Kurahashi, T. (2006) Spinal cord sarcoidosis: A clinical dilemma and informed consent. *Spine & Spinal Cord (Japanese)* Vol. 19, No. 6, pp. 694-701.

Boden, SD.; McCowin, PR.; Davis, DO.; Dina, TS.; Mark, AS. & Wiesel S. (1990) Abnormal magnetic-resonance scans of the cervical spine in asymptomatic subjects. A prospective investigation. *J Bone Joint Surg [Am]* Vol. 72-A, pp. 1178-1184, ISSN 0021-93355

Baruah, JK.; Glasauer, FE.; Sil, R. & Smith BH. (1978) Sarcoidosis of the cervical spinal canal: case report. Neurosurgery Vol. 3, No. 2, pp. 216-218, ISSN 0148-396X

Bogousslavsky, J.; Hungerbühler, JP.; Regli, F. & Graf, HJ. (1982) Subacute myelopathy as the presenting manifestation of sarcoidosis. *Acta neurochirurgica* Vol. 65, No. 3, pp. 193-197, ISSN 0001-6268

Cohen-Gadol, AA.; Zikel, OM.; Miller, GM.; Aksamit, AJ.; Scheithauer, BW. & Krauss WE. (2003) Spinal cord biopsy: A review of 38 cases. *Neurosurgery* Vol. 52, No. 4, pp. 806-816, ISSN 0148-396X

Day, AL. & Sypert, GW. (1977) Spinal cord sarcoidosis. *Annals of Neurology* Vol. 1, No. 1, pp. 79-85, ISSN 0364-5134

Demircan, MN.; Asir, A.; Cetinkal, A.; Gedik, N.; Kutlay, AM.; Çolak, A.; Kurtar, S. & Simsek, H. (2007) Is there any relationship between proinflammatory mediator levels in disc material and myelopathy with cervical disc herniation and spondylosis? A non-randomized, prospective clinical study. *European Spine Journal* Vol. 16, No. 7, pp. 983-986, ISSN 0940-6719

Frank, E. (1995) HLA-DR expression on arachnoid cells. A role in the fibrotic inflammation surrounding nerve roots in spondylotic cervical myelopathy. *Spine* Vol. 20, No. 19, pp. 2093-2096, ISSN 0887-9869

Fried, ED.; Landau, AJ.; Sher, JH. & Rao C. (1993) Spinal cord sarcoidosis: A case report and review of the literature. *Journal of the Association for Academic Minority Physicians* Vol. 4, No. 4, pp. 132-137, ISSN 1048-9886

Ito, T.; Oyanagi, K.; Takahashi, H.; Takahashi, HE. & Ikuta, F. (1996) Cervical spondylotic myelopathy: Clinicopathologic study on the progression pattern and thin myelinated fibers of the lesions of seven patients examined during complete autopsy. *Spine* Vol. 21, No.7, pp. 827-833, ISSN 0887-9869.

Jallo, GI.; Zagzag, D.; Lee, M.; Deletis, V.; Morota, N. & Epstein, FJ. (1997) Intraspinal sarcoidosis: diagnosis and management. *Surgical Neurology* Vol. 48, No. 5, pp. 514-521, ISSN 0090-3019

Joseph, FG. & Scolding, NJ. (2007) Sarcoidosis of the nervous system. *Pract Neurol* Vol. 7, No. 4, pp. 234-244, ISSN 1590-1874

Kanzaki, M.; Mochizuki, H.; Kobayashi, H.; Motoyoshi, K. & Kamakura, K. (2004) Intraspinal sarcoidosis: Clinical features, MR imaging and electrophysiological study. *Neurol Sci* Vol. 25, No. 2, pp. 91-94.

Kayama, S. & Kikuchi, S. (1993) Intramedullary sarcoidosis of the spinal cord. *Spine* Vol. 18, No. 14, pp. 2118-2120, ISSN 0887-9869

Koike, H.; Misu, K.; Yasui, K.; Kameyama, T.; Ando, T.; Yanagi, T. & Sobue G. (2000) Differential response to corticosteroid therapy of MRI findings and clinical manifestations in spinal cord sarcoidosis. *Journal of Neurology* Vol. 247, No. 7, pp. 544-549, ISSN 0340-5354

Longcope, WT. (1941) Sarcoidosis, or Besnier-Boeck-Schaumann disease. Frank Billings lecture. *JAMA* Vol.117, pp. 1321-1327, ISSN 0002-9955

Mathieson, CS.; Mowle, D.; Ironside, JW. & O'riordan, R. (2004) Isolated cervical intramedullary sarcoidosis- a histological surprise. *British Journal of Neurosurgy* Vol. 18, No. 6, pp. 632-635

Mirfakhraee, M.; Crofford, MJ.; Guinto, FC.; Nauta HJW. & Weedon, VW. (1986) Virchow-Robin space: a path of spread in neurosarcoidosis. *Radiology* Vol.158, No.3, pp. 715-720, ISSN 0033-8419

Morita, H.; Hayashi, R.; Tako, K.; Tsukada, N. & Yanagisawa N. (1992) Spinal cord sarcoidosis: MRI findings in response to treatment. *European Neurology,* Vol.32, No.3, pp. 126-129, ISSN 0302-2838

Nagai, H.; Ohtsubo, K. & Shimada, H. (1985) Sarcoidosis of the spinal cord: Report of an autopsy case and review of the literature. *Acta Patholo Jpn* Vol. 35, No. 4, pp. 1007-1022, ISSN 0001-6632

Newman, LS.; Rose, CS. & Maier, LA. (1997) Sarcoidosis *New England Journal of Medicine* Vol. 336, No. 17, pp. 1224-1234, ISSN 0028-4793

Oe, K.; Miyamoto, H.; Doita, M.; Sumi, M. & Kanda F. (2006) Differentiation between cervical spondylotic myelopathy and spinal cord sarcoidosis. *Bessatsu Seikeigeka (Japanese)* Vol.50, pp. 2-8.

Rubinstein, I.; Hiss, J. & Baum, GL. (1984) Intramedulary spinal cord sarcoidosis. *Surgical Neurology* Vol. 21, No.3, pp. 272-274, ISSN 0090-3019

Sakai, Y.; Matsuyama, Y.; Inoue, K. & Ishiguro, N. (2005) Postoperative instability after laminoplasty for cervical myelopathy with spondylolisthesis. *Journal of Spinal Disorder & Technique* Vol. 18, No. 1, pp. 1-5, ISSN 1536-0652

Sakai, Y.; Matsuyama, Y.; Imagama, S.; Ito, X.; Wakao, N.; Ishiguro, N.; Watanabe, H.; Kato, F.; Yukawa, Y.; Ito, K.; Suzuki, K.; Tsuboi, a.; Kanemura, T. & Yoshida, G. (2010) Is decompression surgery effective for spinal cord sarcoidosis accompanied with compressive cervical myelopathy? *Spine* Vol. 35, No.23, 1290-1297, ISSN 0887-9869

Satomi, K.; Nishi, Y.; Kohno, T. & Hirabayashi K. (1994) Long-term follow-up studies of open-door expansive laminoplasty for cervical stenotic myelopathy. Spine Vol. 19, No. 5, pp. 507-510, ISSN 0887-9869

Seichi, A.; Takeshita, K.; Ohishi, I.; Kawaguchi, H.; Akune, T.; Anamizu, Y.; Kitagawa, T. &

Nakamura K. (2001) Long-term results of double-door laminoplasty for cervical stenotic myelopathy. *Spine* Vol. 26, No.5, pp. 479-487, ISSN 0887-9869

Sauter, MK.; Panitch, HS. & Kristt DA. (1991) Myelopathic meurosarcoidosis: Diagnostic value of enhanced MRI. *Neurology* Vol. 41, No. 1, pp. 150-151, ISSN 0028-3878

Soucek, D.; Prior, C.; Luef, G.; Birbamer, G. & Bauer G. (1993) Successful treatment of spinal sarcoidosis by high-dose intravenous methylpredonisolone. *Clin Neuropharmacology* Vol. 16, No. 5, pp. 464-467, ISSN 0362-5664

Stern, BJ.; Krumholz, A.; Johns, C.; Scott, P. & Nissim J. (1985) Sarcoidosis and its neurological manifestations. *Arch Neurol* Vol. 42, No. 9, pp. 909-917, ISSN 0003-9942

Vighetto, A.; Fischer, G.; Collet, P.; Bady, B. & Trillet M. (1985) Intramedullary sarcoidosis of the cervical spinal cord. Journal of Neurology, Neurosurgy, and Psychiatry Vol. 48, No. 5, pp. 477-479, ISSN 0022-3050

Yonenobu, K.; Hosono, N.; Iwasaki, M.; Asano, M. & Ono K. (1992) Laminoplasty versus subtotal corpectomy: A comparative study of results in multisegment cervical spondylotic myelopathy. *Spine* Vol. 17, No. 11, pp. 1281-1284, ISSN 0887-9869

Yukawa, Y. & Kato, F. (1999) Isolated spinal cord sarcoidosis mimicking an intramedullary tumor. *Journal of Spinal Disorder* Vol. 12, No. 6, pp. 530-533, ISSN 1536-0562

Yukawa, Y.; Kato, F.; Ito, K.; Horie, Y.; Hida, T.; Ito Z. & Matsuyama, Y. (2007) Laminoplasty and skip laminectomy for cervical compressive myelopathy. *Spine* Vol. 32, No. 18, pp. 1980-1985, ISSN 0887-9869

Zajicek, JP.; Scolding, NJ.; Foster O.; Rovaris, M.; Evanson, J.; Moseley, IF.; Scadding, JW.; Thompson, EJ.; Chamoun, V.; Miller, DH.; McDonald, WI. & Mitchell, D. (1999) Central nervous system sarcoidosis- diagnosis and management. *The Quarterly Journal of Medicine* Vo.92, 103-117, ISSN 0033-5622

Part 5

Sarcoid-Like Reactions

16

Sarcoid-Like Reactions

Shweta Nag
Meenakshi University,
India

1. Introduction

1.1 History and prevalance

According to a revised definition introduced by the International Conference on Sarcoidosis in 1975, sarcoidosis is a multisystem granulomatous disorder of unknown etiology, most often affecting young adults, in which patients present with hilar lymphadenopathy, pulmonary infiltration, and skin or eye lesions. This definition has been the most accepted till date, although many advancements have been made to understand the pathogenesis of this disease.

Sarcoidosis is a chronic granulomatous disease, which is characterized by the formation of non-caseating granulomas at multiple sites. It is a systemic disorder of unknown etiology, although multiple factors like mycobacterium, viruses like mumps and influenza, beryllium, zirconium, genetic predisposition, autoimmune diseases and also carcinomas, are considered to be responsible for its etiology.

In the first described case of sarcoidosis 120 years ago, it was called "livid papillary psoriasis" by Jonathan Hutchinson. Hutchinson suspected that this was a variant of mumps. The patient presented with purplish skin lesions and gout and later died of renal failure.

Sarcoidosis has been reported to occur in association with malignant tumours, either preceeding or following malignancy. In 1977, a study was conducted on 580 cases of sarcoidosis. Out of these, 7 cases were found to be associated with malignancy. But these authors considered that the association of sarcoidosis to malignant tumour, would be just a co-incidence. (Battesti JP et al., 1977)

By 1987, 23 cases of malignancy following sarcoidosis were reported. It was observed that lung and breast cancer may occur more often than other tumours after sarcoidosis. It was considered that the immunologic abnormalities associated with sarcoidosis may promote the development of certain malignant tumors. (Brincker H, 1987). Patients may rarely present with typical sarcoidosis occurring before, during or after the diagnosis of cancer. Recent studies have documented this type of cases, particularly with lymphomas, testicular and lung cancers, melanomas and hepatocarcinomas. As far as lung cancer is considered, coexistence of sarcoidosis and lung cancer in the same patient is not common, and only 29 such cases have been reported. If bilateral mediastinal lymphadenopathy is found in a case of lung cancer associated with sarcoidosis, surgical tumor resection should be considered.

It has been reported that in patients with malignant diseases, non-caseating epithelioid cell granulomas are occasionally found in lymph nodes draining a region containing the malignant tumor. These non-caseating granulomas are present at single or multiple organ sites without any clinical evidence to establish the diagnosis of sarcoidosis. For such tumour associated sarcoid granulomas, Nickerson in 1937, gave the term 'sarcoid reaction' and first pointed out the difference between sarcoid reaction and sarcoidosis. (Pavic M, 2008) This was accepted later as tumor-associated histologic changes, termed 'sarcoid reactions' (Takaki et al.,2010)

Granulomas may be found as a sarcoid reaction either within the vicinity of the tumour itself or within the regional lymph nodes draining that particular tumour. In some cases, such reactions can be seen in the non-regional lymph nodes. It was reported in 1986, that overall, sarcoid reactions occur in 4.4% of carcinomas, in 13.8% of patients with Hodgkin's disease, and in 7.3% of cases of non-Hodgkin lymphomas.

In 1997, 5 cases of Sarcoid reaction associated with papiollary carcinoma were reported. Brincker reviewed data on 4020 patients with malignant tumors in a broad spectrum. He found that 4.4% patients with carcinomas and one 0.4% of patients with sarcomas had sarcoid reactions. Sarcoid reaction may be slightly more common in patients with squamous cell carcinomas than in those with adenocarcinomas.

Sarcoid reaction has been observed in association with many kinds of primary tumors and particularly in regional lymph nodes, even in the absence of any metastases. But it is observed in studies that sarcoid reaction occurred about four times more often in regional lymph nodes without metastases than in lymph nodes with metastases. Therefore true sarcoidosis may be confused with local sarcoid reactions in cancer patients. This may lead to misdiagnosis and insufficient treatment. In some cases sarcoidosis may also develop by a preceeding treatment of malignancy. Although observed that, sarcoid reaction reported in Hodgkin's disease and gastric adenocarcinomas, may be associated with a better prognosis.

In a case report, association of sarcoid reactions and hepatocellular carcinoma combining early gastric carcinoma was reported was seen which is the first case of its kind (Kojima M et al., 1993). Granulomas may be found as a sarcoid reaction in the vicinity of regional lymph nodes more frequently than within the tumour itself. Sarcoid like reaction has been observed to be 13% in lymph nodes and 5% in spleen in patients with gastric carcinoma. In addition, none of them showed any symptoms or signs indicative of systemic sarcoidosis. (Abdel-Galiil K, 2006).Clinicians need to adapt specific diagnostic techniques to differentiate neoplasia from benign sarcoid reactions. However, biopsies are necessary in most of cases.

With regard to lung cancer patients, Laurberg et al reported that 20 out of 630 patients (3.2%) had sarcoid reactions in the mediastinal lymph nodes. In addition, they can be found not only in the lymph nodes draining a region containing the malignant tumor, but also in the tumor itself or in non-regional tissues. Some studies have shown that sarcoid reactions are observed within the primary tumor in patients with lung cancer. In 2008 there were three reported cases of sarcoid like reactions in head and neck cancer. In 2010, first case of sarcoid like reaction during chemotherapy for recurrent seminoma was reported. A sarcoid-like reaction was suspected in 1.1% of cancer patients, but the diagnosis was confirmed in 0.6%. (Tanizawa K)

In testicular cancer and lymphomas, association of sarcoidosis and sarcoid-like reactions have been reported. They occur either synchronously or metachronously, and may also occur after chemotherapy. In one such case report the importance of considering the diagnosis of sarcoidosis in patients with metastatic disease emphasised the association of sarcoidosis with head and neck cancer.

2. Symptoms

There are no early signs and symptoms of Sarcoidosis. Generalised symptoms are weight loss, fatigue, tiredness, weakness, sluggishness, night sweats, fever, malaise and enlarged lymph nodes. In about 90% of cases, Lungs are involved. Symptoms include, dyspnea, persistent cough and chest pain. Radiographic findings are lung tissue thickening, enlarged chest lymph nodes and small nodules throughout lungs. Eyes are involved in about 20-30% cases, and skin in 20% cases. Skin rashes, red lumps (erythema nodosum), red lumps on the legs (erythema nodosum), purple skin patches.

On the other hand, Sarcoid-like reaction is a localised reaction within tissues in the absence of any respiratory symptoms. A sarcoid-like reaction is often indistinguishable from metastases on radiological studies. Swollen lymph nodes caused by a sarcoid reaction often mimic metastatic lymph nodes. Thus, it is difficult to differentiate sarcoid reaction from lymph node metastases. Except histopathological examination, there is no useful examination for distinguishing them.

Laurberg reported that the frequency of associated sarcoid reactions is 3.2% in patients with pulmonary neoplasms, predominantly in squamous cell carcinomas. Histologically, squamous cell carcinomas show a statistically significant predominance. Sarcoid granulomas are found scattered within the lung parenchyma as well as around the carcinoid tumor. The distribution of this kind of sarcoid reaction is the first description.

3. Diagnosis

1. **ROLE OF IMAGING-** It is required that the clinicians adopt non- invasive diagnostic methods to differentiate neoplasia from benign sarcoid reactions. The 18-fluorodeoxyglucose (18-FDG) PET-scan has not been so successful but the adjunction of a [3-(18) F]-alpha-methyltyrosine ((18) F-FMT) PET-scan could be more useful. FDG-PET has been widely used in the assessment of malignancy. It has been observed that the sarcoid lesions could have increased FDG activity(Daniel RP et al.,1980). Differentiation of sarcoidosis from the sarcoid-like reactions is not an easy step in the final diagnosis. Thus, FDG-PET can be used as a diagnostic tool for the final diagnosis.
2. **ROLE OF CD4 + T LYMPHOCYTES-** The T- and B-lymphocyte disturbances in sarcoid patients may be attributed to the effects of a bacterial or viral infection depressing T-cell function. Mycobacteria or some of its components might be capable of inducing the B-cell immune response and the subsequent pathologic changes.

1.1 **Phytohemagglutinin-** It has been observed that, the cultured lymphocytes from patients with depression of delayed-type hypersensitivity, react poorly to phytohemagglutinin. Thus, it has been used in the diagnosis of sarcoidosis as impaired cellular immunity is observed in these patients.

1.2 **Circulating factors-** Other techniques used to expose immunologic defects in peripheral lymphocytes of patients with sarcoidosis include tests of T and B cell function, rosetie formation and migration inhibition. There are increased circulating immunoglobulin levels, increased circulating antibody levels to Epstein-Barr, herpes simplex, rubella, measles and parainfluenza viruses, increase antibody response to mismatched blood and occasional false-positive Wassermann reactions, but there is no increase in circulating autoantibodies. (Kazuaki Morohashi ,2003)

1.3 Patients with active sarcoidosis, have a depression in systemic cell-mediated immunity manifested by a reduction in the number of circulating T cells and impaired responses of these cells to antigensWhen B cell activity is increased, there is elevated serum immunoglobulins and the presence of autoantibodies and circulating immune complexes.

1.4 Bronchoalveolar lavage has shown that the sarcoid lung is characterized by increased numbers of "activated" T-lymphocytes within the alveolar structures. In contrast to normal control cells, the lung T-lymphocytes of patients with sarcoid release the mediator, monocyte chemotactic factor,which probably contributes to the pathogenesis of sarcoidosis. The recruitment of blood monocytes to the lung provides cellular building blocks for granuloma formation

1.5 Sarcoidosis is recognized to be a multisystem granulomatous disease characterized by activated, cytokine-producing T cells and macrophages at sites of inflammation. Recent work on the molecular structure of T cell receptor genes in sarcoidosis provide evidence that sarcoidosis is characterized by proliferation of T cell population at sites of inflammation. This is consistent with local antigen-mediated immune responses. In addition, cytokine production in sarcoidosis indicates that tissue inflammation is dominated by expression of cytokines such as interferon-gamma and interleukin-12 that regulate the granulomatous response. These studies offer new insight into the molecular mechanisms of granuloma formation in sarcoidosis and provide a framework for developing new therapeutic strategies for the treatment of this disease.

1.6 VEGF has also been reported to enhance the activation and migration of monocytes through the Flt-1 receptor in vitro,6,7 which are key events in granuloma formation. Genetic studies have demonstrated a significant difference in the allele frequency at locus _ 813 between healthy control subjects and patients with sarcoidosis. In sarcoidosis patients, the less common T allele was underrepresented in the sarcoidosis patient population as compared to the C allele which is more common in nirmal patients.(Kazuaki Morohashi ,2003)

3. **KVEIM'S TEST** -Worldwide figures for the Kveim-Siltzbach skin test are presented. They provide evidence of its specificity in various international series. Kveim-Siltzbach reaction is a response to an unknown Ag(s) and there can be causes of non-specific reactions. In an analysis, Kveim-Siltzbach reaction sites was performed using a PCR technique and primers specific for 20 V beta gene families. Results of this analysis demonstrated a pattern of V beta expression dominated by expression of V beta 2, V beta 3, V beta 6, or V beta 8 to levels > 20% of total V beta gene expression in nine of 15 individuals. (Proenca NG, 1982**)** Kveim test performed with G-77 antigen obtained from sarcoid lymph nodes. The antigen was tested in 46 patients with proved or suspected sarcoidosis and in 50 controls. Results were;positive in 85,1%.in patients undergoing treatment for more than two years,only 1out of three was positive. In suspected patients with only on the skin the test was positive in 58,1%.Control group was however negative. (Romer FK,1985)

4. **ROLE OF ACE**-Elevated levels of angiotensin-converting enzyme (ACE) are observed in the sera of patients with clinically active, biopsy-proved sarcoidosis. The specificity of this test lies in the fact that patients with dormant sarcoidosis and those with various other disorders have normal levels. Elevated levels can also be seen in some cases representing sarcoid variants and some cases each of leprosy, carcinoma, tuberculosis,

lymphomatoid granulomatosis, and immunoblastic sarcoma. Although ACE is sensitive to active sarcoidosis, the presence of false-positive findings limits its diagnostic usefulness to an adjunctive role; the assay should be combined with medical evaluation and tissue biopsy in selected cases. (Romer FK,1980)

A review is given on S-angiotensin-converting enzyme (SACE) and its clinical value, based upon 327 sarcoidosis patients and 1,274 patients with various disorders. SACE was elevated in 55% of the sarcoidosis patients, although with a higher frequency in those with active disease. In non-sarcoid patients, elevated SACE was observed in only 10 cases. The sensitivity and specificity were 0.55 and 0.99, respectively, and the positive and negative predictive values were 0.95 and 0.90, respectively. Elevated SACE pointed strongly towards the presence of sarcoidosis, although reservations must be made in patients with liver disorders, diabetes mellitus, hyperthyroidism, asbestosis or silicosis which are rather common disorders also associated with elevated SACE. Normal SACE does not exclude sarcoidosis. (Shultz T, 1979)

Enzyme activity is higher SACE in patients with pulmonary involvement and changes in SACE are correlated to the roentgenological changes. It has been observed that among healthy controls, significantly higher SACE levels were found in children up to 17 years of age (21.2-42.2 U/ml) than in adults aged 18-65 years (12.0-36.8 U/ml). (Kiminobu Tanizawa,2010). In another study, the correlation between S-angiotensin-converting enzyme and disease activity was examined in 185 observation periods in 85 untreated sarcoidosis patients. An agreement between SACE and chest roentgenographic changes was found in 42% of the observations. The most convenient interval between enzyme measurements seems to be 3 months in patients with active disease. Therefore, it can be interpretated that the pattern of enzyme variation may be a prognostic indicator in sarcoidosis. (Yamauchi M et al., 1997)

5. **IMAGING-** Gallium-67 imaging has been widely used in the diagnosis of sarcoidosis. Gallium-67 is usually taken up in lesions with increased blood flow, typically in lesions of inflammatory origin. In sarcoidosis, a characteristic pattern of uptake in the chest has been described as the "lambda sign:" (paratracheal and bilateral hilar uptake) and the "panda sign," caused by uptake in the lacrimal and parotid glands. (J.T.Annema et al., 2005) Conventional monitors of the activity of pulmonary sarcoidosis, such as blood studies, pulmonary function testing, and chest roentgenograms, do not show as much as assessed by bronchoalveolar lavage or by histopathologic studies.
6. **ROLE OF ENDOSCOPY-** In March 2009, a large international randomized clinical study "Trial for the Diagnosis of Sarcoidosis (GRANULOMA)" was started. This phase III study investigates two different diagnostic strategies for patients with suspected stage I/II pulmonary sarcoidosis. Bronchoscopy was done for 121 patients with establishing the definite diagnosis of sarcoidosis in 57 cases (42%). EUS-FNA was used for diagnosis of sarcoidosis and had a yield of 82% and sensitivity of 89–94% by assessing noncaseating granulomas in mediastinal nodes. In 72 cases, EUS-FNA/ EBUS-TBNA was performed, yielding a definite diagnosis in 47 (59%). Endoscopic ultrasound prevented a surgical procedure in more than half of these patients. (Julita Stępień1,2010)

Thus, Endoscopic ultrasound-guided fine-needle aspiration has a high yield in diagnosing sarcoidosis. Endoscopic ultrasound-guided fine-needle aspiration will also reduce the number of mediastinoscopies.

The only abnormal finding in laboratory studies was a slightly elevated ESR (to 14 mm/h, normal range: 0–10 mm/h) In a study by Steinfort et al., which analysed lymph node lesions in patients suffering from non-small cell lung cancer, a sarcoid-like reaction was observed in 8 out of 187 patients who had previously undergone thoracoscopy, lobectomy, or pneumonectomy and in 1 out of 50 patients who had undergone endobronchial ultrasound as part of the diagnostic evaluation for cancer. The authors emphasised that the lymph nodes in which sarcoid tissue was found revealed no tumour cells.

7. **ROLE OF AMYLOID-** A role of serum amyloid A (SAA) in pathogenesis of granulomatous inflammation of sarcoidosis has recently been reported. Serum concentrations of SAA are significantly higher in sarcoidosis patients. The results of some studies have suggested suggest that serum amyloid A could be a suitable marker of sarcoidosis:, the protein is only expressed in gels of sarcoidosis patients and not in healthy subjects, and the SAA1 isoforms could match the biomarker of sarcoidosis reported previously. Further studies on a larger scale are required to understand the effectiveness of SAA as a clinical biomarker of sarcoidosis.(Bässler R,1988) During the past decade, advances have been made in the study of sarcoidosis. The multicenter ACCESS (A Case Control Etiologic Study of Sarcoidosis) trial recruited > 700 subjects with newly diagnosed sarcoidosis and matched control subjects. They were unable to identify a single cause of sarcoidosis, but the Mycobacterium tuberculosis catalase-peroxidase protein has been identified as a potential sarcoidosis antigen. Sarcoidosis remains a diagnosis of exclusion most reliably by a tissue biopsy specimen demonstrating non-caseating granulomas in a patient with additional clinical and radiologic features of the disease. The tumor necrosis factor inhibitors, a relatively new class of agents, have been used in some patients. The diagnosis of sarcoid like reactions may be problematic because other known causes of granulomatous inflammation need to be excluded.

4. Histopathology

Histopathological examination of the involved organ is considered to be the most reliable method of diagnosis of Sarcoid like reaction. Sarcoid granulomas characterictically comprise of collections of numerous epithelioid cells along with many multinucleated giant cells. These giant cells can be of two types; either Langhans giant cells or foreign body type of giant cells. Another pathognomic feature of a sarcoid granuloma is the presence of inclusion bodies within the multinucleated giant cells; lamellated calcified masses named: the Schaumann bodies and the star shaped asteroid bodies.

Tumor-related sarcoid reactions have generally been reported to be in the lymph nodes draining regions with a malignancy disease, or in the parenchyma around the tumor. (Klein M,1994) The induction and evolution of granuloma formation results from a complex interplay between different cell populations, cytokines, and chemokines. Genetic polymorphisms may also influence the clinical expression of the granuloma formation and the prognosis of the disease. Sarcoid reactions in lymph nodes with or without metastasis from a primary malignant neoplasm are well-known. However, it is extremely rare to find these reactions associated with cutaneous solid tumors; only one such case has appeared in the literature. In a patient with cutaneous squamous cell carcinoma sarcoid reactions and metastatic foci in the regional lymph nodes were also associated. The possibilities of systemic sarcoidosis and tuberculosis were excluded after extensive examinations specific for these diseases. Some authors regard the sarcoid reaction to be a sign of a good prognosis on the basis of studies of a few patients with solid tumors. However, systematic analysis of a sufficient number of cases should be carried out to evaluate the clinical significance of this type of reaction. (Okabe T, 2002) In some cases of invasive ductal and lobular carcinoma of the breast multiple epithelioid and giant cell containing granulomas were detected. These granulomas occurred as sarcoid-like lesions in uni- and bilateral primaries, in a recurrent tumour, and also in axillary lymph nodes. Histopathologically, these granulomas are not quite uniform, some of them show classic features of sarcoidosis, while others show marked proliferations of epithelioid or giant cells. The granulomas contain fibrinoid exudate or areas of necrosis and are surrounded by dense infiltrates of mononuclear cells. Pathogenetically, these are reactions in the tumour stroma of varying intensity, and are caused by T-cell mediated immune response to an carcinoma antigen. (Brincker H, Pedersen NT,1991). In sarcoidosis, unknown antigen(s) causes Th1-mediated granulomatous inflammation with cytokines such as IFN gamma and IL-12, initially. Furthermore IL-16, IL-8, IP-10 and RANTES also play a role in the accumulation of CD4+ T cell population. For the chemotaxis of macrophages and monocytes, factors like MCP-1, MIP1-alpha and RANTES are considered responsible.Local proliferation of T cell is induced by IL-2 and IL-15 and that of macrophage/monocyte lineage is done by M-CSF, GM-CSF and G-CSF as in cases of other inflammatory reactions. Removal of the antigen downregulates the immune response via TGFβ and suppresses granuloma formation. Failure of removal of antigen can induce persistence of granuloma and irreversible fibrosis. (Spiteri MA et al., 1989)

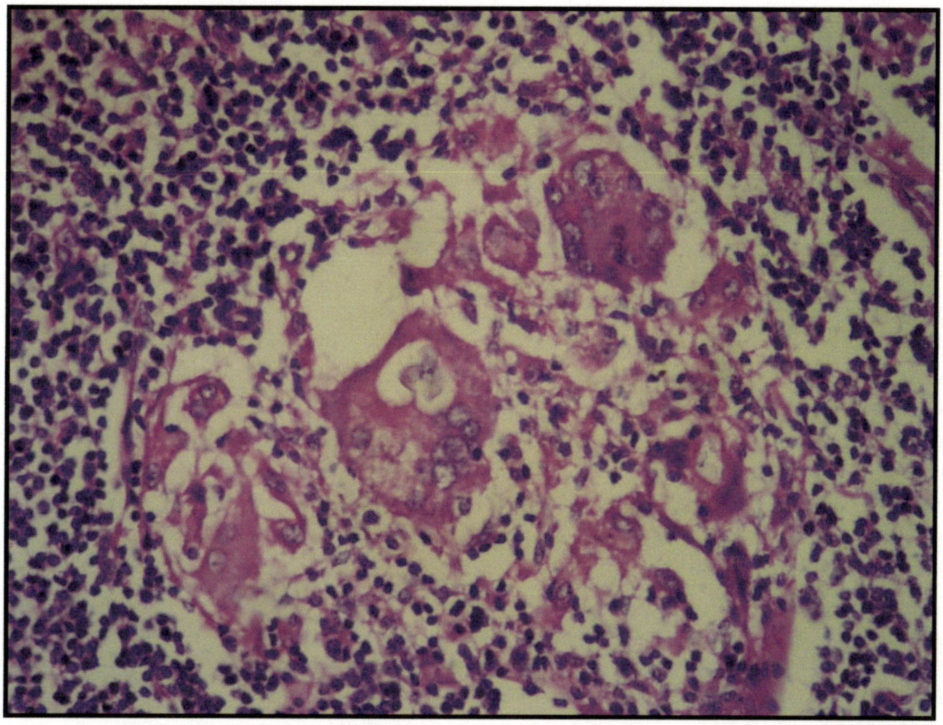

Fig. 1. A Sarcoid granuloma with Schaumann bodies within the multinucleated giant cells.

The pulmonary production of IFN-inducible protein (IP-10), a CXC chemokine that stimulates the directional migration of activated T cells. When compared to control subjects, excessively high levels of IP-10 are demonstrated in the bronchoalveolar lavage (BAL) fluid of patients with pulmonary sarcoidosis . In a study a positive correlation was also demonstrated between IP-10 levels and the number of sarcoid cells in the BAL. Immunochemistry was performed with an anti-human IP-10 polyclonal Ab in lymph nodes showing sarcoid granulomas. It was observed that cells bearing IP-10 were mainly epithelioid cells and CD68+ macrophages located inside granulomatous areas.In addition, alveolar lymphocytes recovered from patients with active sarcoidosis were CD4+ T cells expressing Th1 cytokines (IL-2 and IFN-gamma) and high levels of CXCR3. All these facts suggest the potential role of IP-10 in regulating the migration and activation of T cells toward sites of sarcoid inflammatory process and the subsequent granuloma formation. (Kin T, 1999)

According to a study, granulomas can be divided into two main "families" according to the presence or absence of B cells within the granulomas: one is a B-cell-negative familycomprising of sarcoidosis and mycobacterial infection; the other is a B-cell-positive family comprising of tumor-related sarcoid reactions, toxoplasmosis and other granulomatous lesions of unknown significance.

Sometimes in patients with squamous cell carcinoma of lung, histopathological examination of hilar and mediastinal drainage lymph nodes show many non-caseating epithelioid cell granuloma even in absence of metastasis. Co-existence of sarcoidosis and lung cancer in the same patient is not common, and only 29 cases, have been reported. even if bilateral mediastinal lymphadenopathy is found in a case of lung cancer complicated with sarcoidosis, surgical tumor resection should be considered

One such case of lower esophageal cancer was reported where a lower esophagectomy with a total gastrectomy was performed. A sarcoid-like reaction within lymph nodes can occur even after few year of resection of the tumour.

In some cases, the histological examination may show non-caseous epithelioid granulomas without necrosis in association with moderately differentiated carcinoma without any metastases to the regional lymph nodes; These changes should be considered to be sarcoid reactions, if no other physiological and laboratory findings compatible with systemic sarcoidosis are observed. Such histological findings sugges the possibility that the regional lymph nodes are not involved with the tumor cells at the time of diagnosis of cancer.

The granulomas are present in a lymphatic pattern around bronchovascular structures and, because of this, may show angioinvasion. The bronchial involvement produces a high diagnostic yield for transbronchial and endobronchial biopsies in this disease. Finally, small amounts of fibrinoid necrosis may occur within granulomas of sarcoidosis and do not exclude the diagnosis. A number of cytoplasmic structures/inclusions can be identified within the granulomas of sarcoidosis, including asteroid bodies, Schaumann's bodies, calcium oxalate crystals, and Hamazaki-Wesenberg bodies; the last two of these can cause difficulties in differential diagnosis. Extra-pulmonary sarcoid can be an important factor in prognosis. Involved sites include (in decreasing frequency) skin, endocrine organs, extra-thoracic lymph nodes, neurologic sites, eyes, liver, spleen, bone marrow, cardiac, ear/nose/throat, parotid/ salivary, muscles, bones/joint, and kidney.

The association of soft tissue sarcomas with a granulomatous reaction is very rare, although a case of Kaposi sarcoma containing sarcoid-like granulomas has also been reported. In addition to vascular proliferation, and extravasated erythrocytes numerous spindle cells were observed. These areas were surrounded by non-caseating granulomas. The patient had no clinical or laboratory findings of sarcoidosis. As mentioned earlier the granulomatous reaction is reported to be a good prognostic indicator in several carcinoma types but its importance in sarcomas is not clear.Another unusual type of codition is coexistence of sarcoid-like reaction with synovial sarcoma. There have been no such reported cases in literature. Therefore, understanding this kind of cases and their pathogenesis may help to improve the understanding of the relationship between malignancy and sarcoid-like reactions.

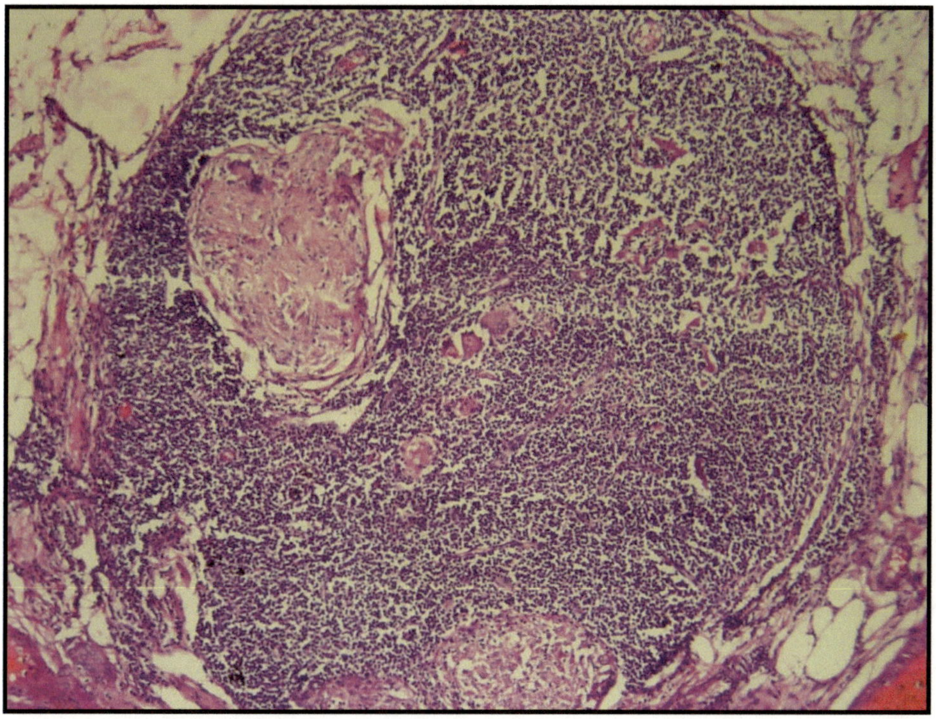

Fig. 2. A cervical lymph node showing non-caseating granulomas comprising of collections epithelioid cells and multinucleated giant cells in the background of Lymphocytes.

The authors report a case of Hodgkin's disease associated with pulmonary and mediastinal sarcoidosis, and the frequency of sarcoid reactions in lymphoma, notably in Hodgkin's disease. The Hodgkin's disease-sarcoidosis association is much less common and sometimes raises difficult diagnostic problems. (Agostini Cet al.,1998)
Electron microscopic examination of epithelioid-cell granulomas of has revealed a morphologic polarization of epithelioid cells, manifesting as 4 zones: crimped [correction of chimp] edge zone, zone of vesicles and vacuoles, basal zone and osmiophilic granules zone. The structure of epithelioid cells in sarcoidosis and in sarcoid reactions are found to be similar. Sarcoid epithelioid cells are believed to be a variant of tissue macrophages, which are derived from circulating monocytes in blood. It is a known fact that formation of monocytes and macrophages is controlled by hematopoietic growth factors, i.e.; colony-stimulating factors in the bone marrow. In the presence of colony-stimulating factors and

vitamin D3, blood monocytes can proliferate and differentiate into epithelioid cells and multinucleated giant cells. Recent observations have shown that sarcoid granulomas themselves produce colony-stimulating factors and vitamin D3 which stimulate the proliferation and differentiation of circulating monocytes into macrophage-epithelioid cells. This also leads to formation of new sarcoid granulomas.

Regarding the association of malignancy with sarcoidosis, various possibilities have been proposed to explain the occurrence of malignancy in sarcoidosis, namely, the occurrence of these two disorders together being a coincidence; sarcoidosis initiating the carcinogenesis or promoting the growth of malignancy via suppression of cellular immunity; and sarcoidosis occurring as a result of host immunological response against malignancy. However, in the absence of systemic involvement, the diagnosis is suggestive of a sarcoid reaction associated with a malignancy, rather than sarcoidosis.

In addition to the pathognomic, asteroid and Schaumann bodies ,reactive hyperplasia within the Lymph nodes can also be observed. This could be explained on the basis of specific cell mediated immune response against the soluble antigenic factors derived from the tumor cells by both activated macrophages and T lymphocytes. Thus the granulomatous reaction and subsequent release of cytokines such as TNF-α, IL-2 and IL-8 might be a marker of an immunologically mediated anti-tumor response.

Three possible mechanisms are offered for the mode of formation of asteroid bodies, namely phagocytosis and partly fused cell membranes; trapping and polymerization of collagen within incompletely fused epitheloid cells; and transformation of epitheloid cells into fibroblasts during the healing of granulomas. The latter possibilityof epithelioid cells being transformed into fibroblasts, is favored but requires more evidence in support of fibroblastic potentiality of epitheloid cells and macrophages

The mechanism of the formation of Schaumann bodies can be explained on the basis of different concepts.Most of the authors who have previously examined these structures have considered them to be products of degeneration of elastic fibrils impregnated with calcium and iron salts. Schaumann advanced the opinion that tubercle bacilli can be transformed into such bodies. It is also believed that these bodies may result from deposition around elastic fibrils, connective tissue fibrils, or hair resulting from disintegrated tubercle bacilli and proposed that they are products of intracellular globulin precipitate.

Sarcoid granulomata result from aberrant immunological reactions initiated by antigen--presenting macrophage--like cells, and maintained by other effector macrophages. These macrophages can be distinguished phenotypically by monoclonal antibodies RFD1 and RFD7 (which recognize dendritic cells and mature macrophages respectively). A study has shown that active sarcoid BAL contains a high proportion of RFD1 + cells (mean 44.7% compared to 12% in normals). Furthermore it has been demonstrated that gamma-interferon, produced in high concentration by activated T-lymphocytes induces not only HLA-DR molecules on cells, but has also been shown in vitro to increase the proportion of RFD1+ cells but suppressing RFD7 expression. Therefore,It seems that the increased proportion of RFD1+ D7+ macrophages seen in active sarcoidosis could arise as a result of an increased induction of RFD1 expression on macrophages which express RFD7. (Sugio K, 1993)

5. Differential diagnosis

The first step in getting correct treatment is to get a correct diagnosis. Granulomas have also been observed within the lymph nodes associated with other granulomatous diseases.

Differential diagnosis list for Sarcoidosis may include: berylliosis, tuberculosis, hypersensitivity pneumonitis (farmer's lung disease), Fungal infections, Rheumatoid arthritis, Rheumatic fever, Lymphoma, Histoplasmosis, Coccidioidomycosis, Idiopathic pulmonary fibrosis, Pneumoconiosis, Syphillis. In 1994, Leibow first described a condition termed; Necrotizing sarcoid granulomatosis (NSG). Based on radiological and clinical features, it was concluded that NSG is the histopathological variant of sarcoidosis, also termed "nodular sarcoidosis. Necrotizing sarcoid granulomatosis has been reported in 1.6% to 4% of patients with sarcoidosis. Although it comprises of sarcoid-like granulomas, they are associated with granulomatous pneumonitis, variable amounts of necrosis and granulomatous vasculitis. Radiographic nodules made up of multiple granulomas are also found.

Common variable immunodeficiency (CVID) is a disorder characterized by hypogammaglobulinemia, poor antibody responses and recurrent bacterial infections. CVID patients have a higher prevalence of autoimmune disease and some of them develop noncaseating granulomas of the lungs, spleen, liver, skin, lymph nodes and eye. In patients with CVID, different types of autoimmune disease could be seen. Therefore, these patients should be carefully evaluated for diseases other than sarcoidosis.

An anti-Kveim monoclonal antibody, IHY-1,was developped which reacts with sarcoid granulomas as well as with epithelioid cells of various granulomatous diseases including tuberculosis. Thus differentiation of Sarcoid grnulomas with granulomas of other conditions was difficult. Recently, 2 new anti-Kveim monoclonal antibodies, IHY-2 and IHY-3 were developed which reacted with epithelioid cells in sarcoidosis but not in tuberculosis. Immunoperoxidase technique was used and it was observed that these antibodies reacted with most epithelioid cells in sarcoid granulomas, confirming the fact that that these cells expressed the antigen present in the Kveim reagent. (Balamurugan S, 2009)

Granulomatous reactions have been reported in association with lymphomas, more often with Hodgkins disease than with Non-Hodgkins Lymphoma. Not many reports are available on the association of anaplastic large-cell lymphoma with sarcoid-type granuloma. It is suggested that a detailed clinical history, careful histological examination and immunohistochemistry helped in attaining the correct diagnosis.

Problems may also arise of distinguishing between tumour-related sarcoid reactions and true systemic sarcoidosis. As mentioned earlier ,the diagnosis of sarcoidosis is based more on exclusion criteria and thorough clinical and radiological investigations are required to differentiate it from sarcoid like reactions. This differentiation is essential for further treatment planning and prevention of recurrence of disease. Most probably, sarcoid reactions are caused by antigenic factors derived from the tumour cells, eliciting an immunological hypersensitivity reaction leading to the formation of epithelioid-cell granulomas. Sarcoid reactions may be a marker of an immunologically mediated anti-tumour response of macrophages activated by T-lymphocytes, and in Hodgkin's disease there is evidence that patients with sarcoid reactions have a better prognosis. Sometimes, sarcoid reactions may be so extensive that they complicate the diagnosis of an underlying malignant disease.

Previous reports indicate that enlarged hilar and mediastinal lymph nodes caused by sarcoid-like reactions may develop after curative resection of cancer. This presence does not indicate recurrence. Reports further suggest that coexisting pulmonary infiltrates in this setting may be related to sarcoidosis. In a study, two patients who had resected lung and gastric cancer and who later developed pulmonary interstitial infiltrate, concurrent with progressive mediastinal lymphadenopathy initially thought to be caused by intrathoracic dissemination of their cancer. These changes were shown by open lung biopsy to be a benign, granulomatous reaction interpreted as sarcoidosis. Thus, it is important to recognize this clinical pattern when pulmonary infiltrates develop after complete treatment of cancer in an otherwise relapse-free patient and to encourage lung or lymph node biopsy in these particular settings in order to confirm a sarcoid-like reaction, thereby avoiding unnecessary chemotherapy for presumed tumor recurrence.

During microscopic examination of sections of lymph nodes, it may give an appearance of a metastatic node with numerous collections of tumour cells. But careful observation may reveal that they are actually epithelioid cells with presence of other pathognomonic features of sarcoid granulomas like, presence of Schaumann bodies and asteroid bodies. Further confirmation of sarcoid like reaction requires ruling out of any systemic involvement by radiographs, ACE level assessment and other investigation procedures which are specific for sarcoidosis.

6. Treatment

A standard treatment with immune suppressants such as glucocorticoids should be started. In some of the patients recover spontaneously without any treatment. In other patients, a treatment is necessary during the follow-up course. Immunosuppressive drugs like hydroxychloroquine and infliximab may be useful in some patients. Treatment should be continued at least for about one year. Initially, patients should receive prednisone or prednisolone at 0.5 to 1 mg/kg daily for 6 to 12 weeks to obtain a complete remission, and then later followed by a gradual dose reduction every 6 to 12 weeks. The follow up should be carried out for about three years. When corticosteroids are contraindicated, methotrexate and azathioprine in low doses are the most useful immunosuppressive drugs. Hydroxychloroquine and chloroquine are indicated in extensive skin lesions or as corticosteroids sparing agents. Recent advancements in the field of Biotechnology has resulted in new treatment stratagies like use of monoclonal antibodies. In patients with sarcoidosis, only the use of monoclonal antibodies that block tumour necrosis factor (TNF) has been studied scientifically and at present, TNF-blockers are used in patients with therapy refractory sarcoidosis

In a Literature review, accessed through MEDLINE (1966-August 2002), OVID (2001-January 2003), and bibliographic searches, the use of infliximab in the treatment of sarcoidosis was evaluated. It was observed that, tumor-necrosis factor-alpha blockade appeared to be a suitable strategy for treating sarcoidosis. Since the evidence for above concept is not sufficient, further data are required to establish the role of infliximab.(Serio PN,2003)

7. Prognosis

of sarcoidosis is often good. About 60-70% cases heal spontaneously within 24-36 months and fatal complications are observed only in 5-10% of patients which may be due to respiratory involvement. Estimated mortality rate for sarcoidosis from prevalence and deaths statistics is 20 per 100,000 overall; 5 in 100,000 white people; 40 out of 100,000 black people; Scandinavia 64 out of 100,000 people. The ratio of deaths to prevalence is 1.1%. As far as sarcoid like reactios are considered, the resection of the tumour to which it is associated and the related surgical treatment of the involved organ and, would be sufficient to restore patient's normal condition. It is considered that granulomatous sarcoid-like lesions are indicative of an immunologically mediated antitumor response of macrophages activated by T lymphocytes. Thus leading to a favorable prognosis.

8. Conclusion

The diagnosis of sarcoidosis, could be difficult; in fact typical laboratory findings of sarcoidosis such as ACE, lysozyme, calcium, sometimes may not be diagnostic. Ultrasonography and CT are important but the diagnosis is mainly established only with the histological examination of suspected lesions. As it is not possible to distinguish sarcoid-like reaction from sarcoidosis only histologically, a thorough investigation of the patient is mandatory to rule out systemic sarcoidosis or other granulomatous diseases. The concept of correlation between various types of malignancies and sarcoid-like reaction and sarcoidosis is still unclear. Further studies are required to explain this concept more accurately.

9. References

Abdel-Galiil K, Anand R, Sharma S, Brennan PA, Ramchandani PL, Ilankovan V.(2006) Incidence of sarcoidosis in head and neck cancer. *Epub* ; 46(1):59-60.

Agostini C, Facco M, Chilosi M, Semenzato G (2001) Alveolar macrophage-T cell interactions during Th1-type sarcoid inflammation. Microsc Res Tech;53(40):278-7.

Agostini C, Cassatella M, Zambello R, Trentin L, Gasperini S, Perin A, Piazza F, Siviero M, Facco M, Dziejman M, Chilosi M, Qin S, Luster AD, Semenzato G.(1998) Involvement of the IP-10 chemokine in sarcoid granulomatous reactions. *J Immunol*;161(11):6413-2.

Artac H, Bozkurt B, Talim B, Reisli I (2009) Sarcoid-like granulomas in common variable immunodeficiency. Rheumatol Int.

Balamurugan S, Rajasekar B, Rao RR (2009) Anaplastic large-cell lymphoma with florid granulomatous reaction: a case report and review of literature. *Indian J Pathol Microbiol.*; 52(1):69-70.

Battesti JP, Turiaf J, Hincky JM, Dournovo P (1977) Sarcoidosis and malignant tumors. *Nouv Presse Med*; 6(14):1213-5.

Bargagli E, Magi B, Olivieri C, Bianchi N, Landi C, Rottoli P (2011) Analysis of serum amyloid A in sarcoidosis patients. *Respir Med.*

Bässler R, Birke F (1988) Histopathology of tumour associated sarcoid-like stromal reaction in breast cancer. An analysis of 5 cases with immunohistochemical investigations. *Virchows Arch A Pathol Anat Histopathol*;412(3):231-9.

Brincker H, Pedersen NT (1991)Immunohistologic separation of B-cell-positive granulomas from B-cell-negative granulomas in paraffin-embedded tissues with special reference to tumor-related sarcoid reactions*APMIS*. ;99(3):282-90..

Brincker H. (1986) Sarcoid reactions in malignant tumours. *Cancer Treat Rev*; 13(3):147-56.

Brincker H (1987). Solid tumors preceding or following sarcoidosis. *Med Pediatr Oncol*;15(2):82-8.

Daniele RP, Dauber JH, Rossman MD (1980)Ann Intern Med;92(3):406-16. Immunologic abnormalities in sarcoidosis.

de Hemricourt E, De Boeck K, Hilte F, Abib A, Kockx M, Vandevivere J, De Bock R.(2008) Sarcoidosis and sarcoid-like reaction following Hodgkin's disease. Report of two cases. Nihon Kokyuki Gakkai Zasshi. 2008 Jun;46(6):505-9.

Giovinale M, Fonnesu C, Soriano A, Cerquaglia C, Curigliano V, Verrecchia E, De Socio G, Gasbarrini G, Manna R (2009) Atypical sarcoidosis: case reports and review of the literature. *Eur Rev Med Pharmacol Sci.* ; 13 Suppl 1:37-44.

Hashem, S A, Sultan, Al-Hussaini M, Hawari F and Yaser.(2010) S Pulmonary sarcoid-like reaction in metastatic synovial sarcoma. *Respiratory Medicine CME.* Article in Press.

Ishioka S, Wiwien HW, Hiyama K, Maeda A, Yamakido M (1999). New monoclonal antibodies against the epithelioid cells in sarcoid granulomas. *Exp Lung Res;* 25(8):663-70.

J.T.Annema, M.Veselic. (2005) Endoscopic ultrasound-guided fine-needle aspiration for the diagnosis of sarcoidosis. *Eur Respir J;* 25: 405–409

Julita Stępień1, Joanna Domagała-Kulawik1, Radosław Chądzyński1, Włodzimierz Kupis, Ryszarda Chazan (2010) Sarcoidal reaction in lung adrenocarcinoma in 50-year old man *Pneumonol Alergol. Pol;* 78(4):302–305.

Kazuaki Morohashi, Toshinori Takada; Kentaro Omori, Eiichi Suzuki, and Fumitake Gejyo (2003) Vascular Endothelial Growth Factor Gene Polymorphisms in Japanese Patients With Sarcoidosis. *CHEST;123:1520–6.*

Kaminsky P, Deibener J, Cocciale MP, DucM(1994) Sarcoid reactions in cystic duct carcinoma. *Chest 106*: 1304.

Kiminobu Tanizawa, Eisaku Tanaka , Seishu Hashimoto, Satoshi Noma, Yoichiro Kobashi, Kazuhiro Okumura,

Toru Shindo and Yoshio Taguchi (2010)Paradoxical Development of a Sarcoid-Like Reaction during Successful Chemotherapy for Seminoma. *Inter Med;* 49: 1423-6.

Kin T, Shimano Y, Shinomiya Y, Nakano H (1999) Double cancers of the lung and esophagus associated with a sarcoid-like reaction in their regional lymph nodes: report of a case. *Surg Today*;29(3):260-3.

Klein JT, Horn TD, Forman JD, Silver RF, Teirstein AS, Moller DR (1995) Selection of oligoclonal V beta-specific T cells in the intradermal response to Kveim-Siltzbach reagent in individuals with sarcoidosis. *J Immunol* ; 154(3):1450-6.

Kojima M, Nakamura S, Fujisaki M, Hirahata S, Hasegawa H, Maeda D, Suito T, Motoori T, Joshita T, Suzuki K, Suchi T.(1999) Sarcoid-like reaction in the regional lymph nodes and spleen in gastric carcinoma: a clinicopathologic study of five cases. *Surg Today;29(6); 549-52.*

Komatsu M, Itoh N, Yazawa M, Kobayashi S, Inoue K, Kuroda T (1997) Sarcoid reaction in thyroid diseases: report of a case of thyroid carcinoma demonstrating sarcoid reaction in regional lymph nodes. *Endocr J;* 44(5):697-700.

Lattaignant JC, Margent P, Arondelle C, Carvaillo D, Groussard O, Battesti JP. (1987) Solid tumours preceding or following sarcoidosis. *Medical and Pediatric Oncology;* 15:2:82-88.

Laurberg P(1975) Sarcoid reactions in pulmonary neoplasms. *Scand J Respir Dis;* 56:20.

Londner C, Zendah I, Freynet O, Carton Z, Dion G, Nunes H, Valeyre D. (2011) Treatment of sarcoidosis. *Rev Med Intern* Feb;32(2):109-113.

Maeda J, Ohta M, Hirabayashi H, Matsuda H (2005)False positive accumulation in 18F fluorodeoxyglucose positron emission tomography scan due to sarcoid reaction following induction chemotherapy for lung cancer. J *Thorac Cardiovasc Surg;* 53(4):196-8.

Morgenthau AS, Iannuzzi MC (2011) Recent advances in sarcoidosis. *Chest;* 139(1):174-82

Okabe T. Origin of epithelioid cells in sarcoid granuloma. *Nippon Rinsho* (2002) Sep; 60(9):1714-9.

Paparel P, Devonec M, Perrin P, et al. (2007) Association between sarcoidosis and testicular carcinoma: a diagnostic pitfall. *Vasc Diffuse Lung Dis.*24; 95-101.

Parra ER, Canzian M, Saber AM, Coêlho RS, Rodrigues FG, Kairalla RA, de Carvalho CR, Capelozzi VL (2004) Pulmonary and mediastinal "sarcoidosis" following surgical resection of cancer. Pathol Res Pract.; 200(10):701-5.

Pavic M, Debourdeau P, Vacelet V, Rousset H (2008). Sarcoidosis and sarcoid reactions in cancer. *Rev Med Interne.* 29(1):39-45.

Proenca NG, Kliemann TA, Muller H (1982) Kveim test performed with antigen obtained from lymph nodes. M*ed Cutan Ibero Lat Am.*10(4):255-60.

Pulmonary sarcoidosis: a disease characterized and perpetuated by activated lung T-lymphocytes. *Ann Intern Med;* 94(1):73-94. No authors listed.

Rajendran R, Sivapathasundharam B (2006) *Shafer's Textbookof Oral Pathology;* (5th edition): Reed Elsevier India Private Limited.

Rømer FK (1980) Angiotensin-converting enzyme in newly detected sarcoidosis. With special reference to enzyme levels in patients with erythema nodosum. *Acta Med Scand.* ; 208(6):437-43.

Rømer FK (1981) Correlation between disease activity, one-year prognosis, and angiotensin-converting enzyme in untreated sarcoidosis. *Acta Med Scand.;* 210(1-2):111-7.

Romer FK (1985) Angiotensin-converting enzyme activity in sarcoidosis and other disorders. *Sarcoidosis;* 2(1):25-34.

Serio RN (2003). Infliximab treatment of sarcoidosis. *Ann Pharmacother.;* 37(4):577-81.

Shultz T, Miller WC, Bedrossian CW (1979) Clinical application of measurement of angiotensin-converting enzyme level. *AMA;* 242(5):439-41.

Sugiyama Y, Oshikawa K (2002) Mechanism of sarcoid granuloma formation--participation of cytokines and chemokines. *Nippon Rinsho;* 60(9):1728-33.

Spiteri MA, Poulter LW, Geraint-James D (1989) The macrophage in sarcoid granuloma formation. *Sarcoidosis;* 6 (1):12-4.

Takaaki Fujii Yuichi Tabe Reina Yajima Soichi Tsutsumi Takayuki Asao Hiroyuki Kuwano. (2010). Adenocarcinoma of Ascending Colon Associated with Sarcoid Reaction in Regional Lymph Nodes. *Case Rep Gastroenterol;* 4:118–23.

Tanizawa K, Tanaka E, Hashimoto S, Noma S, Kobashi Y, Okumura K, Shindo T, Taguchi Y.Paradoxical development of a sarcoid-like reaction during successful chemotherapy for seminoma. *Intern Med; 49(14):1423-6.*

Yamauchi M, Inoue D, Fukunaga Y, Kakudo K, Koshiyama H (1997) A case of sarcoid reaction associated with papillary thyroid carcinoma. *Thyroid* ; 7(6):901-3.

17

Granulomatosis and Cancer

Michel Pavic and Florian Pasquet
Hôpital d'Instruction des Armées Desgenettes,
Internal medicin and Oncoly department,
France

1. Introduction

Sarcoidosis is a granulomatous disease of unknown cause that can virtually affect any organ system. The commonly affected organ areas are thoracic lymph nodes and lungs (90 %). The granulomas appears to be due to an aberant immune response to a persistent antigen in a susceptible host; the antigen, however, is yet to be identified(Shigemitsu, 2008). The diagnosis typically rests on the demonstration of characteristic granulomas in biopsy specimens of one or more organs and exclusion of other causes of chronic granulomatous inflammation(Boffetta et al., 2009; Pavic et al., 2008b). Sarcoidosis affects more frequently young adults. Genetic studies have shown that some major histocompatibility complex alleles and tumor necrosis factor (TNF) polymorphisms are associated with an increased risk of sarcoidosis. The disease is usually characterized by an increased macrophage and CD4 T-cell activation, whereas sarcoidosis patients also show suppressed response to antigen challenges. The coexistent of hyper- and hypoactivity indicates a state of anergy in the immune system(Ji et al., 2009). Relationships betwen granulomatosis and cancers have been suspected for a long time(Askling et al., 1999; Brincker and Wilbek, 1974; Pavic and Rousset, 2008; Romer et al., 1998). Nevertheless, few evidence has been reported until recently. Aside from granulomatosis due to infectious disease (eg: opportunist infections), granulomas can be observed in cancer patients, mainly in two situations. Patients may rarely present with typical sarcoidosis occuring before, during or after the diagnosis of cancer. Secondly granulomas may be found as a sarcoid reaction in the vicinity of the tumour itself ore more frequently in regional lymph nodes(Pavic et al., 2008a). Sarcoidosis has although been reported to occur with some chemotherapeutic agents or immunotherapy such as interferon. The presence of granulomas within the tumor tissue or in regional ganglions is a frequent situation and corresponds to a defense reaction against the tumor-associated antigen (sarcoid like reaction)(Kennedy et al., 2008; Steinfort and Irving, 2009). The precise mechanism of the sarcoid-cancer syndrome is not yet clear, though there are several descriptions in the literature as to the temporal relationship of granulomas developing in cancer and vice versa. The etiology of sarcoidosis and sarcoid reactions in malignancy remains uncertain but some speculations have been made(Trikudanathan et al.): 1/ induction of robust effector T cell response to a tumor antigen or other products of cancer cells either spontaneously or with treatment that result in T helper 1 response along with secretion of TH1 cytokines; 2/ increased vulnerability to a potential infective agent due to immune system imbalance that occurs with cancer; 3/ radiation therapy and antineoplastic agents might enhance granulomatous reactions in tumors; 4/granulomatous reaction could play an important role in the host's defences against metastatic extension. So granulomatous reaction has been associated for some cancers with a better prognosis(O'Connell et al., 1975)

2. Cancer - sarcoidosis syndrome

The literature remained very controversial during many years on the association between sarcoidosis and cancer(Battesti et al., 1977; Brincker, 1989; Brincker and Wilbek, 1974). The association of these two pathologies was first considered as fortuitous(Reich et al., 1995; Romer, et al., 1998; Seersholm et al., 1997). The swedish study of Askling et al. published in 1999 concerns a very large cohort and brings a first objective element of answer to this question(Askling, et al., 1999). This study reported on a retrospective cohort's study analyzing two registers of patients presenting with sarcoidosis (474 and 8541 patients) followed respectively from 1966 till 1980 and from 1964 till 1994. The risk of developping a cancer within these patients's group was studied by crossing the results of the cancer's registers and of the death's registers. The authors investigated the risk of developping a cancer in the sites commonly affected by sarcoidosis. The relative risk of cancer was increased equally in both registers of sarcoidosis (RR: 1,3; CI 95 %: 1,2-1,4). The risk of lung cancer and non-Hodgkin's lymphoma was doubled in the first decade following the diagnosis of sarcoidosis. The relative risk was also increased for the other cancers: melanomas (RR: 1,6; CI 95 %: 1-2,3), other skin cancers (RR: 2,8; CI 95 %: 2-3,8) and unsignificantly for the hepatocarcinomas (RR: 1,4; CI 95 % 0,8-2,2). Le Jeune et al. studied in an English population, the incidence of cancer in patients affected by sarcoidosis (1153 cases) and found a relative risk of 1,65 (CI 95 %: 1,22-2,24)(Le Jeune et al., 2007). Adjusted according to the age, the sex and smoking, the risk was significantly increased for the skin cancers (RR: 1, 86; CI 95 %: 1,11-3,11) and for the lymphomas (RR: 7,04; CI 95 %: 1,54-32,1). Ji et al studied retrospectively 10037 patients having been hospitalized in Germany for a sarcoidosis between 1964 and 2004 and found 1045 cases of cancers occuring in this patients(Ji, et al., 2009). A 40% overall excess incidence of cancer was noted among sarcoidosis patients. Notified cancers were the skin cancers (apart from the melanomas), the renal cancers, the extra-thyroid endocrine tumors, the non-Hodgkin's lymphomas and the leukemias. The increased incidence was confined mainly to the first year after hospitalization. However, for specific cancers, such as squamous cell carcinoma of the skin and non-hodgkin's lymphoma and leukemia, the increases were still significant for patients diagnosed later than 1 year after hospitalization, especially for those with multiple hospitalizations. A late age at hospitalization was associated with a high risk, which calls for clinical attention. All these studies have notified that the association of cancer and sarcoidosis was not fortuitous with an increased incidence (about 40 %) of skin cancers, lymphomas and probably of renal cancers, cancers of the lungs, endocrine tumors and leukemias. Some authors proposed the term of "cancer - sarcoidosis syndrome" to appoint this association(Shigemitsu, 2008). The independant course of the two pathologies are unconsistent to consider sarcoidosis as a paraneoplastic syndrome.

3. Sarcoidosis - lymphoma syndrome

This term was first used by Brincker to describe the association of systemic sarcoidosis and malignant lymphoma(Brincker, 1989). Several cases of lymphomas following various forms of systemic sarcoidosis have been published since then. The increased prevalence of granulomatous disease during the malignant hemopathies is now well established, especially for Hodgkin's disease (14 %) but also for non hodgkin lymphomas (4 in 7 %) (Brincker, 1986a; Brunner et al., 2005). Malignant lymphoproliferative disorders, including B cell lymphomas, Hodgkin's lymphomas, chronic myeloid leukaemias and chronic lymphoid leukaelias, are more often seen among patients affected by sarcoidosis, with an incidence almost 5,5-fold higher than in general population(Apalla et al., ; Brincker, 1986b). Development of lymphoma in an individual with a personal history of sarcoidosis, even though rare, is not considered fortuitous. In the vast majority of reported cases, systemic sarcoidosis precedes the diagnosis of lymphoma by many years. The sarcoidosis - lymphoma syndrome is characterized by a later age of onset of the sarcoidosis (about 41 years, approximately 10 years more than the age of the classical sarcoidosis). Taking into account that the symptoms of sarcoidosis may resemble, or even mask, the symptoms of internal malignancy, physician awareness is considered crucial. Conversely, when a patient presents with a granulomatosis occuring at the end of a malignant hemopathy's treatment, this granulomatosis must be suspected to be linked to an infectious complication (opportunist infection, tuberculosis or other mycobacterias, pneumocystosis, fungal infections). The HHV-8 virus has been incriminated in the genesis of lymphoid pathologies and for some authors of the sarcoidosis, but this remains very controversial. The granulomatous pathology occuring in patients affected by a hodgkin's lymphoma motivated a plentiful literature(Sacks et al., 1978). Approximately 10 % of the patients presenting with a diagnosis of Hodgkin's lymphoma would develop granulomas affecting mainly the spleen and the liver. Some granulomatous vasculitis involving central nervous system have also been reported. Some more unusual sites have also been reported: lymph nodes, bone marrow, testicles, lungs. The granulomatous disease occurs generally concomitantly to the Hodgkin's lymphoma. Nevertheless it also can precede or arise conversely numerous years later. Patients with a history of sarcoidosis develop more often a Hodgkin's lymphoma than the general population with a relative risk of 14,1 (CI 95 %: 5,4-36,8)(Landgren et al., 2006). The antineoplastic treatments (chemotherapy and/or radiotherapy) are sometimes suspected to be causative when the granulomatosis arises with a long delay after the diagnosis of Hodgkin's lymphoma. The organ areas affected by the granulomatous reaction can also contain a neoplastic infiltration which is generally very difficult to determine. Hodgkin's patients presenting with a granulomatous disease have usually a favourable course. Granulomatous disease seems to be a favorable prognosis factor in term of survival and relapse(O'Connell, et al., 1975; Sacks, et al., 1978).

4. Melanomas and other skin cancers

In the swedish study of Askling et al., the relative risk was increased for melanomas (RR: 1,6; CI 95 %: 1-2,3) and other skin cancers (RR: 2,8; CI 95 %: 2-3,8)(Askling, et al., 1999). In a recent work, Sève et al examined the relation between sarcoidosis and melanoma. They identified 7 cases in their population of 1,199 melanoma inpatients(Seve et al., 2009). Including these cases, 20 cases of sarcoidosis have been described in melanoma patients in the literature. Fifteen patients had their sarcoidosis diagnosed after melanoma. In 7 cases, sarcoidosis was related to immunotherapy. Sarcoidosis presented mainly as pulmonary disease without severe organ involvement, with a benign evolution. In this referral center study showed a prevalence of sarcoidosis of 0.58% among melanoma inpatients. By excluding two cases related to immunotherapy, the prevalence was 0.42%, what is close to the prevalence of sarcoidosis found in the general population. This study does not support a strong relationship between malignant melanoma and sarcoidosis. However, clinicians should be aware of the possibility that sarcoidosis may initially manifest or be reactivated in melanoma patients, especially during or after treatment with immunotherapy. Because sarcoidosis is a diagnostic pitfall, biopsies must always be performed before starting an antineoplastic treatment. Although Asking et al. found an increased incidence of other skin cancers presenting with sarcoidosis, very few cases are reported in the literature about this concern(McLoone et al., 2005; Setoyama et al., 1998).

5. Hepatocarcinomas

Sarcoidosis-associated hepatocellular carcinoma (HCC) is rare with only few cases reports(Askling, et al., 1999; Chalasani et al., 2005; Ogata et al., ; Wong et al., 1999). Such a rare association of sarcoidosis with HCC may reflect the presence of relatively weak inflammation or weak hepatocytic regeneration in sarcoid liver disease(Ogata, et al.). Despite a favorable-looking suggesting host immunity against the tumor, its significance on prognosis is unclear.

6. Renal cancers

Only a few publications that mention the presence of granulomatous reaction in renal cell cancer have been published until yet(Bottone et al., 1993; Campbell and Douglas-Jones, 1993; Kovacs et al., 2004; Lucci et al., 2002; Marinides et al., 1994; Moder et al., 1990). In some cases the granulomatous reaction is not related to the cancer but it is a primary process of the kidney, like xanthogranulomatous pyelonephritis, and we must note that cancer and true sarcoidosis may coexist(Kovacs, et al., 2004). According to the few publications that mention cancer associated sarcoid-like reaction, such lesions do not influence the prognosis.
Interferon and interleukin 2 have been usual therapies for the kidney cancers during years. As sarcoidosis induced by interferon or high dose interleukin 2 therapies have been reported in the literature, the role of this agents must be kept in mind(Logan and Bensadoun, 2005; Massaguer et al., 2004; Pietropaoli et al., 1999).

7. Germ cell tumors

I the relevant literature, several case reports and small case series have described a total of 67 patients with "sarcoidosis" or "sarcoidosis-like reaction" and testicular germ-cell tumors (GCT) so far (Dick et al., ; Paparel et al., 2007). The phenomenon is clinically relevant, because the finding of granulomatous lesions in patients with cancer may lead to difficulties of interpretation resulting in appropriate treatment of both the granulomatous disease and the malignancy. Some data in the literature have raised the question of an increased incidence of sarcoidosis in GCT. It is suggested that the incidence of sarcoidosis could be increased following testicular cancer with an estimated incidence of 1.1% (Pandha et al., 1995; Rayson et al., 1998). Analysis of data from 1 center suggested that the incidence of testicular cancer in patients with sarcoidosis was 100 times the expected rate(Rayson, et al., 1998). Sarcoidosis is associated with different types of testicular cancer, with seminoma being the most common. In 80% of the cases with concomitant sarcoidosis, the sarcoidosis regresses simultaneously. The coexistence of sarcoidosis and testicular cancer doesn't change the overall prognosis(Paparel, et al., 2007). Epidemiological studies of sarcoidosis and malignancy have potential confounding factors; both maximal incidences of testicular cancer and sarcoidosis occur at the same age. It is known that sarcoidosis is often a latent disease and is more easily discovered when the clinical survey is tight as in patients treated and followed for cancer. Thus, a great attention has to be paid to the group used to compare the incidence of sarcoidosis. The coexistence of sarcoidosis and testicular cancer presents potential pitfalls for oncologists during initial staging and follow-up of patients. Clinicians who deal with testis cancer should always consider one of the "great imitator" granulomatosis in the differential diagnosis of patients with GCT. An usual distribution of metastatic spread or coincident findings such as the rash of erythema nodosum demands further investigation. Conventional cross-sectional imaging and functional imaging with FDG PET can be unreliable, and histological assessment remains the only reliable way of confirming the diagnosis(Dick, et al.).

8. Lung cancers

Several cases of the occurence of sarcoidosis and lung cancer have been reported (Kobayashi et al., ; Yamasawa et al., 2000). In most of these cases, sarcoidosis was present for some years preceding the development of lung cancer, but in some cases both diseases were detected simultaneously. It is sometimes difficult to determine whether non-caseinting epithelioid cell granulomas coexisting with lung cancer represent sarcoid reaction or true systemic sarcoidosis. Epidemiologically, the causal relationship between the two diseases is controversial. Some reports supported the theory of an association between the 2 diseases(Brincker and Wilbek, 1974; Yamaguchi et al., 1991) but some reports did not(Romer, 1982; Seersholm, et al., 1997). Either causality or coincidence, lung cancer, a condition that can be observed in patients with sarcoidosis, should be considered in the differential diagnosis when suspicious findings of it are discovered(Kobayashi, et al.).
Tumor-related sarcoid reactions may be found in lymph nodes draining an area containing malignant tumor, in the tumor itself, or even in non regional tissues(Segawa et al., 1996). The association of sarcoidal reaction and cancer makes the cancer patient with lymphadenopathy a diagnostic dilemma: malignant involvement of the lymph nodes is common, but benign diagnoses are possible and must be considered(Hunt et al., 2009). Sarcoidal reactions in the setting of lung cancer (NSCLC) have been identified in two Japenese studies of lung cancer, with an incidence rates of 1,2% and 1,3% (Kamiyoshihara et al., 1998; Tomimaru et al., 2007). Steinford et al found in a recent Australian work an overall incidence of sarcoidal reactions occuring in regional lymph nodes of NSCLC patients of 4,3%(Steinfort and Irving, 2009). The findings were confined to patients with Stage I disease, with in an incidence in this group of 7,7%. In 1975, Laurberg reported an incidence of 3,2% among 734 Danish patients with lung malignancy, noting that sarcoidal reactions were seen only in patients with Stage I disease(Laurberg, 1975). Other authors have also noted a significantly increased incidence in Stage I disease, though very rare occurrence in Stages II and III disease has been reported(Kamiyoshihara, et al., 1998; Tomimaru, et al., 2007). Most of the authors have noted no association with histological sub-type. Laureberg noted a preponderance of squamous cell tumours and postulated that the slower growth and higher tendency to necrosis of this tumour type may result in a more vigorous and longer-lasting stimulation of the regional lymph nodes(Laurberg, 1975). A significant proportion of the sarcoidal reactions in regional lymph nodes of lung cancers are radiologically and metabolically occult. It appears that metastatic involvement by NSCLC is not seen in lymph

nodes exhibiting sarcoidal granulomatous reactions. The sarcoidal reaction do not influence the prognosis, and may be a local reaction or resistance to cancer cells(Kamiyoshihara, et al., 1998). Sarcoidosis must be considered in the differential diagnosis of patients with a history of malignancy who develop lymphadenopathy. It is imperative to obtain a tissue diagnosis before instituting therapy for presumed cancer recurrence(Hunt, et al., 2009).

9. Breast cancers

Lower et al reviewed the medical records of 629 women with sarcoidosis followed in the Interstitial Lung Disease Clinic at the University of Cincinnati for findings associated with breast disease(Lower et al., 2001). In addition, three women with breast cancer who had granulomas in proximity to their tumors were also examined. Abnormal breast examinations or mammograms were reported in 15 patients with sarcoidosis (2% of women with sarcoidosis). Breast biopsy revealed granulomas consistent with sarcoidosis in six. One of them developed breast cancer five years later. Breast cancer was identified in twelve further patients, therefore a total of thirteen patients with breast cancer were identified. Ten were diagnosed with breast cancer plus sarcoidosis: sarcoidosis preceded breast cancer in three, followed breast cancer in five, the two diseases appeared simultaneously in two. Three additional women with breast cancer were also evaluated and classified as patients with sarcoid-like reaction. Review of the mammographic and physical findings could not distinguish between sarcoidosis in the breast and breast cancer. The autors concluded that sarcoidosis patients develop breast cancer at the expected frequency. The breast cancer diagnosis may precede or follow that of sarcoidosis. There is no relationship between stage of sarcoidosis or treatment and the development of cancer. Because physical examination and mammography findings are unable to distinguish between sarcoidosis and malignancy, biopsy of all suspicious lesions in sarcoidosis is recommended.

10. Digestif tract cancers

The incidence of a sarcoid reaction in surgical specimens, derived from 319 Japenese gastric cancer patients, was first reported to be 5% (Takeuchi et al., 1982). To clarify the occurence of sarcoid-like reaction in the spleen of the gastric carcinoma patients, 100 consecutive specimens from gastrosplenectomy were examined(Kojima et al., 1997). Sarcoid-like reaction was observed in the lymph nodes of 13 cases (13%) and the spleen of five cases (5%). None of them showed any symptoms or signs indicative of systemic sarcoidosis. It seems that the cases with sarcoid-like reaction in the spleen ocurred more frequently in an advanced stage of the gastric cancer than those without this phenomenon. Epithelioid cell granulomas (EPGs) appeared to arise in the periarteriolar lymphoid sheaths of the spleen histologically, but were never found in red pulp or germinal centers. None of the 13 cases contained EPGs in the primary tumor. This study indicates that sarcoid-like reaction in the spleen is possibly not a rare phenomenon in the gastric cancer and more frequently seen in the advanced stage of the gastric cancer. Sarcoid-like reactions of the regional lymph nodes are more frequently seen in the patients with EPGs in the spleen than in those without. The incidence of sarcoid-like reactions in the spleen seems to be closely related to those in pancreaticosplenic nodes and/or nodes of the hilus of the spleen. Granulomatous gastritis is a rarely observed pathological diagnosis. This condition often mimics gastric adenocarcinoma clinically, resulting in gastric resection. However, granulomatous gastritis has long been viewed as a benign process not observed in association with adenocarcinoma of the stomach. Newton et al. described a patient with granulomatous gastritis occurring in close proximity to an area of superficially invading gastric adenocarcinoma. The findings in this patient did not support a diagnosis of Crohn's disease, tuberculosis, sarcoidosis, syphilis, histoplasmosis, berylliosis, or foreign-body reaction. This unique case suggests a possible association between isolated granulomatous gastritis and metaplastic mucosal changes(Newton et al., 1998). Sarcoid reactions in colorectal is considered to be quite rare. There has been some case reports in the Japenese literature on colorectal cancers with sarcoid reactions in the dissected lymph nodes or continous to the tumor(Nozoe et al., 1999). In these cases, the most outstanding common clinicopathologic feature was the lack of metastatic carcinoma in the dissected lymph nodes despite the large size of the tumors.

11. Possible role of antineoplastic treatments in the pathogenesis of granulomatosis

Immunotherapy such as interferon (IFN) and interleukine-2 (IL-2) has been reported to induce systemic sarcoidosis probably by reproducing some physiological mechanisms involved in sarcoidosis(Logan and Bensadoun, 2005; Massaguer, et al., 2004; Pietropaoli, et al., 1999; Raanani and Ben-Bassat, 2002). Although no specific etiology has been implicated in the pathogenesis of the sarcoidosis, inflammatory mediators such as IL-2 and IFN are probably involved(Raanani and Ben-Bassat, 2002). IFN is released spontaneously from lung T lymphocytes and alveolar macrophages of patients with sarcoidosis. Moreover, quiescent macrophages of these patients are activated by exposure to IFN. Therefore, IFN given in pharmacological doses could cause macrophage activation especially in patients with a certain predisposition and thus might induce the clinical development of sarcoidosis. IFN γ appears to play a major role as a mediator responsible for macrophage activation. IFN g is released from lung T-lymphocytes and alveolar macrophages when these cells are obtained from normal subjects ans are exogenously stimulated(Robinson et al., 1985). It has been demonstrated that the same cells from patients with sarcoidosis release this cytokine spontaneously. Quiescent macrophages from patients with inactive sarcoidosis are activated by exposure to IFN γ. There is little published evidence implicating any of the other IFNs in the pathogenesis of sarcoidosis. IL-2, a T helper 1 (Th1) also plays an important role in the pathogenesis of the granulomatous inflammation in sarcoidosis(Logan and Bensadoun, 2005; Ziegenhagen and Muller-Quernheim, 2003). It has been postulated that a Th1 predominant pattern may be more important in promoting granulomatous inflammation while a Th2 predominant pattern may be more involved in the development of fibrosis. There is usually a chronological link between the occurrence of the granulomatosis and the beginning of the immunotherapy. The association can so rapidly be suspected. The occurrence of granulomatosis attributed to the classic antineoplastic chemotherapies is exceptionally reported in the literature.

To date, alpha interferon appears to be the most common agent that causes sarcoidosis in patients treated for malignancies, although many other agents such as cisplatin have also been reported(Shigemitsu, 2008).

12. Diagnostic strategy

Clinicians in charged with tumoral pathology would be interested in a non-invasive test allowing him to avoid a systematic a biopsy to distinguish cancer and benign pathology. Nevertheless clinicians have to keep in mind that neoplastic tissue and sarcoidosis can coexist.

Differenciation between malignant and benign pulmonary nodules is a common probleme encountered by radiologists which has provided the impetus to explore alternative imaging techniques(Chang et al., 2006). Accurates diagnosis can reduce unnecessary thoracotomies in patients with benign diseases. Metabolic imaging with 2-(18F)-fluoro-2-deoxy-D-glucose positron emission tomography (PET) is being used more and more to differentiate benign from malignant focal lesions and it has been shown to be more efficious than conventional chest CT. Howewer, fluorodeoxyglucose (FDG) is not a cancer-specific agent, and false positive findings in benign diseases have been reported in active inflammation or infection, causing false-positive results. Active granulomatous conditions with agregation of inflammatory cells in sarcoidosis results in accumulation of FDG and it has been suggested that the intensity of FDG uptake may reflect disease activity(Brudin et al., 1994). A retrospective study was conducted by Chowdhury et al. to evaluate the prevalence of sarcoid-like reaction to malignancy detected using integrated 18 FDG PET/CT in patients undergoing staging or restaging of solid-organ malignancy(Chowdhury et al., 2009). Sarcoid-like reaction was initially suspected in 23 of the 2048 (1.1%) FDG PET/CT examinations, with the diagnosis confirmed histologically or by clinico-radiological follow-up in 13 of the 23 cases (57%). Sarcoid-like reaction was more commonly seen in patients undergoing FDG PET/CT for restaging of suspected recurrence rather than for primary tumour staging (77% versus 23%; p=0.05). The mean maximum standardized uptake value (SUV(max)) of confirmed hilar and mediastinal sarcoid-like reaction was 7.3 (range 3.1-13.6). Symmetric hilar uptake was demonstrated in 11 of the 13 (85%) and all 13 had additional mediastinal nodal uptake. Pulmonary uptake was seen in seven of the 13 cases (54%). Extra-thoracic involvement was present in eight of the 13 (61.5%), including nodal, splenic, and hepatic lesions. Sarcoid-like reaction was suspected in 1.1% of cancer patients at FDG PET/CT examination, with confirmation of the diagnosis in 0.6%. With the increasing use of FDG PET/CT in cancer patients, it is important to be aware of the prevalence of this uncommon, but important, disease entity and to consider this diagnosis in appropriate cases in order to avoid a false-positive interpretation of metastatic disease. Some authors have suggested that early metabolic response to systemic corticosteroid treatment may be used as a tool in the establishment of final diagnosis when sarcoidosis is suspected in a cancer patient and could be capable of differentiating cancer from sarcoidosis in the case of coexisting diseases(Aide et al., 2009). New radiopharmaceutical probes are under development and will improve the performance of PET(Bonardel et al., 2011).

Hence clinicians must be aware that a florid sarcoid-like reaction can camouflage tumor recurance and hence, should preferably perform multiple sections of the tissues or perform multiple biopsies at different sites in addition to continually following these patients for tumor recurrence(Trikudanathan, et al.). This is particularly true for Hodgkin's lymphomas and non-Hodgkin's lymphomas. So when a patient presents with an atypical sarcoidosis (age of beginning > 50 years, change of the general health status, no involvement of the lung or of the mediastinum, personal history of cancer), physicians must take the diagnosis of sarcoidosis very cautiously. The pathologist will have to look the whole block of inclusion with a particular attention. He also will have to look for cytokeratin expressions and to search a clonality. In this context, a corticotherapy must be avoided not to erase later the possibility of bringing to light lymphoma's cells.

13. Conclusion

Thanks to recent epidemiological studies the links between sarcoidoses and cancer are finally demonstrated. Nevertheless the over-risk of cancer after sarcoidosis remains modest.

The clinician has to remain particularly watchful when he is in front of an atypical sarcoidosis. In this situation he has first to suspect a possible lymphoma or an infectious pathology. This approach can avoid to delay an adapted specific treatment.

- **Infections:**
  - Fungal: Histoplasma, Coccidioides, Blastomyces, Sporotrichum, *Pneumocystis jirovecii*, Cryptococcosis
  - Mycobacterial: *Mycobacterium tuberculosis*, Atypical mycobacterial infections (*Mycobacterium avium complex, Mycobacterium gordonae, Mycobacterium kansasii*)
  - Bacterial : Brucella, Chlamydia, Tularemia
  - Spirochaeta : Treponema (Pallidum, *Pertenue carateum*)
  - Parasites: Leshmaniasis, Toxoplasmosis
  - Virus (Cytomegalovirus, Immune Reconstitution Inflammatory Syndrome during HIV)
- **Occupational and environmental exposures:**
  - Hypersensitivity pneumonitis: Farmer's lung, Bird fancier's, Other (> 50 types)
  - Chemical/drugs: Silica, Calcium carbonate or oxalate, Metals (Chronic beryllium disease, titanium, zirconium, aluminium), Glass fibers, Hydrocarbons, Methotrexate, BCG therapy, Interferon…)
- **Immunologic:**
  - Sarcoidosis, Wegener granulomatosis, Crohn disease, Rheumatoid arthritis
- **Immunodeficiency :**
  - Common Variable Immune Deficiency…
- **Malignancy:**
  - Radiation and chemotherapy
  - Neoplasia (carcinoma, seminoma, sarcoma, lymphoma)
  - Sarcoid-like reaction

Table 1. Main diseases (affecting preferentially the lungs) associated with granulomas on histologic examination

- Granulomatous reaction in loco-regional adenopathy
- Unfortuitous association between cancer and sarcoidosis but without paraneoplastic characteristics
- Opportunist infection
- Antineoplastic therapy

Table 2. Main contexts of granulomatosis during cancers

Features	Local sarcoid reaction	Multisystem sarcoidosis
Organ(s) involved	Single	Multiorgan
Age	Any	Middle age
Associated disease	Malignancy	None
Pathogenesis	May be local immune response	Unknown
Chest radiograph	Normal	Abnormal
Delayed hypersensitivity	Normal	Usually depressed
Elevated serum ACE	Rare	Common
Kveim-Siltzbach test	Negative	Positive
BAL lymphocytosis	Absent	Present
Slit lamp examination	Normal	Abnormal in 15-20%
Hypercalcemia	Absent	Common
Gallium body scan	Localized uptake	Multisystem uptake

ACE, angiotensin-converting enzyme ; BAL, bronchoalveolar lavage. Reproduced from Shigemitsu, 2008.

Table 3. Difference between a local sarcoid reaction and systemic sarcoidosis

14. References

Aide, N., Allouache, D., Ollivier, Y., de Raucourt, S., Switsers, O., and Bardet, S. (2009). *Mol Imaging Biol* 11, 224-8.

Apalla, Z., Karakatsanis, G., Koussidou, T., Sotiriou, E., and Chaidemenos, G. *Eur J Dermatol* 20, 651-3.

Askling, J., Grunewald, J., Eklund, A., Hillerdal, G., and Ekbom, A. (1999). *Am J Respir Crit Care Med* 160, 1668-72.

Battesti, J. P., Turiaf, J., Hincky, J. M., and Dournovo, P. (1977). *Nouv Presse Med* 6, 1213-5.

Boffetta, P., Rabkin, C. S., and Gridley, G. (2009). *Int J Cancer* 124, 2697-700.

Bonardel, G., Carmoi, T., Gontier, E., Lecoules, S., Cambon, A., Foehrenbach, H., and Algayres, J. P. (2011). *Rev Med Interne* 32, 101-8.

Bottone, A. C., Labarbera, M., Asadourian, A., Barman, A., and Richie, C. (1993). *Urology* 41, 157-9.

Brincker, H. (1986a). *Cancer Treat Rev* 13, 147-56.

Brincker, H. (1986b). *Br J Cancer* 54, 467-73.

Brincker, H. (1989). *Sarcoidosis* 6, 31-43.

Brincker, H., and Wilbek, E. (1974). *Br J Cancer* 29, 247-51.

Brudin, L. H., Valind, S. O., Rhodes, C. G., Pantin, C. F., Sweatman, M., Jones, T., and Hughes, J. M. (1994). *Eur J Nucl Med* 21, 297-305.

Brunner, A., Kantner, J., and Tzankov, A. (2005). *J Clin Pathol* 58, 815-9.

Campbell, F., and Douglas-Jones, A. G. (1993). *Sarcoidosis* 10, 128-31.

Chalasani, P., Vohra, M., and Sheagren, J. N. (2005). *Ann Oncol* 16, 1714-5.

Chang, J. M., Lee, H. J., Goo, J. M., Lee, H. Y., Lee, J. J., Chung, J. K., and Im, J. G. (2006). *Korean J Radiol* 7, 57-69.

Chowdhury, F. U., Sheerin, F., Bradley, K. M., and Gleeson, F. V. (2009). *Clin Radiol* 64, 675-81.

Dick, J., Begent, R. H., and Meyer, T. *Urol Oncol* 28, 350-4.

Hunt, B. M., Vallieres, E., Buduhan, G., Aye, R., and Louie, B. (2009). *Am J Surg* 197, 629-32; discussion 632.

Ji, J., Shu, X., Li, X., Sundquist, K., Sundquist, J., and Hemminki, K. (2009). *Ann Oncol* 20, 1121-6.

Kamiyoshihara, M., Hirai, T., Kawashima, O., Ishikawa, S., and Morishita, Y. (1998). *Oncol Rep* 5, 177-80.

Kennedy, M. P., Jimenez, C. A., Mhatre, A. D., Morice, R. C., and Eapen, G. A. (2008). *J Cardiothorac Surg* 3, 8.

Kobayashi, N., Nakamura, R., Kurishima, K., Sato, Y., and Satoh, H. *Acta Medica (Hradec Kralove)* 53, 115-8.

Kojima, M., Nakamura, S., Fujisaki, M., Hirahata, S., Hasegawa, H., Maeda, D., Suito, T., Motoori, T., Joshita, T., Suzuki, K., and Suchi, T. (1997). *Gen Diagn Pathol* 142, 347-52.

Kovacs, J., Varga, A., Bessenyei, M., and Gomba, S. (2004). *Pathol Oncol Res* 10, 169-71.

Landgren, O., Engels, E. A., Pfeiffer, R. M., Gridley, G., Mellemkjaer, L., Olsen, J. H., Kerstann, K. F., Wheeler, W., Hemminki, K., Linet, M. S., and Goldin, L. R. (2006). *J Natl Cancer Inst* 98, 1321-30.

Laurberg, P. (1975). *Scand J Respir Dis* 56, 20-7.

Le Jeune, I., Gribbin, J., West, J., Smith, C., Cullinan, P., and Hubbard, R. (2007). *Respir Med* 101, 2534-40.

Logan, T. F., and Bensadoun, E. S. (2005). *Thorax* 60, 610-1.

Lower, E. E., Hawkins, H. H., and Baughman, R. P. (2001). *Sarcoidosis Vasc Diffuse Lung Dis* 18, 301-6.

Lucci, S., Rivolta, R., Fazi, M., Iorio, L., Raschella, G. F., Merlino, G., Giordano, R., and Redler, A. (2002). *G Chir* 23, 75-8.

Marinides, G. N., Hajdu, I., and Gans, R. O. (1994). *Nephron* 67, 477-80.

Massaguer, S., Sanchez, M., and Castel, T. (2004). *Eur Radiol* 14, 1716-7.

McLoone, N. M., McKenna, K., Edgar, D., Walsh, M., and Bingham, A. (2005). *Clin Exp Dermatol* 30, 580-2.

Moder, K. G., Litin, S. C., and Gaffey, T. A. (1990). *Mayo Clin Proc* 65, 1498-501.

Newton, C., Nochomovitz, L., and Sackier, J. M. (1998). *Ann Surg Oncol* 5, 407-10.

Nozoe, T., Matsumata, T., and Sugimachi, K. (1999). *J Clin Gastroenterol* 28, 377-9.

O'Connell, M. J., Schimpff, S. C., Kirschner, R. H., Abt, A. B., and Wiernik, P. H. (1975). *Jama* 233, 886-9.

Ogata, S., Horio, T., Sugiura, Y., Shimazaki, H., Saito, H., Aiko, S., Nakanishi, K., and Kawai, T. *Acta Med Okayama* 64, 407-10.

Pandha, H. S., Griffiths, H., and Waxman, J. (1995). *Clin Oncol (R Coll Radiol)* 7, 277-8.

Paparel, P., Devonec, M., Perrin, P., Ruffion, A., Decaussin-Petrucci, M., Akin, O., Sheinfeld, J., and Guillonneau, B. (2007). *Sarcoidosis Vasc Diffuse Lung Dis* 24, 95-101.

Pavic, M., Debourdeau, P., Vacelet, V., and Rousset, H. (2008a). *Rev Med Interne* 29, 39-45.

Pavic, M., Le Pape, E., Debourdeau, P., Rabar, D., Crevon, L., Colle, B., and Rousset, H. (2008b). *Rev Med Interne* 29, 5-14.

Pavic, M., and Rousset, H. (2008). *Rev Med Interne* 29, 1-2.

Pietropaoli, A., Modrak, J., and Utell, M. (1999). *Chest* 116, 569-72.

Raanani, P., and Ben-Bassat, I. (2002). *Acta Haematol* 107, 133-44.

Rayson, D., Burch, P. A., and Richardson, R. L. (1998). *Cancer* 83, 337-43.

Reich, J. M., Mullooly, J. P., and Johnson, R. E. (1995). *Chest* 107, 605-13.
Robinson, B. W., McLemore, T. L., and Crystal, R. G. (1985). *J Clin Invest* 75, 1488-95.
Romer, F. K. (1982). *N Engl J Med* 306, 1490.
Romer, F. K., Hommelgaard, P., and Schou, G. (1998). *Eur Respir J* 12, 906-12.
Sacks, E. L., Donaldson, S. S., Gordon, J., and Dorfman, R. F. (1978). *Cancer* 41, 562-7.
Seersholm, N., Vestbo, J., and Viskum, K. (1997). *Thorax* 52, 892-4.
Segawa, Y., Takigawa, N., Okahara, M., Maeda, Y., Takata, I., Fujii, M., Mogami, H., Mandai, K., and Kataoka, M. (1996). *Intern Med* 35, 728-31.
Setoyama, M., Nishi, M., Uchimiya, H., and Kanzaki, T. (1998). *J Dermatol* 25, 601-5.
Seve, P., Schott, A. M., Pavic, M., Broussolle, C., Gilis, L., and Thomas, L. (2009). *Dermatology* 219, 25-31.
Shigemitsu, H. (2008). *Curr Opin Pulm Med* 14, 478-80.
Steinfort, D. P., and Irving, L. B. (2009). *Lung Cancer* 66, 305-8.
Takeuchi, H., Suchi, T., Suzuki, R., and Sato, T. (1982). *Gann* 73, 420-8.
Tomimaru, Y., Higashiyama, M., Okami, J., Oda, K., Takami, K., Kodama, K., and Tsukamoto, Y. (2007). *Jpn J Clin Oncol* 37, 90-5.
Trikudanathan, G., Philip, A., and Hegde, U. P. *Conn Med* 74, 403-6.
Wong, V. S., Adab, N., Youngs, G. R., and Sturgess, R. (1999). *Eur J Gastroenterol Hepatol* 11, 353-5.
Yamaguchi, M., Odaka, M., Hosoda, Y., Iwai, K., and Tachibana, T. (1991). *Sarcoidosis* 8, 51-5.
Yamasawa, H., Ishii, Y., and Kitamura, S. (2000). *Respiration* 67, 90-3.
Ziegenhagen, M. W., and Muller-Quernheim, J. (2003). *J Intern Med* 253, 18-30.